THE
PERFECT
PRESCRIPTION

THE PERFECT PRESCRIPTION

Godly Wisdom on Public Health

REIGH SIMUZOSHYA

Copyright © 2019 by Reigh Simuzoshya.

ISBN Softcover   978-1-951469-69-6

All rights reserved. No part of this book may be reproduced or transmitted in any form or by any means, electronic or mechanical, including photocopying, recording, or by any information storage and retrieval system without express written permission from the author, except in the case of brief quotations embodied in critical reviews and certain other non-commercial uses permitted by copyright law.

Printed in the United States of America.

To order additional copies of this book, contact:
Bookwhip
1-855-339-3589
https://www.bookwhip.com

Dedication

To my parents who gave me life and were the first ones to introduce me to the Lord Jesus Christ, and to my own nuclear family, those resolute team-mates in the race that is set before us, this book is dedicated.

Acknowledgment

This book is a product of many years of interacting with different people from all walks of life. During the process of my academic career and general life experiences that led to the writing of this book, I became a recipient of the support, wisdom, and goodwill of so many individuals, organizations, and communities to whom I am deeply indebted. It would be difficult to acknowledge all of them.

My spiritual journey and academic career would be incomplete without the encouragement and wisdom of many teachers and professors. I would especially like to mention the following: Miss W. Cheney, Dr. H.P. Africa and Sister O'Leary. I also would like to especially thank Dr. K. Miller, Dr. W. Nordlund, Dr. J. L. Connors, Dr. D. Stein, and Dr. M. Sharma.

While writing this book, I came into contact with many people who evaluated my work and provided the advice I needed. I admired and respected these individuals' worldview, academic prowess, and spiritual insight. Among them I would like to mention particularly Dr. R. Snuffer who was the first person to read the manuscript and provide priceless input to help smoothen its rough edges. Then there are those literary giants whom I have never had the opportunity to meet face-to-face but whose work inspired me to keep on writing my book. Their names are too many to be listed on this page, but most of them appear in the endnotes of this book. However, I would like to mention the following: Mary-Jane Schneider, Philip Yancey, Rex Russell, S.I. McMillen, and David E. Stern.

I would also like to thank my husband for his unwavering support throughout my entire career as well as during the time I was writing this book. I am also grateful for my children and grandchildren for sharing me generously with this work. They never complained about my failure to participate in some of the family activities and games during the time I was writing this book.

Finally, I am eternally grateful for the leading of the Holy Spirit in this project; for the Holy Scriptures, that endless mine of wisdom and counsel which addresses all human needs, but particularly spiritual and physical health. Thank you, Lord.

Table of Contents

Foreword..11
Introduction...13
Chapter 1: Health—A Fundamental Commodity........17
Chapter 2: Public Health—Overview 21
Chapter 3: Functions of Modern Public Health..........25
Chapter 4: A Closer Look at the Global Burden of Disease...43
Chapter 5: Air Pollution and Health 47
Chapter 6: Safe Drinking Water 55
Chapter 7: Alcohol Consumption 63
Chapter 8: Waste Disposal and Sanitation..............85
Chapter 9: Infectious Diseases......................101
Chapter 10: Deadly Infectious Diseases................117
Chapter 11: Quarantine..............................129
Chapter 12: Incest 135
Chapter 13: Rape...................................145
Chapter 14: Stress 161
Chapter 15: Mental Illness...........................173
Chapter 16: Mold and Fungus in Buildings.............189
Chapter 17: Sexually Transmitted Diseases 201

Chapter 18: HIV/AIDS............................215
Chapter 19: Child Sex Trafficking....................227
Chapter 20: Health and Diet........................245
Chapter 21: Chronic Diseases—I.....................261
Chapter 22: Chronic Diseases—II....................271
Chapter 23: Smoking..............................293
Chapter 24: HIV Infection and Circumcision............307
Chapter 25: Elder Abuse...........................323
Chapter 26: Asthma...............................337
Chapter 27: Cost Saving in Healthcare:
            A Biblical Perspective....................357
Endnotes 371

FOREWORD

The Perfect Prescription: Godly Wisdom on Public Health is a must-read for health professionals, social workers, and individuals who want to take control of their health using time tested and tried principles as old as the Bible itself. If everyone in America would implement the health principles found in the Bible, which are reflected in this book, the health crisis that looms over this nation would diminish greatly. Reigh Simuzoshya meticulously outlines useful and realistic ideas that have the potential to revolutionize the health care industry. Her religious convictions do not come across as judgmental; rather, Dr. Simuzoshya compassionately builds her case line by line, chapter by chapter. She convincingly uses a balance of Scripture, common sense, and contemporary data in her presentation.

In practical matters, this book squarely faces off against substance abuse, poor diet, and sexual promiscuity. While health care professionals, social workers, and government leaders debate how to address the economic issues related to our health crisis, the answers are all right here. While these leaders debate how to address social and medical issues related to our health crisis, the answers are all right here. While debates rage on in how to deal with prescription drug abuse, venereal disease, obesity, alcoholism, and drug abuse, this book offers preventative measures that could revolutionize our society.

One of the greatest sources of health problems in this nation is clearly related to diet. Instead of raw vegetables, whole grains, and healthy meats, we consume canned foods, sugary baked goods, and processed meats. Our food has been depleted of nutrients, probiotics, and antioxidants in its over-processing. Instead of energizing whole foods, we stuff ourselves with empty calories. No wonder cancer rates, heart disease, obesity, and neurological diseases are out of control. Dr. Simuzoshya's principles (or should I say the biblical principles that she outlines?) offer real hope for real and positive change for a society in desperate need.

Finally, a word of encouragement for those who would dismiss this book based on religious grounds. Dr. Simuzoshya does not use this paper and ink to proselytize. Rather, she offers practical answers to practical problems. If the health care industry and its related fields could work towards new policies with these principles in mind, a real measurable difference could be made. Set your religious or anti-religious biases aside and take a fresh look at age-old wisdom that could change the world. At least be open minded enough to let it change your world.

Ryan Snuffer, D. Min.

> Everybody is a genius but if you judge a fish by its ability to climb a tree, it will live its whole life believing it is stupid.
>
> (Albert Einstein)

Dr. Snuffer is a prolific author whose literary work includes *Love Your Neighbor*, a book he co-authored with Dr. Norman L. Geisler in which they tackle pertinent ethical questions of our day. Dr. Snuffer also taught philosophy and religious studies at Mountain State University. He is currently the Director of Appalachian Community Mission, a non-profit organization committed to alleviating suffering among the less advantaged.

INTRODUCTION

The Bible has always been fascinating to me. Every time I read it, it is reading me. It is saturated with simple yet infinite wisdom. It is also replete with guidelines for everyday living. Its uncompromising stance against all forms of evil is intriguing. It also warns what the wages of sinful living are and stipulates the blessings that accompany obedience. The God of the Bible and his Son, the Lord Jesus Christ, became real to me.

Each time I read the Bible, it was like entering into a different realm with peculiarly familiar undertones; like a long-lost homeland. After reading it, I always feel like an exile stranded in a foreign land. Therefore, I decided to study it further with much depth to try and connect with the realm it so fondly talks about. I discovered that the Christian faith is not an apron to be worn and discarded depending on the task being performed.

The Lord Jesus Christ, the founder of the Christian faith, must either be Lord of all areas of my life or he is nothing at all. His love for me and all human beings exemplified in his ultimate sacrifice to reconcile us to the Father won my heart to him and all he stands for. I discovered that God is interested not only in my salvation but in every minute detail of my life. He has even counted the hairs on my head. As such, he must also be interested in my health. That is the reason why he put in place different laws to protect and promote it.

Since then I have learned how much God cares for his creation; how he put laws in place to protect our health and wellbeing as individuals and as communities. Most of these laws, I discovered, still undergird the laws that govern our health care systems.

I have discovered that the Bible is an infinite mine of wisdom and instructions about life. The Bible revealed to me that God, the Creator, has the owner's manual for each person he created. I also found out that our health is of uttermost importance to him. That is the reason he instituted laws to protect it. But he will not coerce us into obedience. Graciously, he has endowed us with the power of choice. We can break these laws at will. But that is always to our detriment, for he will not bend them to accommodate our rebellious inclinations. The fact that he knows me so intimately that he has even numbered the hair on my head is an astounding discovery. Even more astonishing is the fact that he is interested in my health as an individual and also in the corporate health of his people that he carefully designed guidelines to enhance it.

Good health is one of the greatest gifts that can ever be bestowed on us in this life. Good health contributes significantly to our quality of life. This is why from time immemorial, mankind has been locked in a mortal struggle with disease. Some diseases have been astoundingly virulent, wreaking havoc in their wake. Others have been novel diseases that have stumped biomedical science and decimated large portions of the global population. It almost seems as if the more advanced the biomedical discoveries the greater the virulence with which some of the diseases have attacked mankind.

For over thirty years now we have been contending with the HIV/AIDS pandemic and other re-emerging diseases that have become drug resistant for varied reasons. Diseases have often underscored the reality of our mortal nature. Disease prevention efforts such as research, immunization campaigns, and screening initiatives for early detection of disease continue to claim a significant percentage of national budgets in many nations.

International organizations such as the World Health Organization (WHO) have been established to function as watchdogs of global health. By them and through them multiple pilot programs have been designed and implemented to combat diseases wherever they have threatened the very survival of mankind. Health promotion and wellbeing programs have been enacted by individual nations, sometimes in collaboration with international organizations, for certain population groups such as children and women's health programs.

Sometimes physicians have adopted biblical laws in their fight against disease. For example, in 1847, Dr. Ignaz Semmelweiss introduced the hand-washing practice for doctors, students, and midwives in chlorinated water after conducting an autopsy or after delivering a baby to reduce the incidence of puerperal fever. The practice significantly lowered the percentage of deaths among the patients. Hand washing continues to be a demonstrably effective preventive measure against infectious diseases. A recent adoption of biblical principles has mitigated the impact of HIV/AIDS on mankind. For instance, health professionals engaged in the fight against HIV/AIDS and other sexually transmitted diseases have adopted some biblical principles to prevent infection such as abstinence and fidelity.

The Bible is replete with health-promoting guidelines and directives—from childbirth to infectious diseases and chronic diseases and many others. A great part of Jesus' ministry was devoted to healing diseases. That is how important our health is to God. As such, it is only logical to examine more carefully the efficacy of the laws he established way before the Germ Theory and other biomedical discoveries in the continued struggle against diseases. This book is an attempt to demonstrate how biblical principles still undergird our personal and public health laws.

All Scripture is from the Revised Standard Version

Chapter 1

Health—
A Fundamental Commodity

Beloved, I pray that all may go well with you and that you may be in health...

(3 John 1:2)

If you will diligently hearken to the voice of the Lord *your God, and do that which is right in his eyes, and give heed to his commandments and keep all his statutes, I will put none of the diseases upon you which I put upon the Egyptians; for I am the* Lord, *your healer.*

(Exodus 15:26)

The quest for optimum health has been inextricably connected to mankind from time immemorial. The desire to attain and maintain good health outweighs all other desires and drives most modern research projects. Time and again we are bombarded with advertisements, books, documentaries, and other publications proclaiming the discovery of a "fountain of youth and anti-aging remedies," which promises not only agelessness but a reprieve from debilitating disease.

The battle against disease, which is the fending off of the onslaught of a myriad of diseases, as well as the pursuit of optimum health, is relentless at individual, community, national, and international levels.[1] We understand good health to be a fundamental human right that determines the quality of life of an individual, to a large extent; although this right continues to be elusive in most cases. Good health is also one way to save money on doctors' visits and drugs. Good health has connotations of enjoying life and being free from pain. Everybody wants to be in good health, because good health is closely linked to physical, mental, and emotional soundness and longevity.

A deliberate neglect of the choices that lead to good health can lead to a poor quality of life and reduced life expectancy. But it takes energy, time, financial resources, skilled human labor, and a committed, concerted effort at every level of human society to achieve good health. Pursuing good health involves making choices that promote a healthy existence for every phase of life. It requires the involvement of individuals, non-governmental agencies, and government departments in proactively designing, establishing, and enforcing evidence-based laws, regulations, practices, and standards aimed at disease reduction and prevention. Good health plays a key role in the economic growth, vibrancy, and prosperity of any nation. But without proper and accessible guidelines, it is almost impossible for individual members of the general public to make informed health-promoting choices for themselves.

In modern times, governments and other agencies have assumed the responsibility for providing health guidelines, services, and education for the general public in order to promote general health and to reduce health expenditure. Often health-promoting guidelines incorporate recommendations for lifestyles, dietary habits, and behavioral choices that enhance health and wellbeing, primarily, at an individual level.

Thomas Jefferson, the third president of the United States and principal author of the Declaration of Independence, aptly remarked in 1787 that: "Without health there is no happiness. And attention to health then should take the place of every other object."[2] This underscores the assertion by Redwanur Rahman, an author who recognizes that health is a fundamental human right and should be recognized as an expedient of human development.[3]

WORLD HEALTH ORGANIZATION AND HEALTH

Rahman further stresses that the World Health Organization perceives health as an essential and basic human right. This assertion is affirmed by the Universal Declaration of Human Rights (UDHR), which perceives health as an instrument of welfare and general wellbeing. These viewpoints are consistent with those of the International Covenant on Social, Economic, and Cultural Rights (ICSECR).

All the above organizations emphasize that governments should recognize health as an indispensable human right and that they should endeavor to design and implement policies that enhance access to health resources and services. The definition of health by the World Health Organization (WHO) is that it is "a state of complete physical, mental and social well-being," and not merely the absence of disease.[4] Governments are further urged by the WHO and other related international organizations that function as watchdogs for the health of the general public to have sound resource distribution programs so that they can bridge any healthcare gaps between the rich and poor, males and females, and also between children from low socioeconomic statuses and those from affluent socioeconomic statuses.

Governments are further encouraged to design programs aimed at providing healthcare for everybody at every phase of their lives as a means of protecting, respecting, and fulfilling their citizens' right to health. By providing health for its citizenry, a government is not doing them a favor. Rather, it is merely meeting its obligation and responsibility toward them. Poor health is usually associated with suffering and loss of productivity, while good health is associated with high energy levels, vibrancy, abundant living, pursuance of dreams and goals.

Good health is wealth and ill health can be synonymous with poverty. Good health is associated with an ability to perform and accomplish activities of daily living, production, education as well as social and economic growth, and ill health is an impediment to all these activities.

BIBLICALLY BASED PERCEPTION OF HEALTH

The Bible teaches us a lot about health promotion and enhancement measures. The Bible is the oldest book to incorporate public health principles in its teachings. It provides unique counsel for promoting health and reducing the burden of disease wherever this counsel is properly applied. Although biblical principles incorporate individual responsibility for achieving optimum health, they are also mainly a population-based approach to achieving good health and well-being for entire communities.

The primary emphasis of biblical health principles is the achievement of optimum community health. This is consistent with the operations of modern-day public health. Similar to public health tenets, biblical health laws are guidelines for avoiding infectious diseases, contagious diseases, sexually transmitted diseases, mental illness, addictions, chronic and degenerative diseases such as heart diseases, obesity-induced diabetes and many others, to benefit not only individuals but whole societies as well.

Chapter 2

Public Health—Overview

For I will restore health to you, and your wounds I will heal, says the LORD.

(Jeremiah 30:17)

The Association of the Schools of Public Health defines public health as "the science and art of protecting and improving the health of communities through education, promotion of health styles and research for disease and injury prevention."[5] Public health involves the process of exploring the health of different population groups. It is also the practice of making evaluations that lead to diagnosing the prevailing health profiles of different population groups in order to pinpoint areas that need improvement and to identify issues that impact it, negatively or positively.

"Healthcare is vital to all of us some of the time, but public health is vital to all of us all of the time," said former United States Surgeon General C. Everett Koop when addressing the Public Health Functions Steering Committee in 1994. Public health embraces all communities regardless if they are composed of a handful of people or large multitudes from diverse nations or continents.

The discipline of public health is galvanized by concern for people's overall health and wellbeing and not merely a desire to satisfy a social responsibility. A close scrutiny of the tenets of modern public health reveals that it is mainly founded on the principles found in the Bible about promotion of overall health. These are also known as biblical health laws.

Both biblical health laws and public health focus on preventive rather than curative or therapeutic aspects of health. They are mainly concerned about community-based health issues. They both warn against adoption of destructive lifestyles and injurious habits and behavioral practices such as illicit drug use, tobacco use, poor hygiene, sexual promiscuity, poor dietary habits, and sedentary lifestyles.

Scientists McGinnis and DeGraw provide the following information about the health benefits of adopting a health-promoting lifestyle. They particularly focus on the public health benefits of avoiding tobacco use:

> If tobacco use was stopped entirely today throughout the nation, an estimated 390, 000 fewer Americans would die before their time each year. If all Americans reduced their consumption of foods high in fat to well below current levels and engaged in physical activity no more strenuous than sustained walking for 30 minutes a day, additional results of a similar magnitude could be expected. If alcohol were never carelessly used in our society, about 100, 000 fewer people would die from unnecessary illness and injury. Together, deaths from these causes comprise a sizeable share of the 2.1 million deaths that occur annually and are examples of the impact of personal lifestyle choices on the health destiny of individual Americans and the future of the nation.
>
> (McGinnis & DeGraw, 1991)[6]

The Perfect Prescription

It is clear from the above quotation that if entire communities were to refrain from tobacco use, the health benefits would be astounding and positively palpable. This is consistent with God's method of dealing with disease, that is, he warns his people and urges them to abstain from different types of self-destructive behavioral choices to protect their health. Although the Bible is not a textbook about healthcare, about one-third of its laws are relevant in regards to the prevention of disease, good hygiene and proper diet, all of which are critical components of public health activities.[7] A strict adherence to these laws can have great individual and public health benefits because of their strong emphasis on prevention and prophylactic activities.

The germ theory was virtually unknown to the people of Bible times. In those times, people completely relied on the Lord God to prevent occurrence of diseases and to heal them whenever diseases afflicted them. Therapeutic interventions were not very popular either. Instead, people and communities adopted and applied the preventive biblical health laws that forbade them from utilizing and ingesting harmful substances or indulging in deleterious and risky behavioral activities. People also adhered to prescribed strong moral guidelines.

They were frequently warned against engaging in certain activities and eating certain foods as prevention against myriads of diseases. By observing these laws, people in Bible times enjoyed good health and longevity. Scriptures tell us that "Moses was a hundred and twenty years old when he died; his eye was not dim, nor his natural force abated" (Deuteronomy 34:7 RSV). If these laws could be applied vigilantly and successfully in modern times, the work of public health professionals would be much easier, as the result would be a general upsurge in the health and wellbeing of the general public worldwide. This is not to say that everybody should be converted to Christianity in order to enjoy the health benefits of these laws. By merely adopting them and incorporating them in one's life, one can benefit greatly from them.

The Bible speaks about physicians only in isolated instances. In 2 Chronicles 16:12 we are told that "In the thirty-ninth year of his reign Asa was diseased in his feet, and his disease became severe; yet even in his disease he did not seek the Lord, but sought help from physicians."

The implication is that if King Asa had sought help from the Lord God, he would have given him counsel to prevent the progression of the disease and to heal him. Tragically, King Asa placed his confidence in the wrong place. He trusted the physicians of his time who probably did not know what disease he had. Almost every ailment has a preventive variable that can easily be adopted and applied to mitigate its progression and virulence. Some of the biblical health laws have been found to have had a dual function: ritual purity and health promotion. For example, the main reason given for maintaining high sanitation standards was "Because the Lord your God walks in the midst of your camp…" (Deuteronomy 23:14).

But it has also been scientifically proven that good sanitation practices enhance health by eliminating exposure to disease-carrying agents or pathogens. Like other biblical health laws, this is a law that has universal health benefits. According to Margaret Chan, Director of World Health Organization, "Sanitation is a cornerstone of public health…Improved sanitation contributes enormously to human health and well-being" (World Health Organization, 2008).[8]

Chapter 3

Functions of Modern Public Health

And the Lord will take away from you all sickness.
(Deuteronomy 7:15)

Public health is a multipronged discipline that incorporates a myriad of functions in its population-based approach to health promotion. Dr. Mary-Jane Schneider, author of *Introduction to Public Health* observes that the goal of public health is achieving maximum health for everybody and finding the means by which that goal can be achieved.[9] Unlike medicine, which usually focuses on the individual, public health is population-based. Its main thrust is prevention of disease and associated disability.

In a nutshell, Schneider further asserts that "public health diagnoses, and treats the community's ills by way of assessment, policy development, and assurance." The following list constitutes some of the functions of modern-day public health as they have been stipulated by the Public Health Functions Steering Committee:

Public health:

1. Helps prevent pollution of our air and land by enforcing regulatory controls and managing hazardous wastes;
2. Works to ensure that our drinking and recreational waters are safe;
3. Controls and prevents infectious diseases and outbreaks such as measles, HIV/AIDS; tuberculosis, cholera, malaria and the Ebola virus;
4. Facilitates community empowerment and education to improve mental health, reduce substance abuse and social violence;
5. Promotes healthy lifestyles that prevent development of chronic diseases such as cancer, heart disease, and obesity;
6. Educates at-risk population groups in order to reduce the incidence and prevalence of sexually transmitted diseases, teen pregnancy, and infant mortality;
7. Ensures access to cost-effective healthcare. It also provides assurance of availability of a skilled and competent workforce;
8. Evaluates the effectiveness of clinical and community-based interventions;
9. Reduces death and disability due to unintentional injuries through the formulation of policies designed to protect the safety of the public, such as seatbelt laws and worker safety laws;

The above nine functions of public health are incorporated into the following three categories:

1. Assessment of the health of the public;
2. Development and enforcement of policies, regulations and laws that protect the health of the public.

3. Assurance of the provision of healthcare when and where it is needed.

(Public Health in America, 2011)[10]

THE ROLES OF BIBLE TIMES RELIGIOUS LEADERS AS PUBLIC HEALTH PROFESSIONALS

Although the Bible should not be treated as a public health textbook or a textbook for nutritionists, in it God has outlined key health principles that can help us make appropriate, informed choices for promoting health and preventing disease. In Bible times, apart from being religious leaders, priests were ascribed roles that were equivalent to those of modern-day public health officers.[11] They were responsible for educating the people about the basic individual and community health-promoting principles the Lord gave them through Moses and for enforcing them. They also supervised the food quality and enforced dietary laws. They ensured that there was a supply of fresh, clean water. They also made sure that waste was properly disposed of. The priests enforced the Sabbath rest as a way of promoting physical, mental, and spiritual health. The priests and Levites set the pace for the establishment of the national health policy in Israel as they received instructions from God through Moses. The Lord God told Israel that they could avoid the curse of disease if they obeyed the commandments and statutes he gave them:

> "If you will diligently hearken to the voice of the LORD your God, and do that which is right in his eyes, and give heed to his commandments and keep all his statutes, I will put none of the diseases upon you which I put upon the Egyptians; for I am the LORD, your healer."
>
> (Exodus 15:26)

The commandments and statutes referred to in the above Scripture contain powerful tools that are necessary for prevention of disease even in our day. Prevention is always preferable to therapeutic treatment because it is less expensive and without side effects. For example, we know that most infectious and contagious diseases are often contracted through contacts with body fluids such as blood, semen, milk, vaginal secretions, tears, and nasal discharges. This is the reason we now have an approach known as universal precautions, which is an infection control strategy.

This approach was established because some blood and other body fluids-borne infectious diseases are not easy to identify, as carriers are often asymptomatic for a number of years. This is the reason why clinicians in our day are required to wear gloves whenever they are in contact with people's bodily fluids. In a preventive measure, long before the establishment of the universal precautions strategy, God knew about all this and commanded that those who came into contact with certain bodily discharges and fluids should wash their clothes and bodies.

People who came into contract with discharges were deemed unclean until evening, which meant they were separated from the rest of the people. For instance, after copulation in which bodily discharges are inevitable, a couple was deemed unclean until evening, and they were also required to wash their clothes (Leviticus 15:18).

This was both a hygienic as well as preventive measure. Additionally, in Leviticus 15:2-10, Scripture provides a step-by-step process of how the individual who had either an incident of a bodily discharge or a chronic discharge was to be treated and cleansed so that he could be restored to the broader community. He was not to allow anyone to come into contact with anything he had sat on or touched. Whatever he spat on was deemed unclean. Every individual who came into contact with the unclean person or his property became unclean. He, too, had to wash his clothes and bathe his entire body and still remain unclean for the rest of day, until evening time, as depicted in the text below:

> "Say to the people of Israel, When any man has a discharge from his body, his discharge is unclean. And this is the law of his uncleanness for a discharge: whether his body runs with his discharge, or his body is stopped from discharge, it is uncleanness in him. Every bed on which he who has the discharge lies shall be unclean; and everything on which he sits shall be unclean. And any one who touches his bed shall wash his clothes, and bathe himself in water, and be unclean until the evening. And whoever sits on anything on which he who has the discharge has sat shall wash his clothes, and bathe himself in water, and be unclean until the evening. And whoever touches the body of him who has the discharge shall wash his clothes, and bathe himself in water, and be unclean until the evening…And whoever touches anything that was under him shall be unclean until the evening; and he who carries such a thing shall wash his clothes, and bathe himself in water, and be unclean until the evening."
>
> (Leviticus 15: 2-5, 10)

The priests were to ensure that these commandments were strictly observed. It was also the priests' responsibility to designate as unclean any person who had a contagious disease that was characterized by lesions on the skin or rashes such as might be caused by measles, small pox, or leprosy. They diligently supervised the isolation of these individuals from the rest of the community by declaring them unclean as is indicated in the Scripture below:

> "When a man has on the skin of his body a swelling or an eruption or a spot, and it turns into a leprous disease on the skin of his body, then he shall be brought to Aaron the priest or to one of his sons the priests, and the priest shall

examine the diseased spot on the skin of his body; and if the hair in the diseased spot has turned white and the disease appears to be deeper than the skin of his body, it is a leprous disease; when the priest has examined him he shall pronounce him unclean."

(Leviticus 13: 2-3)

The priests emphasized the necessity of quarantining the affected individuals and their property. Sometimes the property was to be washed in clean water. Other times it was to be destroyed completely to protect the entire community from disease outbreaks.

CONTRIBUTING FACTORS TO ETIOLOGY OF DISEASE

A critical contributing factor to the rise in the burden of disease in modern times is ignorance of some of these laws and many other health promoting principles. This makes the fight against disease a tedious, uphill battle. Douglas S. Winnail writing in Tomorrow's World asks poignant questions regarding the apparent loss of the battle against disease "But how do you banish ignorance? How do you change human behavior? How do you motivate people to think and act differently? How can you eliminate disease and consequences of poverty?"

Although we know that efforts by health planners, government officials, public health professionals, medical doctors, and economists have yielded some benefits in the fight against disease, they still have not yet completely freed mankind from disease. It may come as a shock to some people to learn that religious leaders have the potential to defeat or reduce the burden of disease by providing public health education to the multitudes of people who frequent their congregations every week.

Comforting the bereaved and the sick and giving clothing and food to the poor and needy are all great and commendable undertakings, but these are not the only roles religious leaders should focus on. Religious leaders need to be sensitized to the important role of teaching health behavioral choices among the people. Unfortunately, many religious leaders believe that the God-given directives for optimizing the health of the general public were exclusively for the nation of ancient Israel at that particular period of time.

However, it is noteworthy that when these biblical principles were adopted during certain epidemics in more recent historical settings, the spread of disease was stemmed and hundreds of people's lives were saved. Dr. J. C. Geiger, a medical doctor writing for the official journal of the California Medical Association, claimed that "The Plague disappeared from London about 1703…the disappearance was attributed to the quarantine regulations" (Geiger, 1933).[12] This was a practice that had its foundation in Scripture.

Role of Religion in Promoting Health

In modern-day public health, the success of any form of intervention is dependent on the compliance of the target population group. One way to secure this compliance in an intervention strategy is to have the consent of the target population group. This can be gained by convincing them that the intervention is in their best interest. The compliance can also be secured easily and effectively if public health professionals can have easy access to the target population groups through local community and religious leaders and work with them to implement evidence-based health community education campaigns.

Religious leaders can also incorporate biblical health laws in their sermons and help educate the people about the health benefits of adopting these laws. Such a concerted effort can have far-reaching positive outcomes in relation to disease prevention.

Biblical health laws can provide the bedrock or foundation for designing intervention strategies aimed at reducing unnecessary disease outbreaks and suffering in modern societies.

The Bible has provided us with a template for health promotion for all mankind, and we only ignore it to our detriment. These are the same laws that stemmed the fatal epidemic that plagued mothers after delivering babies during Dr. Ignaz Semmelweis' time. Dr. Semmelweiss discovered that puerperal fever among new mothers could be reduced by vigorous hand washing among attending physicians, which was an application of the biblical law that required that a person should carefully wash their hands and body after dissecting a cadaver and before coming into contact with another human being (see Numbers 19:11-13). This affirms the universal benefits provided by observance of some of these laws. The details of Dr. Semmelweiss' work are discussed in greater detail later in chapter 9 of this book.

Certain religious groups have developed a specific subculture for their denominations characterized by distinct lifestyles. Adoption of these lifestyles is fluid, which means that although these lifestyles have been designed by members of these denominations, they are not exclusive to their membership. Any individual outside the denominations who wishes to adopt these lifestyles and enjoy their benefits is free to do so without being pressured to join the ranks of the denominations in question.

Prominent among these denominations are Mormons and Seventh-day Adventists. These denominations have taken up the challenge of living by the dictates of biblical health laws as much as possible and are committed to teaching others about the benefits derived from these laws. They uphold strict dietary and health standards for their membership not as a means to salvation but as a means of promoting health. The leadership of the Seventh-day Adventist church is responsible for educating the laity and the broader community about the benefits of avoiding ingestion of substances that adversely affect health.

The Perfect Prescription

Seventh-day Adventists practice a lifestyle that encourages total abstention from alcohol, tobacco, and other harmful and mind-altering substances based on the understanding that their bodies are the temple of the Holy Spirit: "Do you not know that your body is a temple of the Holy Spirit within you, which you have from God? You are not your own; you were bought with a price. So glorify God in your body" (1 Corinthians 6:19, 20).

They have also set up health centers and hospitals running along these convictions in areas that desperately need them. Most Seventh-day Adventists are lacto-ovo-vegetarians. Others are vegans. Lacto-ovo-vegetarians are individuals who do not eat animal flesh but consume dairy and egg products. Vegans do not use or consume any type of animal products. Those who are not vegetarians among them eat only clean meat as stipulated in the Bible in Leviticus chapter 11. To assess the efficacy of these biblical dietary laws, Mills and associates conducted a research study among 34,000 non-Hispanic Seventh-day Adventists in California between 1976 and 1982 to monitor the incidence of cancer among this population group.[13]

The researchers compared rates of the incidence of cancer between the participants and an external reference population group in their area "by calculating standardized morbidity ratios (SMRs) for all cancer sites." The researchers also measured relative risks by analyzing data from the questionnaire completed by the participants regarding their lifestyle. The results of this research study demonstrated that Seventh-day Adventists had "a lower risk of developing cancer at most of the major sites..." This was consistent with the findings of a study conducted by Philips between 1960 and 1972.

The study by Philips endeavored to measure mortality among California Seventh-day Adventists. The results of this study also demonstrated that the risk of death from cancer among Seventh-day Adventists was lower than in other populations groups.[14] This low mortality rate was found to be persistent when Seventh-day

Adventists were compared with similar non-smoking population groups, which was indicative of the fact that other aspects of the lifestyle adopted by Seventh-day Adventists accounted for the low mortality rates among them.

Similarly, a study on the lifestyle and reduced mortality rates among white California Mormons conducted between 1980 and 2004 by Enstrom and Breslow revealed that Mormons who were actively involved in their faith had an unusually low standard mortality ratio (SMR). Mormons observe a healthy lifestyle, which highlights a strong family foundation, abstention from liqueur, and emphasis on education.

The Mormon "Doctrine and Covenants" which is known as the "Word of Wisdom" strictly exhorts Mormons to abstain from utilizing tobacco products, illicit drugs, alcohol, tea, coffee, and emphasizes adoption of a well-balanced diet as well as strong family units, high moral standards, and education. Another research study by Enstrom explored the health practices in relation to cancer mortality rates among active Mormons in California.[15] The results also demonstrated low standard mortality ratios (SMRs) for Mormons in comparison with the general population of the United States.

When religious leaders take up the responsibility to guide and educate the laity about behavioral choices that promote healthy lifestyles, the results are positive health outcomes and low health expenses. The efforts of religious leaders can yield remarkable positive results because these individuals can have access to at-risk population groups that healthcare professionals might not be able to have access to. An observation by the Congregational Health Ministries of the United Methodist Church reveals that:

> The church is the only community-based organization that is found in virtually every community in this country. It is able to reach people of all ages, races, and economic backgrounds, and it can strongly influence people's values and personal life choices. Because the church is

generally more integrated into the life of individuals and communities than our modern medical establishment, it can better enable people to assume responsibility for their own health.

(Health and Welfare Ministries)[16]

From the above quote, it is obvious that the religious leadership has an opportunity to provide a holistic understanding of the concept of health to the laity as laid down in Scripture; an understanding that an individual's health profile should integrate body, mind, and spirit, and that good health can only be optimized by emphasizing and adopting preventive measures. Religious leaders should not wait for a health crisis to arise before addressing the issue of health, as was the case with the HIV/AIDS crisis.

There should be an ongoing health-promoting initiative and strategy in churches. The fact that the church, as a religious body, is perceived as having credibility and is generally entrenched in the community gives it the clout to make a positive impact on the health of the community. The United Nations Children's Fund (UNICEF) acknowledges that religious leaders have a lot of influence in promoting community health and shaping social values of their communities as well as steering these communities toward adopting preventive health choices. The church has the ability to successfully promote adoption of responsible behaviors that enhance health and uphold the dignity and sanctity of human life. The church can educate the public about disease in general.

AIDS AND THE AFRICAN AMERICAN CHURCH IN THE UNITED STATES

In the United States, African Americans are reported to be disproportionately affected by HIV/AIDS.[17] The African American church in the United States has historically played a pivotal role as an institution that has successfully advocated for social justice and psychosocial wellbeing of the black community.

The African American church has also been an ideal place for promotion of health education activities. However, for a long time after the advent of the HIV/AIDS disease, the African American church hesitated to address the disease because of a reluctance and bashfulness to deal with issues of homosexuality and sexuality in general. Some religious leaders in African American communities found it uncomfortable to openly discuss sex. They also had difficulties about how to relate to the issue of people from different sexual orientations in their congregations as well as dealing with the problem of drug abuse and its relationship to HIV/AIDS infection.

But with the changing demographics of people who contracted HIV within the church, the church's perception of the disease began to shift positively. As more and more heterosexual individuals became infected with HIV and the general public became more tolerant to people with HIV/AIDS, the stance of the church, in general, also softened. They began to adopt a less demure stance and became more compassionate toward those who were ill. The church began to design programs that allowed it to become more involved in AIDS ministries and outreach programs. Because approximately 75 percent of HIV transmission occurs through sexual intercourse, it is imperative that the church takes on the responsibility of educating its members, particularly the youth about sexual responsibility.

In Uganda, church leaders and leaders of other faiths have learned the necessity of abandoning their phobia of discussing sex and sexuality and have begun to incorporate sexual responsibility as well as personal integrity and ethics in the sermons they deliver to their congregations. They are also becoming more involved in counseling sessions with members of their congregations. In Bible times, religious leaders always had the unique role of confronting difficult, sensitive, and uncomfortable issues among the people to provide them with guidance. Modern religious leaders ought to emulate them.

In commenting on the dangers of religious leaders shying away from their responsibility to their church members, especially adolescents and young adults, the United Nations Children's Fund (UNICEF) Report of 2003 in conjunction with the World Conference of Religions for Peace and the Joint United Nations Programme on HIV/AIDS (UNAIDS) observed that "If the Christian family cannot give the answers to its teenagers…the family will lose them to someone who can. If the church in turn is silent, the church will lose them too."[18] Teenagers in the church are as curious about sex as teenagers in the world. Therefore, there is need for the church to address the issue of sexuality by developing Bible-based theological programs, which should serve as a foundation for designing practical strategies that parents and religious youth workers can utilize in teaching teenagers about sexual responsibility.

It is an issue that must be confronted with biblical truths, and it should be done in a way that makes it less intimidating and scary. Circumventing and avoiding the issue due to bashful embarrassment only serves to pique the interests of teenagers and young adults in our communities. This can even force youngsters to seek and look elsewhere even outside the church for information about sexuality. The problem with teenagers and young adults seeking information about a sensitive subject such as sex from someone else other than a member of their nuclear family or church family is that they might find wrong information from dubious characters who might lead them astray.

How Religion Influences Positive Health Outcomes

Dr. Koenig, founder and former director of Duke University's Center for the Study of Religion, Spirituality and Health, and currently Director of Duke's Center for Spirituality, Theology and Health, has extensively studied and conducted research on the influence of religion and religious lifestyles on people's physical and mental health. Dr Koenig informs us that hundreds of studies affirm religion's preventive quality as one of its benefits. He claims that

> If the religious congregations in America all had health programs, then two-thirds of the U.S. population would be exposed to disease detection, disease prevention, and health promotion efforts. Since persons of all ages participate regularly in religious congregations, this means that health education efforts would occur at all ages, from the young (focused on substance abuse prevention and character development) to the middle aged (focused on healthy eating, exercise, stress-reduction, etc.) to the elderly (focused on volunteering, mentoring and generative types of activities).
>
> (6th Annual Health & Wellness Fair, 2009)[19]

As mentioned earlier, the main thrust of biblical health principles is preventive health. A systematic and diligent study and observance of these laws is a sure way to reduce the burden of disease across cultures. The church cannot leave the issues pertaining to the health of the public to chance or to government programs alone. It should do its uttermost to preserve the health of the public by endeavoring to empower its membership to make right decisions and choices daily, such as exercising restraint and temperance in all aspects of their lives. If more people would adopt healthier lifestyles, personal and national health care expenditure would be reduced drastically.

Dr. Harold Koenig further claims that the findings from a 1983 review and evaluation of numerous previous health studies by the National Institute for Healthcare Research in Rockville (NIHR), Maryland, found that 77 percent of these studies confirmed the positive effects of religion and its tenets on general health.[20]

This undertaking by NIHR evolved into a research study guide that has become known as *The Faith Factor*. *The Faith Factor* elicited increased general interest in the role of religion and health among different organizations as well as individuals. When people walk in step with their Creator, optimization of spiritual, emotional, and physical health and wellbeing becomes inevitable.

Here is a promise from the Creator himself that confirms it: "If you will diligently hearken to the voice of the LORD your God, and do that which is right in his eyes, and give heed to his commandments and keep all his statutes, I will put none of the diseases upon you which I put upon the Egyptians; for I am the LORD, your healer" (Exodus. 15: 26).

The Egyptians relied on plants and oils to cure disease and, although the Israelites spent centuries under Egyptian bondage being exposed to Egyptian remedies for disease, these remedies are not mentioned or recommended in the Bible. Some of the Egyptian remedies for disease were not wrong. It is just that the Bible is more focused on prevention of disease rather than on curative therapies or remedies.

Dr. Roderik Saxey enlightens us that "Egyptian medical practice had become a complex blend of reason and superstition" and that treatment of pediatric illnesses included "ingestion of skinned dead mice ... and potions which were sometimes more toxic than the disease" (Saxey, n.d.).[21] God took a completely different approach for Israel and the spiritual as well as the health profile of this nation would be an exemplar to other nations; a showcase highlighting the benefits of God's health laws, so that these other nations would also be motivated to adopt the same health principles.

Ancient Israel was charged with a mission to be "a light to the nations" (Isaiah. 42:6; Isaiah 60:3). They were called, among other things, to provide the rest of the nations with moral, spiritual, and healthy lifestyle leadership: "Keep them and do them; for that will be your wisdom and your understanding in the sight of the peoples, who, when they hear all these statutes, will say, 'Surely this great nation is a wise and understanding people'" (Deuteronomy 4:6). The Egyptian health remedies were concoctions made by human beings, but the biblical health laws were given by the one who created the human body and intricately designed its functions.

Dr. Jordan Rubin in his book, *The Great Physician's R$_x$ for Health & Wellness,* further reveals to us that the Jews were protected from many forms of virulent diseases by the hygiene they learned from the health laws given to them by God through Moses so that "when the bubonic plague swept through Europe in the Middle Ages and wiped out more than a quarter of the population, many small pockets of observant Jews escaped the Black Death" (Rubin, 2005).[22]

Regular church attendance and involvement in worship and service to others keeps people mobile and physically active. For the elderly, this mobility and physical activity is a preventive factor against negative health outcomes characteristic of a sedentary lifestyle. Physical mobility also reduces levels of being isolated from the rest of the community, which can be a precursor for health conditions such as depression and anxiety.

This can lead to general functional decline. By being involved in church attendance and activities, the elderly people can become members of a vibrant social network. These networks often evolve into spiritual families, which take it upon themselves to look out for these elderly people's wellbeing. As they break bread together, they share each other's burdens and needs, which provides a sense of relief. Some religious groups across denominations have special committees that are specifically set aside to monitor the physical and spiritual wellbeing of their elderly members. They bear each other's burdens so that no one has to feel lonely and unwanted. Other churches teach their members about topics that include the health and longevity benefits of being temperate in their eating and other habits.

Church-going people across different Judeo-Christian denominations believe that their bodies are the temples of the Holy Spirit and that there is a divine presence living within them. Therefore it is imperative that they treat these bodies with respect. Human beings are the crowing act of God's creation since unlike any other created animals they alone are made in the image of God and after his likeness: "So God created man in his own image, in the image of God he created him; male and female he created them," (Genesis1:27). To knowingly put harmful products of any kind in them or to involve them in any form of immoral conduct or criminal activities is to betray that sacred image. People who live by these beliefs tend to do their best to ensure that their bodies and environments are properly cared for. They strive to engage their bodies only in life-enhancing, health-promoting activities.

After a diligent study and reflection upon the biblical health laws, especially the Old Testament laws on health, Dr. Roderik Saxey, concluded that the contribution of these laws embody "an affirmation of life and the importance of healthy bodies as mortals relate to God…a reason for compassionate service and reverence for life by recognizing the divine in human beings" (Saxey, n.d.). Overall, the above functions of modern public health enumerated by the Association of the Schools of Public Health are echoes of the biblical health principles God gave mankind through the nation of Israel to promote health and well-being.

CHAPTER 4

A CLOSER LOOK AT THE GLOBAL BURDEN OF DISEASE

I have heard your prayer, I have seen your tears; behold, I will heal you...

(2 Kings 20:5)

Although statistics might have slight variations from year to year, currently in developed countries, cancer and cardiovascular diseases continue to be the leading causes of death. According to statistics from the National Vital Statistics Report of April 2009, as reported in 2009 by the Centers for Disease Control and Prevention (CDC), in the United States, 632,636 people died from heart disease. This was 26 percent of all deaths that took place during that year. In the same year, cancer claimed 559,888; about 23.1 percent of all deaths in that year. Stroke killed 137,119 people. Chronic lower respiratory diseases claimed 124,583. The list goes on and on.[23]

The report from the World Health Organization (WHO) Fact sheet indicates that cancer "accounted for 7.6 million deaths world-wide in 2008 alone" (World Health Organization, 2010).[24]

Massive investments are being made to find the prevention and cure for these deadly diseases. In spite of the commendable efforts being forged by the World Health Organization and other health organizations to eradicate disease, the dream of health for all still remains a mirage, an illusion that keeps receding further and further away in the distance with the emergence of new diseases and the re-emergence of old ones with more virulence.

These diseases seem to defy technological and medical advancement. In developed nations, remarkable longevity has been achieved thanks to science and medical breakthroughs, but a new host of age-related challenges has emerged such as Alzheimer's disease. Huge financial investments and unprecedented policy adjustments are being made to enhance research and development for more effective therapies. It is obviously a vicious cycle of discovering remedies for novel diseases only to be assailed by new ones again.

As Winnail further observes, this indicates that "leaders in government and the medical community are beginning to realize that medicines, money, research and legislation alone cannot win the battle against disease" (Winnail, 2002).[25] Winning the battle against disease may require incorporating every tool that is at our disposal including practical biblical counsel and principles.

In developing nations, infectious diseases continue to ravage both young and old. Sometimes they threaten to decimate entire generations. These diseases leave more problems in their wake such as large numbers of orphans for which local governments are ill prepared. Malaria, the age-old killer disease that helped topple the Roman Empire, continues to kill thousands every day in developing nations.

According to a 2003 report by the World Health Organization (WHO), 3,000 African children die every single day from malaria alone.[26] This means that an African child dies from malaria every 30 seconds. This is a great loss of human capital for Africa and for the global community. Tuberculosis still grips much of Africa and Asia and is spreading rapidly to Russia and Eastern Europe.

Additionally, the World Health Organization Fact Sheet claims that in tropical climatic zones, 2.5 billion people are at risk of contracting dengue fever, another mosquito-borne disease. Every year there are 50 million cases of dengue that result in 50,000 fatalities. The WHO report further claims that over 60 million individuals are at risk of being infected with sleeping sickness and about 500,000 people actually suffer from it in some developing nations annually.

More than 500 million people are at risk of being infected with schistosomiasis (bilharzia, snail fever), and 200 million actually get afflicted by the disease. HIV/AIDS has literally paralyzed and crippled Africa's emerging social and economic development and growth, leaving the continent reeling in astonishment under the ruthless attack of the disease with no hope of a cure or even an effective vaccination in sight. In 2008, there were 33.4 million people living with HIV/AIDS and two million AIDS deaths each year. Because of climatic conditions that are conducive for breeding and existence of different disease-carrying agents, and a public and medical health care system that is still in its infancy, Africa has borne a very grievous burden of disease, many times more than any other continent.

Unfortunately, most diseases, particularly infectious ones, are endemic in low income and poor communities in which there is not enough food with the necessary nutritional value needed to prepare the body to resist disease. Villages, migrant farm areas, and urban slums continue to bear the heavier burden of disease. These areas constitute population groups known as hard to reach by public health and other health professionals. The reason is lack of proper transportation system and paved roads to allow for accessibility.

As a consequence, these population groups have no access to comprehensive preventive and curative resources. Their dwelling places are often characterized by crowding, poor sanitary resources, lack of clean water, or protection from vectors or other disease-carrying agents. Most of them have never had any access to public health educational or preventive programs, and so they still do not know how some diseases such as HIV or tuberculosis or leprosy are transmitted from one person to another or that consumption of foods rich in saturated fats, calories and sugar can lead to cardiovascular disease, cancer, and diabetes.

Sometimes they are not aware of the fact that it is critical for health and well-being to wash their hands every time they handle food or after using the restroom. As such, they often develop a fatalistic attitude toward disease. The church, in these locations, is in a strategic position to provide the necessary disease prevention education stipulated in Scripture. By carefully studying Scripture, the clergy in these areas can tap into a rich mine of disease-preventive strategies, which they can share with their congregations. Biblical principles could have a direct and positive impact in curtailing many communicable diseases in these areas.

Chapter 5

Air Pollution and Health

The Lord God took the man and put him in the garden of Eden to till it and keep it.

(Genesis 2:15)

Over the last few decades, air pollution has escalated to alarming proportions in some societies and has become a source of concern for individuals, community-based organizations, and governments. Increase in levels of air pollution was aggravated by the Industrial Revolution of the eighteenth century, which was characterized by heavy manufacturing activities that replaced agricultural activities as a source of a livelihood. Because these activities were concentrated in cities, people seeking a means of livelihood emigrated from rural areas that were characterized by agrarian lifestyles to emerging cities to seek employment.

The result was a demand for more housing, public utilities, and other amenities that exceeded supply. The heat that was needed for industrial activities was produced by using solid fuel, which emitted huge clouds of smoke, ashes, and other pollutants, often blowing toward residential areas and saturating them with health-damaging soot. The problem of air pollution was further intensified by the invention of automobiles. Cities began to be besieged by smog emanating from exhaust pipes. This further increased air pollution, which threatened the health of the people.

In the United States, air pollution became such a prevalent and pervasive problem that in 1940s, the federal government had to get involved to establish environmental regulations.[27] In 1950 in Poza Rica, Mexico, twenty-two people died after being poisoned by hydrogen sulfide that was released in the air by a city plant that was engaged in processing natural gas.[28]

Two years later, in London, over 4,000 people died from bronchitis, pneumonia, respiratory, and cardiac problems that were caused by a five-day smog over the city. In Bhopal, India, a Union Carbide pesticide plant accidently emitted a highly poisonous gas.[29] As a result, over 4,000 people died instantly from methyl isocyanate poisoning, while many thousands were disabled permanently. The Indian government claims that an estimated 15,000 subsequent deaths can be traced to the Bhopal gas leak. Since the Industrial Revolution, air pollution has evolved into a discipline of its own kind. It has continued to be a threat to individual and community health even as governments continue to grapple with the issue by enacting laws to try to reduce air pollution.

Modern-day urban areas bear the brunt of air pollution. People continue to be exposed to particulate matter (PM) resulting in frequent emergency visits due to asthmatic attacks, bronchitis, and other respiratory problems. Others are subjected to loss of productivity and absenteeism at work and school. Particulate matter is a mixture of natural or manmade solid and liquid particles that are constantly suspended in the air and which can be easily inhaled.[30]

Sources of particulate matter include diesel-operated and non-diesel operated automobiles, power plants, industrial boilers, and combustion activities. Automobiles produce 50 percent of PM in urban areas. In rural areas, PM comes, largely, from biomass burning. When inhaled, particulate matter can lodge itself in the lungs and cause health problems over a period of time. A global estimate of the burden of disease attributable to pollution indicates that 1.4% of total mortality, 0.4% of total disability-adjusted years (DALYs), and 2% of all cardiopulmonary health problems are a result of outdoor air pollution.[31]

According to World Health Organization (WHO), disability-adjusted life years are the lost years of a healthy life. "The sum of these DALY across the population, or the burden of disease, can be thought of as a measurement of the gap between current health status and an ideal health situation where the entire population lives to an advanced age, free of disease and disability" (World Health Organization, 2010).[32] Mortality rates resulting from exposure to particulate matter are usually higher in vulnerable populations consisting of the elderly, infants, children, and people with compromised immune systems than in the general population.

Frank Raes of the Institute for Environment and Sustainability in Europe claims that the global demand for energy has continued to be sustained mainly by fossil fuel.[33] The combustion of this fossil fuel has been emitting greenhouse gases such as carbon dioxide, methane, nitrous oxide, and chlorofluorocarbons. When these gases accumulate in the atmosphere, they act like glass covering the roof and walls of a building so that they are able to allow sunlight to penetrate but block infrared radiation from escaping the earth's surface with heat back into space.

Local concentrations of greenhouse gases play a significant role in increasing local heat, reinforcing differences between hotter and colder regions and making weather patterns more extreme. Environmentalists claim that as the gases continue to accumulate over a number of years, the average temperature of the planet begins to rise, resulting in what is termed as global warming. Combustion of fossil fuels produces other air pollutants that include carbon monoxide, carbonaceous aerosols or soot sulfur dioxide, and nitrogen oxides.

When some of these compounds saturate the atmosphere, they begin to form secondary pollutants such as ozone and particulate sulfate, which can have adverse effects on the ecosystem. Dr. Jeffery Chanton of Florida State University, Department of Oceanography, asserts that "The 10 warmest years on record have been since 1983 and the 7 warmest years on record have been since 1990" (Canton, 2002), and that if the current rate of consumption of fossil fuel continues, the level of carbon dioxide in the air will have doubled by the year 2100.[34]

In her document on climate change, Naomi Oreskes observes that controversy continues to rage over the issue of global warming as individuals whose corporations' revenue stands to be adversely affected if stringent measures to control emissions of carbon dioxide were to be adopted by the international community. These people continue to argue that there is no scientific consensus about greenhouse gases emissions being associated with global warming.[35] Oreskes dismisses their claim and contends that

> The scientific consensus is clearly expressed in the reports of the Intergovernmental Panel on Climate Change (IPCC). "Created in 1988 by the World Meteorological Organization and the United Nations Environmental Programme, IPCC's purpose is to evaluate the state of climate science as a basis for informed policy action, primarily on the basis of peer-reviewed and published scientific literature" and that "In its most recent assessment, IPCC states unequivocally that the consensus of scientific opinion is that Earth's climate is being affected by human activities."
>
> (Oreskes, 2004)

INDOOR AIR POLLUTION

Air pollution is no longer limited to outdoors. The United States Environmental Protection Agency (EPA) claims that indoor air pollution has become a significant menace to health as well. In societies that have shifted from agrarian economies to modern urban lifestyles that require working indoors such as in homes, offices and other enclosures, indoor air pollution poses as a great threat to health. The EPA further asserts that, currently, a significant percentage of people spend 90 percent of their time indoors where they are constantly exposed to indoor air pollution caused by mechanical heating and cooling systems, cooking and cleaning activities that utilize mostly ammonia-based products.

Other products that cause indoor pollution include tobacco, air fresheners, kerosene, gas, coal and wood. Asbestos, damp and old carpeting and furniture are additional sources of indoor air pollution. A basic antidote for this type of pollution is an increase in the flow of air from outside into the home. Other suggested solutions to this problem include a significant reduction in the use of harmful products. In 2000, the WHO reported that indoor air pollution was responsible for more than 1.5 million deaths, worldwide, and 2.7 percent of the global burden of disease.[36] But deaths and disability-adjusted life years (DALYs) resulting from indoor air pollution are unevenly distributed across nations.

A study was conducted by Gregory A. Wellenius and associates to evaluate a potential association between elevated levels of ambient particulate air pollution and admissions to various hospitals for congestive heart failure in seven selected cities of the United States.[37] In this study, the researchers specifically assessed the association between the daily levels of respirable particulate matter with aerodynamic diameters of less than or equal to 10 μm (PM_{10}) and the rate of emergency room visits due to exacerbation of congestive heart failure between 1986 and 1999.

The results of this study demonstrated that a mere 10 ug/m^3 increase in particulate matter (PM_{10}) was associated with a rate increase of 0.72% hospital admissions for individuals suffering from congestive heart failure. The results of this study indicate that an increase in particulate matter in ambient air even below the limits set by the United States Environmental Protection Agency (EPA) can have adverse health outcomes, as was the case with the participants in the study who had congestive heart failure.

Other epidemiological studies conducted over time have confirmed associations between air pollution and high levels of morbidity and mortality. "Indeed, in addition to the classical risk factors such as serum lipids, smoking, hypertension, aging, gender, family history, physical inactivity and diet, recent data have implicated air pollution as an important additional risk factor for atherosclerosis" (Bhatnagar, 1006 and Brook, 2008).[38][39]

Small particulates are generally measured in micrometers according to their size. In the state of Virginia, there are two types of particulates monitored by the US EPA and the Virginia Department of Environmental Air Quality (DEQ). One type includes those particulates that have a diameter under 10μ; the second one includes particles with a mean diameter of less than 2.5μ. Both types are harmful to respiratory health.

BIBLICAL COUNSEL ASSOCIATED WITH POLLUTION

The Bible does not specifically address air pollution. There were no industrial fumes or any gas emissions to threaten the health of the people or the purity of the air then. The only main substance that could pollute the air would have to be human excrement carelessly dumped and exposed close to the encampment and left to poison and pollute the air.

It is obvious from the Scripture found in Deuteronomy 23:12-13 that God did not only want to protect His people from infectious diseases but also from breathing in foul air emitted by fresh and decomposing sewage. The principle is still the same. Anything that had the potential to pollute the air had to be dealt with. Hence the command that "You shall have a place outside the camp and you shall go out to it; and you shall have a stick with your weapons; and when you sit down outside, you shall dig a hole with it, and turn back and cover up your excrement" (Deuteronomy 23:12-13).

Whenever people live together in large communities, there is an inevitable production of great loads of human waste and other garbage that is likely to threaten community health and wellbeing. These waste products need to be properly treated to avoid disease as well as atmospheric and air pollution, over time, similar to that which occurred during the industrial revolution when large amounts of raw sewage and other animal and industrial wastes were deposited and left openly to rot in the streets. This waste and its foul odor were released in the air, fouling the environment. The waste also became breeding ground for pathogens, flies, and other disease-carrying insects. The biblical imperative is to take care of our environment so that we can enjoy optimum health.

Mankind has been entrusted with stewardship of God's creation. That is, he has been given the responsibility of caring for the earth and its substance because it is necessary for his survival and the survival of future generations: "Thou hast given him dominion over the works of thy hands; thou hast put all things under his feet" (Psalm 8:6). As stewards, our responsibility is not limited to fundraising. Stewards understand that whatever they own is a gift from God: "No one can receive anything except what is given him from heaven" (John 3: 27). Additionally, in Psalm 24:1 we are told that "The earth is the LORD's and the fulness thereof, the world and those who dwell therein." Polluting the earth through thoughtless exploitation and without regard for the wellbeing of other people's lives is not only a breach of this trust but it is also detrimental to health including the health of the perpetrator. Depletion of the earth's resources, inevitably, places the lives of future generations in a predicament.

CHAPTER 6

SAFE DRINKING WATER

If anyone thirst, let him come to me and drink.

(John 7: 37)

"Pray give me a little water to drink from your jar." She said, "Drink, my lord"; and she quickly let down her jar upon her hand, and gave him a drink.

(Genesis 24: 17, 18)

Water is an indispensable life-sustaining substance. It makes up over two thirds of the weight of the human body. Without water, human beings can live no longer than a few days. The *United Sates Geographical Survey* report informs us that the human brain is composed of approximately 70% water; lean muscle is about 75% water, blood is 83% water, and lungs about 90%.[40] Loss of water in our bodies even by as little as 2% could result in severe dehydration. Other adverse health conditions emanating from loss of water in our bodies include problems with focusing on computer-related tasks and problems with performing basic math calculations.

To function effectively, the human body requires a constant supply of water. However, in order for the water to be of benefit to the body, it must be clean and safe. An inadequate supply of clean water is always a threat to health. Some of the indispensable benefits and functions of water have been stipulated by *Water Treatment Solutions* and *Hall Center-University of Washington* as follows:

> Water transports nutrients and oxygen to the cells of our bodies. These blood cells absorb the water that passes through the bone marrow structure to help them perform their functions of diffusion;
>
> Water keeps the lungs moist in order to facilitate the process of respiration. Without the right amount of water in the lungs, the process can be severely disrupted, endangering the general health of the organism;
>
> The kidneys excrete waste such as uric acid and urea. This waste must be dissolved in the water for the kidneys to be able to remove it;
>
> Water assists in the process of metabolism. The chemical reactions in the body that facilitate this process of metabolism rely on water;
>
> Water helps the organs of the body absorb nutrients better and effectively;
>
> Water helps regulate the temperature of the body through perspiration, which eliminates excess heat and cools our bodies;
>
> Water assists in the process of detoxification. For water to achieve this process of waste removal, it must be in its purest form otherwise it can easily worsen the situation by saturating the body with more waste;
>
> Water also functions as a moisturizer for our joints. The tissues of the cartilages in the body keep a lot of water, which works as a lubricant and assists in the movements of the joints;
>
> When the body is dehydrated, the energy generated by the brain decreases resulting in depression and chronic fatigue syndrome
>
> (Water Facts and Trivia, 2009)[41]

If any of the above functions are disrupted for a prolonged period of time, the health of the individual can be seriously threatened. Every cell in the entire human body needs clean and safe water. Unsafe drinking water can be a depository of and a transmitter of a myriad of diseases. Unfortunately, access to safe drinking water continues to elude millions of people worldwide today. A significant burden of disease can be attributed to lack of adequate safe drinking water.

Over 2.5 billion people worldwide live in areas where there is inadequate water supply for essential activities such as sanitation. It is these people who bear the larger burden of water-related diseases.[42] It is estimated that one tenth of diseases worldwide can be prevented by improving water supply, proper sanitation, and by observing rigorous hygiene standards.

The World Health Organization claims that 1.6 million people die each year from diarrheal-related diseases.[43] Most of these deaths occur in developing nations, and 90% of them occur among children. An estimated 2.5 billion people still lack access to safe drinking water. Usually people in these places draw their drinking water from contaminated open wells and lakes in which they also do their laundry and swim.

Drinking water systems can be contaminated by waste matter such as urine and feces, especially in cases where the water comes directly from water surfaces, such as rivers, creeks, and lakes where human and animal waste is likely to be deposited.

INTERNATIONAL YEAR OF FRESHWATER

On December 12, 2003, the International Year of Freshwater was launched at a ceremony that was held at the United Nations offices in New York by the United Nations Educational, Scientific and Cultural Organization (UNESCO). The main thrust of the event was to highlight the importance of preserving, managing, and protecting freshwater as well as raising the awareness of the indispensability of clean freshwater for human health and wellbeing.[44]

At the meeting, the Director-General of UNESCO, Koïchiro Matsuura, observed that "water can be an agent of peace, rather than conflicts, and UNESCO is looking at ways that will allow this century to be one of 'water peace' rather than 'water wars.' By developing principles and methods to manage this resource efficiently and ethically, while respecting related ecosystems, we move a step closer to the goal of sustainable development" (Matsuura, International Year of Freshwater, 2003).

The highlight of the launching of this significant event was the 3rd Water Forum that would later be held in Kyoto, Japan. The forum coincided with the World Water Day held every year on March 22 in Japan. The United Nations Educational, Scientific and Cultural Organization (UNESCO) hosted the International Year of Freshwater (IYFW) in Japan and the World Water Assessment Programme (WWAP), which is a collaboration of 23 United Nations agencies for freshwater presented its World Water Development Report.

The report was the first of the series of presentations that revealed the extent of water stress worldwide. The IYFW is a program that aims to achieve the United Millenium Declarion Goal on Water pledging "to halve, by the year 2015, the proportion of the world's people unable to reach, or to afford, safe drinking water…to stop the unsustainable exploitation of water resources" (United Nations Millennium Declaration, 2000).[45]

WATER CONTAMINANTS AND HEALTH

The Centers for Disease Control and Prevention (CDC) claim that clean water is an indispensable component of life. When it is contaminated, the consequences can be disastrous. Contaminated water can undermine sanitation, leading to hygiene-related health problems that include salmonellosis, cholera, diarrhea and shigellosis, malaria, schistosomiasis, and many others.

In fact, as mentioned earlier, most of the diseases that afflict humanity, especially in the developing world, can be traced back to polluted water supply systems. In Bangladesh alone, about 35 million people are constantly exposed to high levels of arsenic in their drinking water, which is not only a threat to their health but shortens their life expectancy as well.

Similarly, water supply systems that are in close proximity to landfills, runoff, sewer pipes, and residential areas can be contaminated and become a source of constant health problems, often leading to being underweight. Pruss-Ustum and associates from World Health Organization claim that about 35% of all deaths of children under the age of 5 in developing nations occur in children who are underweight.[46] Fifty percent of this problem of being underweight in children is a result of nematode infections or diarrhea caused by drinking unsafe water, poor hygiene, and insufficient sanitation.

Substances found in biomedical waste can also pollute water and cause gastrointestinal infections such as cholera, typhoid, and dysentery, ascariasis, as well as polio. Some biomedical waste might even contain tuberculosis bacteria, HIV, and hepatitis B and C, and other virulent viral agents that can easily place whoever comes into contact with it at great risk of contracting some of these serious diseases.

Dr. Mukesh Yadav describes biomedical waste as "the rubbish containing human tissues, body fluids, excreta, unused drugs, swabs, disposable syringes and sticky bandages" (Mukesh, 2001).[47] Therefore, stringent sanitation and proper hygiene practices ought to be observed to protect the health of not only health professionals but the general public as well.

God instilled into the minds of ancient Israelites the importance of safe drinking water and set some guidelines by which the safety of water could be maximized. For example, God forbade the Israelites from drinking from vessels or from stagnant water in which a dead animal had fallen. It was only about one hundred years ago that medical science discovered that stagnant water can become a breeding ground for disease-carrying insects and a source of typhoid and cholera.

Running water is good for washing and bathing. Commenting on the command to avoid drinking water in which a dead animal had fallen, Dr. Thomas L. Constable claims that "those objects that water would cleanse could be reused, but those that water would not cleanse could not. In this case, neither the container nor the water became impure; only the person who fished the dead animal out would be. However, if one of these creatures fell into a spring or cistern, an exception was made" (Constable, 2010).[48]

The following is an excerpt from Scripture:

> These are unclean to you among all that swarm; whoever touches them when they are dead shall be unclean until the evening. And anything upon which any of them falls when they are dead shall be unclean, whether it is an article of wood or a garment or a skin or a sack, any vessel that is used for any purpose; it must be put into water, and it shall be unclean until the evening; then it shall be clean. And if any of them falls into any earthen vessel, all that is in it shall be unclean, and you shall break it. Any food in it which may be eaten, upon which water may come, shall be unclean; and all drink which may be drunk from every such vessel shall be unclean. And everything upon which any part of their carcass falls shall be unclean; whether oven or stove, it shall be broken in pieces; they are unclean, and shall be unclean to you. Nevertheless a spring or a cistern holding water shall be clean; but whatever touches their carcass shall be unclean.
>
> (Leviticus. 11:31-34)

This counsel from God's word still stands: water must be clean for it to be of benefit to health and wellbeing. Contaminated water is a source of a myriad of diseases worldwide. Millions of lives are being lost due to lack of access to life-promoting clean water supplies.

Chapter 7

Alcohol Consumption

Woe to the proud crown of the drunkards of E'phraim, and to the fading flower of its glorious beauty, which is on the head of the rich valley of those overcome with wine! The proud crown of the drunkards of E'phraim will be trodden under foot.

(Isaiah 28:1-3)

Alcohol is a type of drink that contains ethanol. Ethanol is commonly referred to as alcohol. There are three types of alcoholic beverages: wines, spirits, and beers. Many findings from various archaeological excavations have demonstrated that alcohol is one of man's oldest and widely diffused intoxicating beverages.[49]

From time immemorial, every culture and social system has wrestled with health and socioeconomic issues associated with alcohol consumption. Intoxicating drinks were often incorporated in community celebrations and religious rites worldwide. Probably due to their intoxicating capacity, alcoholic beverages have always been perceived across cultures as special commodities consumed at special occasions by certain population groups. For instance, alcohol has often been withheld from children and infants.

Over the years, alcohol-related health and social issues have become a worldwide concern. With the increase in construction work demanding operations of machinery, concern over alcohol consumption has increased. Similarly, the coming of factory work and vehicle operation activities that require protracted levels of focus and concentration has ushered in new concerns about alcohol consumption. Alcohol consumption undermines levels of alertness necessary for this nature of work by reducing the span of concentration and reaction time characteristic in these duties.

The World Health Organization (WHO) was first established in Geneva, Switzerland, on April 7, 1948, as the First World Health Assembly.[50] April 7 is now observed worldwide as World Health Day. Shortly after this it became known as the World Health Organization (WHO) and almost from its inception, the WHO realized that it had a role to play in alcohol-related problems. Because alcohol-related problems pervade the general public's critical areas of wellbeing such as social, economic and psychological functions, the WHO is committed to reducing and preventing a wide range of alcohol abuse-related problems. The easy availability of alcoholic beverages has precipitated a global atmosphere that is replete with alcohol-related problems. Alcohol consumption contributes significantly to morbidity and mortality of different population groups. The World Health Organization's intervention strategies are focused more on preventing alcohol-related problems than on trying to repair the associated damages.

This approach is an echo of the Scriptural approach, which warns us about the destructive nature of alcohol abuse and admonishes us to avoid it in the book of Proverbs:

> Who has woe? Who has sorrow? Who has strife? Who has complaining? Who has wounds without cause? Who has redness of eyes? Those who tarry long over wine, those who go to try mixed wine. Do not look at wine when it is red, when it sparkles in the cup and goes down smoothly. At the last it bites like a serpent, and stings like an adder.

Your eyes will see strange things, and your mind utter perverse things. You will be like one who lies down in the midst of the sea, like one who lies on the top of a mast. "They struck me," you will say, "but I was not hurt; they beat me, but I did not feel it. When shall I awake? I will seek another drink."

(Proverbs 23: 29-35)

Scripture further tells us that "Wine is a mocker, strong drink a brawler; and whoever is led astray by it is not wise" (Proverbs 20:1).

The above are only two examples in which Scriptures give us warning against abuse of intoxicating drinks in order to optimize our health. Intoxicating drinks eliminate inhibition and self-restraint, thereby promoting callous and destructive behaviors. Looking down the corridor of time, God foresaw how the effects of abuse of alcoholic drinks would destroy the beautiful human machine he had created as well as the social system necessary for nurturing these same human beings.

The harmful effects of intoxicating drinks are evident in many global communities. Public health professionals are working frantically with medical communities, non-governmental organizations as well as governments to design effective intervention strategies for this 100% preventable tragic epidemic, which contributes to many other evils such as rape, domestic violence, and incest, to mention just a few.

Researchers at the Center for Social Research on Alcohol and Drugs in Stockholm claim that research that has been based on the epidemiology of the role of alcohol in health and illness has demonstrated that there is a significantly complex and multidimensional relationship between alcohol consumption and health outcomes.[51]

Alcohol abuse is reported to be causally related to an estimated sixty medical conditions. Currently, approximately over 4% of the global burden of disease can be ascribed to alcohol abuse. Alcohol abuse also accounts for the same rates of morbidity and mortality as those caused by tobacco and hypertension although the range and intensity of alcohol-related problems may be different from one country to another.

MEDICAL PROBLEMS CAUSED BY ALCOHOL ABUSE

In a research study, conducted by Glucksman, it was discovered that approximately 40% of all hospitalizations in the United Kingdom are related, either directly or indirectly, to alcohol consumption.[52] This is an alarmingly high percentage of preventable health challenges for any society to bear. Different researchers present us with a list of specific health conditions that are likely to be caused by alcohol abuse. The conditions listed below can severely hamper the body's everyday functions:

> Cardiomyopathy: In the *American Journal of Pathology* of 2005, scientists reported that chronic abuse of alcoholic drinks may instigate drastic changes in the functions of major organs of the body such as the heart. The damages caused to the heart can be in form of dilated cardiomyopathy, which can be fatal. Cardiomyopathy "is characterized by reduced contractility, ventricular dilatation, cardiomyocyte apoptosis, and fibrosis, often progressing to heart failure."[53]
>
> (Keith, 2005)

According to the Mayo Clinic, an individual who has cardiomyopathy has a heart that does not function normally because it is enlarged, abnormally thick, or is not able to transmit electrical impulses in the normal way.[54] Although some people can live long lives without being aware that they have cardiomyopathy because they are asymptomatic, others can develop serious complications that can progress to abnormal heartbeats and sudden death. Cardiomyopathy is reported to be the most common cause of untimely death among young athletes.

> Hepatitis is the inflammation of the liver, resulting in liver cell damage and destruction. Alcoholic hepatitis is a complex problem and is a precursor to chronic liver disease and cirrhosis. If an individual develops alcoholic hepatitis and stops drinking, the inflammation is often reversible over time.
>
> However, if the individual has already developed cirrhosis, the liver disease can progress rapidly to liver failure. The individual with alcoholic hepatitis may be admitted to the hospital or treated on an outpatient basis. Abstinence from alcohol is essential for reversing the hepatitis. This is a complex problem that may require an alcohol treatment program. There is no medication to cure alcoholic hepatitis; therefore, treatment involves reducing the symptoms and halting the progression of the disease.[55]
>
> (Health Encyclopedia, 2012)

Usually the livers of individuals who have developed alcoholic hepatitis are enlarged and tender. There is no particular type of alcohol that is especially associated with alcoholic hepatitis. This means that any type of alcohol could be causative if it is abused over a long period of time. Individuals who have been diagnosed with alcohol-related hepatitis should refrain from further consumption of alcohol in order to mitigate the progression of the disease.

However, if excessive alcohol consumption continues, the disease can progress into liver cirrhosis. During this phase, the liver becomes hard like a rock so that blood cannot easily flow through it.[56] The patient then develops a distended belly and has difficulty breathing. As the illness progresses, the blood is forced to bypass the damaged liver and instead flows through the esophagus and other veins, causing these veins to swell.

When these veins rupture due to pressures from the blood, the individual starts vomiting large amounts of bright red blood. Without proper medical intervention, the bleeding could be fatal. The liver is an organ whose function is to metabolize fats, proteins, and carbohydrates. It is also responsible for other functions that include bile secretion and excretion, detoxifying and purifying blood, as well as enzyme activation. These functions are disrupted when liver failure sets in.

Alcohol-Related Dementia is another condition that can be caused by protracted alcohol abuse. Long-term consumption of alcohol has always been associated with negative health outcomes. Usually, the most commonly identified health problems include liver failure.

In a study reported in a journal called *New England Journal of Medicine*, the researchers demonstrated that long-term alcohol consumption is also significantly associated with cognitive decline or deficit.[57] Even individuals who report drinking alcohol only at social events can exhibit "signs of regional brain damage and cognitive dysfunction" (Harper, 2009).[58]

Excessive alcohol consumption, therefore, causes significant harm to the brain, hampering essential overall body functions and activities. Alzheimer's Australia, which provides information about living with dementia, claims that symptoms of alcohol-related dementia may include difficulties learning new things, significant and noticeable changes in personality, having trouble with short-term memory, having difficulties maintaining balance, and exhibiting bad social skills.[59]

It is not unusual for some individuals who have been abusing alcohol over a long period of time to develop this condition, although it is more prevalent among men aged 45-65 who have had a long-term alcohol consumption habit. If alcohol consumption is not reduced or eliminated, the condition is likely to progress. However, elimination of alcohol consumption can curtail the progression of the health condition.

Pancreatitis: As stated earlier, alcohol abuse is a global problem that spans socio-economic statuses. Excessive alcohol consumption can be a risk factor for pancreatitis. In his article the *Pathophysiology of Alcoholic Pancreatitis*, professor Parimal Chowdhury and his associate Priya Gupta inform us that approximately 30% of acute pancreatitis cases in the United States are induced by consumption of alcohol and between 60% to 90% of individuals with pancreatitis have a history of chronic alcohol consumption, meaning that the risk of developing this disease increases with not only the amount consumed but the duration of consumption as well.[60]

Chowdhury and Gupta further assert that consumption of more than 2.75 ounces of alcohol every day for a period of between 6 and 12 years is likely to produce symptomatic pancreatitis. The pancreas is an organ that lies behind the stomach. It is responsible for producing enzymes that assist in food digestion. A defective pancreas cannot perform this function well.

Pancreatitis is characterized by inflammation of the pancreas. In acute pancreatitis, the inflammation is severe although it develops over a short period of time. With chronic pancreatitis, the inflammation develops over a long period of time and is persistent, but it is not as intense as in acute pancreatitis. Symptoms of pancreatitis include abdominal pain, poor digestion, and nausea.

ECONOMIC COST OF ALCOHOL ABUSE

The National Institute of Alcohol Abuse and Alcoholism (NIAAA) news report indicates that, between 1985 and 1992, the direct and indirect economic cost of problems related to alcohol abuse amounted to $148 billion.[61] The National Institute of Alcohol Abuse and Alcoholism further claimed that the economic cost of alcohol had increased to $184.6 billion in 1998.

Most of this cost is incurred through services such as alcohol abuse treatment and resources, alcohol abuse preventive intervention programs, research into causes and effects of alcohol abuse, lost productivity due to alcohol-induced illness or disability, lost productivity caused by premature deaths, medical expenses, costs of alcohol-related automobile crashes, and social welfare administrative expenses.

ALCOHOL-RELATED SOCIAL PROBLEMS

The National Association for Children of Alcoholics (NACA) estimated that 43% adults in the United States have been affected one way or another by alcohol consumption in their families.[62] Approximately 62% of high school seniors reported having been drunk at some point in their lives. Driving while intoxicated is pervasive among young adults even though it places the driver and others on the road at great risk for accidents. Other significant social problems associated with alcohol consumption are enumerated below:

> Alcohol-Related Sexual Assault: Heavy alcohol consumption has been implicated as the main contributor to sexual assault. A research study conducted among inmates demonstrated that a significant number of men self-reporting as heavy drinkers were also more likely to report having committed sexual assault.
>
> (Abbey, 2001)[63]

Alcohol is reported to increase sexual desire, especially in men, because inebriation causes them to feel more powerful, masculine, in control, belligerent, and uninhibited. By arousing these factors, alcohol makes it easier for an individual to sexually assault another person. Alcohol consumption also has a tendency to distort interpersonal communication in which a female peer's friendliness, especially in a social setting, can easily be misinterpreted by the perpetrator to be sexually motivated.

Any resistance afterward is viewed as a mere farce, which further incites the perpetrator to ensure that his mission needs to be accomplished. Although alcohol consumption may lead to more sexual aggression scientists have discovered that persistent alcohol abuse is actually associated with sexual dysfunction.[64] In a study conducted among one hundred male subjects who were admitted to a De-addiction Centre of the National Institute of Mental Health And NeuroSciences (NIMHANS), Bangalore, India, who were diagnosed with Alcohol Dependence Syndrome with Simple Withdrawal Symptoms, seventy-two percent of them were found to have one or more sexual types of dysfunction. The dysfunctions included a significantly reduced desire for sex, difficulty to have an erection or to maintain it, failure to achieve orgasm and recurrent premature ejaculation. According to Mendelson and Mello (1979), alcohol abuse is the main causal factor of impotence and other forms of sexual dysfunction.[65]

> Homelessness: Although the problem of homelessness is multidimensional and complex, the European Federation of National Organizations Working with the Homeless (FEANTSA) reports that alcohol consumption is a common underlying problem among the homeless population group.[66] Most of these individuals are chronic alcohol consumers and the proportion of homeless people adversely affected by excessive alcohol consumption is higher compared to the general population. Therefore, alcohol is perceived to be a significant contributor to homelessness, and alcohol dependence tends to keep people homeless.
>
> (FEANTSA, 2011)

During my tenure at a faith-based community clinic, which catered for individuals who had not health insurance, our patient base included people who were in alcohol rehabilitation programs. They were usually very grateful for the clinic. Sometimes some of them told stories about their personal experiences. Billy (not his real name) was one of the individuals who decided to share his experience. His alcohol consumption had escalated to a point of becoming homeless. Billy had sustained back injuries as a construction worker, which hindered his ability to continue working.

As a result, he became eligible for disability benefits. Billy received a check for his condition every month, which meant that he could buy the food he needed. He also paid for his rent and amenities although his budget was limited. He had enough money left over to buy cigarettes. Often he would stock up on food for the whole month. Life looked quite manageable, but then he began to feel a little bored. All he did when he woke up in the morning was sit around and watch TV while he drank some alcohol.

The drinking started off slow at first, but it got worse with time, and soon Billy discovered that buying alcohol was the first thing he wanted to do whenever he received his disability check. Before long, he started feeling depressed, and sometimes he would just sit in his home and drink. It seemed that was the only thing he could do.

So he drank more and more alcohol in order to forget about the boredom and depression that plagued him. He no longer wanted to hang out with his friends or to have them come home to visit with him. He just wanted to drink and forget about the challenges of life. He was in the grip of alcohol. Billy could no longer clean his home. Soon it started to have a stale smell.

His landlord was not impressed with the whole situation, and he told Billy to clean up or risk losing his accommodation. The landlord was getting tired of Billy trashing his property. Finally, he actually got rid of Billy. His debauchery and drunkenness had escalated to a destructive level. He did not care anymore if he ate or not. He started feeling ill, but he thought it was a minor illness his body could easily shake off.

The Perfect Prescription

Finally, he decided to go to a local clinic where they told him his liver was showing signs of swelling and that he had some internal bleeding. They warned him that if he continued drinking at the same rate, he would not be around too long. Sometimes Billy slept under the bridges and other times on benches in the park. At some point, he mustered enough courage to seek help and get treatment for his alcoholism.

He found some programs that promised to help him. One program seemed to be sobering him up. But as soon as they let him go, he started drinking all over again. This happened with every other program he joined. It became a vicious cycle. He finally found a program that refused to give up on him. The support and love was so excellent that Billy did not want to disappoint the people in charge. They told him he was created for a special purpose—that God does not make junk. Billy felt a spark of hope ignite from deep within him—a spark he had not felt in a long time. He began to think that maybe he could really be somebody one day after all. Those guys at the program were interested in *him*; they actually believed in him. He resolved not to let them down.

The thing about being created for a special purpose stuck with him. No one had ever said that to him, not even his own parents. This was something new. Slowly he began to control the amount of alcohol he consumed. He was beginning to win the battle slowly. Finally, the urge to drink alcohol began to decrease until it was finally gone. Now Billy is completely dry. He has not tasted alcohol for three years! During this time he found his calling. He began helping others, especially young adults, understand the dangers of excessive drinking and he told them that they were created for a special purpose. Nevertheless, Billy is remorseful that he wasted the most productive years of his life. He regularly shares his story particularly with the youth to warn them against self-destructive choices such as alcohol consumption.

Although not everybody has or will experience what Billy experienced, nevertheless his story is instructive. It is a story, which reveals the subtlety with which seemingly moderate alcohol consumption can escalate to a point where it becomes deleterious to the health and general well-being of the individual. It is a warning to the dangers lurking in an innocent-looking glass of alcohol. The story also highlights the fact that alcohol can steal a significant portion of its victim's life. That loss is irretrievable. Some people might not be as fortunate as Billy was in finding a Bible-based, God-fearing program to restore them to what God intended them to be. We gain wisdom by taking a leaf from another person's experience.

> Aggressive Behavior: Researchers Moeller and Dougherty claim that a significant link exists between excessive alcohol consumption and aggressive behavior because of the capacity of alcohol to reinforce antisocial personality disorders characterized by disregard of other people's rights and preferences.
>
> (Moeller & Dougherty, 2001)[67]

These researchers further assert that excessive alcohol consumption can significantly alter the activities of several brain chemicals, including g-aminobutyric (GABA) and serotonin, which are neurotransmitters linked to several types of aggressive behavior in humans and animals. In the 2010 *Personality and Social Psychology Bulletin*, scientists reported that the findings of two experimental studies testing the link between alcohol consumption and aggression "demonstrated that mere exposure to alcohol-related cues can increase aggressive thoughts and behaviors" (Subra, et al., 2010).[68]

In other words, sometimes people may only need to be exposed to alcohol-related cues for aggressive thoughts to be aroused in them. Further, where expression of aggressive behavior by participants was allowed in the above Subra study, exposure to alcohol-related cues was enough stimulus to invoke not only aggressive thoughts in the participants but to cause actual expression of aggressive behavior as well.

Alcohol-related aggressive behavior is not only directed toward others. Studies have demonstrated that two-thirds of people who have been involved in self-destructive behaviors have done so while under the influence of alcoholic drinks.[69] Elevated blood alcohol concentrations are known to have been found in most individuals who have attempted to commit suicide as well as those who have actually committed suicide.

Legal Problems:

A myriad of legal problems are associated with excessive alcohol consumption. Inebriated individuals often find themselves in violation of the laws of the societies where they live. Some of the alcohol-related legal violations are indicated below.

> Alcohol-Related Driving Offenses: These offenses and their associated negative outcomes are 100% preventable. Nevertheless, alcohol-related driving offenses remain a serious public health problem worldwide. In the United States, an estimated 11,773 individuals were killed in alcohol-related motor vehicle accidents and crashes in 2008.[70]

Researcher Mercer and his associates indicate that these figures represent one third of all traffic-related fatalities that occurred during that year. In addition, an estimated 1,347 traffic-related fatalities involving young children aged 0-14 occurred in the same year; one in six of these deaths was linked to a driver under the influence of alcohol.

Additionally, each day 32 people lose their lives in automobile crashes involving alcohol-impaired drivers in the United States.[71] Approximately every 45 minutes someone dies from an alcohol-related accident. In 2000, alcohol-related crashes cost the nation over $51 billion.[72] These fatalities involved drivers whose blood alcohol levels exceeded the legal amount. These are sobering figures considering the fact that they are 100% preventable.

> Alcohol-Related Homicide: Alcohol intoxication is a significant factor in many homicides. In Europe, homicides are more endemic in locations where heavy drinking takes place which is consistent with the assessment by social scientists and other health professionals that excessive alcohol consumption tends to increase the rate of homicides.[73]

A 2003 study by Makkai and Payne, examining alcohol consumption patterns among Australian prisoners including those incarcerated for homicide demonstrated that 22% of the prisoners serving time for homicide had been addicted to alcohol at the time they committed the crime.[74] Aggressive behavior leading to violence and homicide is more likely to take place in beer halls and bars where patrons are often belligerent and less inhibited. In these circumstances people are likely to express violent behavior due to being under the influence of alcoholic drinks.

Intoxicated individuals tend to have a distorted view of themselves and their environment. For example, they may perceive themselves as strong enough to fight and subdue any of their opponents. Their main concern is about the present, not the future or the consequences of their actions.

Alcohol certainly weakens cognitive functions and diminishes the ability to resolve conflicts amicably. The more alcohol an individual consumes, the greater the risk for aggressive and violent behavior. According to the United States Department of Justice, Bureau of Justice Assistance, there is a close cultural and historical link between alcohol consumption and violence in the United States.[75] This connection could have been "through battles fought over the taxation of alcohol, such as the Whiskey Rebellion of 1794, or through the tradition of hard-drinking, bar-brawling frontiersmen of the early days of the nation's existence, alcohol and violence have been closely connected and deeply tied into American custom. This link is highly destructive" (U.S Department of Justice, 2006).

> Damage to Property: Although some intoxicated adults do occasionally damage and vandalize other people's property in their communities, this behavior is more common among young adults, mostly in colleges and universities, according to a survey by Perkins (2005).

Research among college students has found that about 8% of students participate in damaging their institution's property when intoxicated.[76] College parties characterized by binge drinking exacerbate the situation. Furthermore, in these settings, some students usually incur damage to their personal property caused by intoxicated peers. There is usually a tragic interconnection between alcohol use and aggressive behavior especially among adolescents and young adults in these settings.

DEATHS:

The Morbidity and Mortality Weekly Report (MMWR) of January 2012 indicated that "Binge drinking accounts for more than half of the estimated 80,000 average annual deaths and three quarters of $223.5 billion in economic costs resulting from excessive alcohol consumption in the United States."[77]

A separate report claims that "In 2009, a total of 24,518 persons died of alcohol-induced causes in the United States... This category includes deaths from dependent and nondependent use of alcohol, and also includes accidental poisoning by alcohol. It excludes unintentional injuries, homicides, and other causes indirectly related to alcohol use, as well as deaths due to fetal alcohol syndrome."⁷⁸ Its contribution to 100,000 deaths each year makes it the third leading cause of preventable death in the United States with tobacco and diet and activity patterns topping the list at number one and two, respectively. The Glucksman (1994) study mentioned above further demonstrated that in the United Kingdom, alcohol consumption is responsible for 50,000 deaths annually and about 500,000 hospitalizations.

The Bible has a lot of counsel on the evils associated with addiction to alcohol, which can be applied to other current mind-altering substances. In recent years we have witnessed the emergence of other mind-altering substances in addition to alcohol such as cocaine, crystal methamphetamine, and some types of painkillers and tranquilizers that lead to dependence or addiction. Although the Bible does not mention cocaine, heroin, and other drugs, their effects on health are the same and most times worse than those of alcohol. They, like alcohol, lead to shameful and destructive behavioral patterns.

The addiction is often slow and insidious. Abuse of any of these substances can ruin not only families but entire communities. Sometimes they cause irrevocable loss and damage to individuals, families, and societies. A report by Youngers and Rosin claim that for the past twenty-five years the United States has been fighting a war on drugs across the nation as well as across the entire hemisphere.⁷⁹

Multi-faceted efforts involving police officers, social workers, medical personnel, soldiers, and counselors have relentlessly been made to eradicate drug trafficking and drug abuse. It continues to be an uphill battle, but much has been achieved in the form of enacting drug control policies and laws such as the United States policy of "zero tolerance for drug crops which has led to eradication of coca and opium poppy crops" (Youngers & Rosin, 2004).

The illicit drug trade and the ensuing violence it generates have ravaged the western hemisphere. Drug trafficking has been responsible for fueling inconceivable criminal and violent activities that have resulted in a senseless loss of lives. Sometimes government officials, law enforcement officials, and judiciaries have compromised their responsibilities and betrayed the people they are meant to serve by falling prey to the temporary monetary benefits of the drug trafficking trade.

No wonder Scripture warns us against consuming that which alters the structure and functions of the neurons and promotes poor judgment. The Bible informs us that Lot committed incest twice after being intoxicated in Genesis 19:33-35 and that Noah forgot about discretion in his drunken stupor in Genesis 9:20-21. Finally, specific Scriptural warning against alcohol consumption is given to those who are placed in leadership positions because alcohol perverts judgment (see Proverbs 31:4-5).

EFFECTS OF ALCOHOL ON CHILDREN AND FAMILIES

A link has been established by scientists between excessive alcohol consumption and episodes of intimate partner violence (IPV).[80] In a research study by Kaufman and Strauss examining the belief that physical abuse of wives is strongly influenced by drunkenness found that more than 20% of male subjects and about 10% of their female counterparts had consumed significant levels of alcohol before engaging in their most recent violent fights.[81]

Among college students, perpetrators of IPV and other forms of sexual violence were under the influence of alcohol in 50% of the cases. Health care practitioners have confirmed that a significant association exists between alcohol consumption and episodes of IPV. A similar finding has been established by health professionals in rural health clinics. Alcohol-related violence against intimate partners has serious physical, emotional, and psychosocial consequences for all its victims, including children.

Alcohol abuse results in compromised parenting and other negative familial occurrences.

Children caught up in alcohol-related intimate partner violence (IPV) situations usually experience short-term as well as long-term adverse health outcomes. Children of individuals who consume alcohol tend to exhibit propensities toward delinquency and attention deficit disorder. They also suffer from internalized health disorders such as anxiety and low self-esteem. Alcohol abuse during pregnancy is associated with diseases that manifest themselves in adulthood but have their origin in the fetal stage.[82]

Children of alcohol abusers tend to view themselves as the main cause of their parents' drunkenness and carry that guilt with them most their lives. Wherever they are they worry about their situation at home. This creates an atmosphere of tension and anxiety for all affected. The children cannot freely invite their friends to their home because of what is happening at home. It is possible for a parent who is an alcohol abuser to be kind and loving when sober, but as soon they consume alcohol, they become angry and hateful, often screaming incoherently at their family members. These parents have no regular schedule for family activities necessary for providing a nurturing environment for their children. Family activities such as bedtime story reading or family mealtimes are almost nonexistent. This instills in the children a sense of helplessness and hopelessness since they are powerless to change the situation.

Sometimes, the child may develop resentment against the parent who drinks and also against the one who does not drink for allowing that kind of environment to continue and for failing to protect the children in the home. People who abuse alcohol can hurt everybody they are connected with, including parents, children, spouses, other close relatives, friends, workmates, and bosses. Often the hurt takes many years of therapy to heal. Most people carry the scars of their hurt most of their lives.

FETAL ALCOHOL SYNDROME

Fetal alcohol syndrome is one of the most common harmful effects of alcohol consumption during pregnancy. In western countries Fetal Alcohol Syndrome (FAS) is the leading cause of mental retardation.[83] Alcohol is a teratogen, which means that it is a substance that can adversely affect the development of a fetus.[84] Since there is no known established amount or type of alcohol that is safe for a pregnant woman to drink, the Centers for Disease Control and Prevention (CDC) advise that women should refrain from drinking alcohol during pregnancy altogether.

Additionally, the CDC urges all women planning to get pregnant to avoid all manner of alcoholic drink. Alcohol consumption during pregnancy has been implicated as a leading cause of preventable birth defects in the United States.

When a pregnant woman consumes alcohol, the alcohol enters the bloodstream and finds its way to the placenta and to the baby via the umbilical cord. Therefore, it is true that when a pregnant woman consumes alcohol, her fetus does the same. A lot of lifelong damages can ensue if this practice continues. These damages are called fetal alcohol spectrum disorders (FASDs). Disabilities include functional abnormalities, growth deficiency such as low birth weight, poor coordination, learning ability impairment, and brain structure abnormalities.

The health expenses associated with such defects cost approximately $1.4 million per child throughout that child's lifetime.[85] Since there is no effective treatment for the effects of fetal alcohol syndrome, prevention is the best intervention method. The health expenses of a child with FASDs include early intervention to help the child develop social and educational skills. This is an interdisciplinary effort involving a number of specialists. The costs of such therapies can be prohibitive for some people from low socioeconomic statuses who have financial needs.

Dr. Stern, co-author of the book *None of These Diseases*, with Dr McMillen, tells of a story of a forty-two-year-old patient of his who went to his office with a case of jaundice.[86] The patient told Dr. Stern he was experiencing excruciating abdominal pain. His mother, with whom he lived, told the doctor that her son had not eaten any solid food in the previous fourteen months.

His diet was composed of a daily dose of 3,000 calories of beer. The doctor found that the patient had a significantly swollen and tender liver, obviously as a result of his drinking habit. The jaundice was a result of a backup of his bile. The patient had suffered nerve damage that made it difficult for him to walk properly. He was not even able to feel his feet. Dr. Stern recommended hospitalization, which the patient downright rejected. He also turned down the physician's recommendation to stop drinking altogether, opting instead to try and reduce the amount of alcohol he consumed. The physician warned him that he was near death and that stopping alcohol consumption was his only hope. But he refused to take the doctor's advice and instead asked for pain medication.

Dr. Stern could not comply with the request because it would not be effective as a therapy. The doctor also hoped that the continued pain would finally force the patient to stop drinking and look for help. The patient went back to his mother's home, and after another month of continuous alcohol consumption, he went into a coma. His mother finally had him hospitalized. During the period of his hospitalization, his liver began to heal and regain its ability to function well. He was discharged from the hospital with a positive report. However, as soon as he got home, he bought himself a six-pack of alcohol. He was back to square one. There are numerous similar stories out there with tragic endings that could have been prevented.

Treatment of Alcohol Dependence

The best antidote for alcohol-related negative health outcomes is to abstain from alcohol altogether. But should an individual who is addicted to alcohol require help, numerous rehabilitation and treatment modules are available that can place the individual on the way to recovery. Treatment of alcohol abuse can be achieved by conducting early intervention in primary care as well as other behavioral and pharmacological interventions. These treatment regimens are usually incorporated into the discipline of public health as a response to alcohol abuse problems. A general health practitioner is usually in a strategically appropriate position to identify individuals who abuse alcohol.[87]

In such cases, the physician may initiate or recommend counseling by other allied health professionals so that the condition may not progress to the point of incapacitating the individual by triggering other health disorders. The counselor defines the goals for the individual during the assessment process, and strategies are often implemented for meeting those goals. Other intervention strategies may include the involvement of the individual's family members to provide the needed social support. The support and understanding shown by those closest to the person are very critical for the intervention strategies to be efficacious. Alcohol treatment centers are also available to teach alcohol abusers self-discipline and other skills to guide them in breaking the cycle of alcohol abuse.

CHAPTER 8

WASTE DISPOSAL AND SANITATION

> *You shall have a place outside the camp and you shall go out to it; and you shall have a stick with your weapons; and when you sit down outside, you shall dig a hole with it, and turn back and cover up your excrement.*
>
> (Deuteronomy 23: 12, 13)

Waste management is a critical issue in our day. An inadequate waste management system can undermine health in numerous ways. Writing about the Bible as the foundation of good personal and public health, author William F. Dankenbring observes how the unsanitary and deplorably filthy conditions of seventeenth-century cities became breeding grounds for flies and other vectors that transmit pathogens to human beings.[88]

Because there was no comprehensive sanitation system in place, excrement, urine, and garbage lay exposed all over in streets. In the nineteenth century, cholera and other infectious diseases ravaged Europe simultaneously for the same reason.[89] People did not comprehend the etiology or causes of such diseases. Meanwhile, human excrement in the streets continued to decompose, polluting the air with its foul smell and threatening the health of the general public. It acted as a reservoir for various pathogens.

A few large tunnels had been dug under the streets to accommodate sewage. But they were not properly managed due to a lack of a proper drainage system. Sanitary workers attempted to empty these tunnels every five years or so. They would load the sewage into wagons and transport it to farms where farmers applied it to their crops as fertilizer. Crops that were grown using untreated human excrement were sold for consumption, establishing a vicious cycle of spreading disease.

During the nineteenth century, as cholera and other fatal infectious diseases ravaged societies, public hysteria grew, forcing the Prime Minister of England to establish a Royal Commission of Enquiry on the Poor Laws; Edwin Chadwick, who had spent over a decade studying the diseases of England, was chosen to be one of the assistant commissioners to collect information about disease trends among England's poor.[90]

Other infectious and contagious diseases that plagued Europe at that time besides cholera included typhus, fever, small pox, whooping cough, and tuberculosis. The poor working class people were disproportionately affected by these diseases, and morbidity and mortality rates were alarmingly high among them. The reasons for this, according to Chadwick's report of the Royal Commission of Enquiry on Poor Laws, were "atmospheric impurities produced by decomposing animal and vegetable substances, by damp and filth, and close over-crowded dwellings..." (Del Col, 2002).

These conditions were typical of the residential areas of the poor population class. The Chadwick Report proposed "removal of noxious physical circumstances, and the promotion of civic, household and personal cleanliness..." (Del Col, 2002). As a follow up to the recommendations of his report, Chadwick carefully examined the city of London in order to find a strategy he could use to design a viable sewage system that would ultimately remove all the human waste from the city.

This sewage system would be separate from the drinking water system, since the existing sewage system sometimes spilled its contents in drinking water sources. Chadwick's report prompted some positive public health changes in Europe. By 1853 his sewage system proposal was in motion. Tons of sewage was removed from residential areas housing susceptible population groups.

Chadwick's efforts paved the way for an era that became known as "the sanitary movement" during which water supply, drainage, and sewage systems underwent remarkable improvements and the Public Health Act of 1848 was passed. This Act prompted the setting up of a General Board of Health to oversee these health reforms. Unfortunately, this incited indignation among the affluent, who viewed Chadwick's efforts as a waste of resources. Consequently, Chadwick was put on forced retirement because of his "revolutionary" ideas. Nevertheless, the seed had been sown and England was on its way to better sanitary conditions.

Many preventable infectious diseases continue to be of concern to the World Health Organization, particularly in developing nations. The diseases are transmitted from one person to another via various routes. A report by Pruss-Ustum and associates from the World Health Organization (WHO) about infectious diseases indicates that intestinal nematode infections such as ascariasis, trichuriasis, and hookworm are transmitted through soil contaminated by fecal matter.[91] These preventable diseases, similar to those that plagued Europe in the 19th century, are still highly prevalent in some parts of the world today. These diseases can be prevented by proper sanitation and hygiene practices.

BIBLICAL WASTE DISPOSAL METHOD

A close examination of the biblical laws concerning cleanliness, washing, and other forms of hygiene practices reveal to us that they were not merely ceremonial rituals. These laws were given to Israel to protect them and whoever adopted them from infectious diseases, contagious diseases, plagues, and chronic diseases.

Over three millennia ago, God gave Israel one of the fundamental principles for safeguarding their health: "You shall have a place outside the camp and you shall go out to it; and you shall have a stick with your weapons; and when you sit down outside, you shall dig a hole with it, and turn back and cover up your excrement," (Deuteronomy 23:12-13). This was a comprehensive law that, from a public health perspective, addressed hygiene, environmental pollution, and sanitation. If properly applied, universally, this would contribute significantly to an unprecedented global reduction in the burden of infectious diseases. After carefully studying the Book of Leviticus, Dr. Atkinson expressed his insights about its contents as follows:

> One has but to read the book of Leviticus carefully and thoughtfully to conclude that the admonitions... contained therein are, in fact, the groundwork *of most of today's sanitary laws*. As one closes the book, he must, regardless of his spiritual leanings, feel that the wisdom therein expressed regarding the rules to protect health are superior *to any which then existed in the world and that to this day they have been little improved upon.*
>
> (Atkinson, 1950)[92]

Modern cities especially in developing nations face a repeat of what transpired in the seventeenth century because of inadequacy of sanitation services caused by increasing urban population congestion, littering, and pollution. Periodic strikes by sanitation employees only serve to increase the possibility of chronic and serious outbreaks of infectious diseases such as cholera. Currently, about 2.6 billion people worldwide lack access to basic sanitation.[93]

According to the United Nations Press Release of 2008, the International Year of Sanitation (IYS) was officially launched by the United Nations in November 2007 to address the issue of the 2.6 million people who have no adequate sanitation.[94] The IYS focused on the following objectives:

The Perfect Prescription

1. Increasing awareness and commitment of interested parties and participants at all levels of society and achieving the millennium development goal (MDG) to reduce by half the world's current population that has no sustainable access to proper sanitation;

2. Mobilizing governments, financial institutions, research institutions, non-governmental organizations, major interest groups, private sectors and United Nations Agencies to form a concerted effort to achieve the MDG;

3. Securing real commitments from participating parties to design and implement proposed sanitation programs, and assigning specific responsibilities to relevant parties to ensure that the programs are achieved at national and international levels;

4. Applying bottom-up strategies for communities and health practitioners to work together to seek and identify sustainable, demand-driven, traditional solutions to the sanitation problem;

5. Because every program requires financial support, the IYS endeavors to secure funding from national budgets, donations and development partner allocation programs; all necessary for implementing and sustaining the programs;

6. Developing and reinforcing institutional and human capacity by understanding and realizing that, at all levels, any progress toward the MDGs is a multipronged process incorporating hygiene, existing household, school, and public amenities such as toilets and washing facilities; collection, transportation and disposal of wastewater and sewage. Community mobilization involving recognition of the key roles played by women in achieving MDGs is regarded as an indispensable strategy;

7. Enhancing the sustainability and efficiency of existing sanitation solutions to enhance positive health outcomes; ensuring cultural and social acceptance of existing sanitation solutions; ensuring the technological and institutional suitability of proposed sanitation projects; and ensuring environmental protection and;

8. Promoting and capturing the type of learning that enhances evidence-based knowledge about sanitation in order to increase advocacy and to promote necessary investments for the sanitation programs.

(United Nations International
Year of Sanitation Global Launch, 2007)

Lack of proper toilet facilities in some societies renders women and girls vulnerable to violence and exposes them to sexual predators. Because of lack of proper sanitation facilities, the only time for the women and girls that seems safe for them to defecate is at night in the darkness of the woods and brushes in hidden and secluded locations. But predators who know about these practices lurk in these areas to pounce on unsuspecting and vulnerable women and abuse them.

Proper sanitation can provide the women with the privacy they need and enhance their safety and dignity. The launching of the IYS motivated the formation of a coalition whose membership included more than 50 different kinds of organizations. These organizations included multilateral organizations, non-governmental organizations (NGOs), bilateral organizations, research institutions, and governmental organizations to form what was termed as the Sustainable Sanitation Alliance (SuSanA). The Sustainable Sanitation Alliance drew up a blueprint for promoting sustainable sanitation systems. SuSanA provides resources and a platform for knowledge exchange among stakeholders focused on improvement of sanitation and waste management.

MEDICAL WASTE DISPOSAL

Another modern-day sanitation problem involves the management of medical waste. With the re-emergence of dangerously infectious diseases, medical waste has become hazardous. The problem of biomedical management was first acknowledged as an issue of global concern when the WHO's European Regional Office convened a meeting in Bergen, Norway, in 1983 to address the subject of waste management from hospitals and other healthcare facilities.[95] Medical waste wash-ups fouled beaches in New Jersey, New York, Rhode Island, and Massachusetts areas in the summers of 1988 and 1998.[96]

The waste, which included used needles and syringes and other bio-medical waste, highlighted the seriousness of improper biomedical waste management practices and their threat to health. The Environmental Protection Agency of the United States investigated the beach wash-ups problem at the time. The findings led to the passing of the Medical Waste Tracking Act (MWTA) in 1998. Because biomedical or medical waste constitutes agents that are harmful to health, it needs to be collected, transported and disposed of with the uttermost care.

The Bible expressly commands that any type of substance that threatens health should be properly disposed of so that no human being should come into contact with it again. Animal refuse likely to putrefy and cause a foul smell and to attract disease-carrying agents had to be burned in a designated place away from the encampment or community: "But the skin of the bull and all its flesh, with its head, its legs, its entrails, and its dung, the whole bull he shall carry forth outside the camp to a clean place, where the ashes are poured out, and shall burn it on a fire of wood; where the ashes are poured out it shall be burned" (Leviticus 4: 11-12). Similarly human excrement was also to be disposed of away from the encampment (Deuteronomy 23:12-14).

Waste Management in Industrialized Nations

The biblical injunction of burning and burying deadly waste remains one of the most effective methods for disposal of waste today. With technological advancement this method has been improved and is being practiced on a wider scale to benefit larger communities. Burying waste is also a way of protecting the environment and keeping it safe as long as the process is properly designed. The modern type and volume of waste has changed, but its threat to the health of the public is still the same if not worse. Waste management has become a global problem of significant proportions. However, because of the changes in the volume and nature of the garbage being produced over the years, different disposal strategies are being designed and explored so that a permanent viable solution to the lingering problem of waste management and disposal can be found once and for all.

The United States alone produces approximately 210 million tons of municipal solid garbage annually.[97] This garbage is composed of durable and nondurable goods, packaging materials, food scraps, waste from residential areas as well as commercial, industrial, and institutional waste. Other garbage needing proper disposal includes industrial waste, automobile scrap bodies, and municipal sludge.

Prior to the 1970s, there was no cohesive plan for household garbage disposal in the United States. Residents were at will to dispose of their garbage in open dumps or to burn it in the open or in incinerators. Other times it was deposited in rivers, lakes, and oceans. But as the volume of the garbage increased, garbage-disposal related problems increased. The garbage deposited in rivers and lakes began to contaminate water supplies. Garbage deposited in oceans and rivers became a threat to marine life, and some of it washed-up on beaches in recreational locations.

The garbage that was burned in incinerators produced black smoke, noxious gases, and foul smells. The open dumps soon became homes for vermin and other disease-carrying agents. As the garbage began to rot in theses dumps, it started producing liquids that leached into the soil and polluted ground water. Environmental laws had to be enacted to control these practices. The environmental laws that were passed included the Clean Air Act, the Clean Water Act, and the Marine Protection, Research and Sanctuaries Act of 1972. These laws stimulated methods of disposing of garbage in a manner that took into account the protection of the general public. Henceforth garbage would be disposed of only in allowable places such as in sealed landfills whose structures minimized infestation by vermin.

Waste disposal became a national issue when, in 1987, a barge carrying garbage could not find a place to unload its cargo. According to Schneider "Carrying more than 3,000 tons of commercial trash banned from the local landfill in Islip, NY, the barge's vain search for a disposal site somewhere along the Atlantic or Gulf coasts, Belize or the Bahamas, made national news over a five-month period. Finally, the barge returned to New York, and the trash was incinerated" (Schneider, 2004). This scenario demonstrates how critical the issue of garbage disposal had become.

Landfills as a Method of Garbage Disposal

Public health and environmental health professionals were responsible for designing guidelines for appropriate landfill construction and operations. These guidelines recommend that landfills should be constructed in a dry place away from residential areas. A landfill is a large hole dug in the ground for garbage disposal. The public health and environmental guidelines state that the landfill should be layered first with clay and then with a plastic lining over the clay lining before the process of dumping garbage can be allowed to begin.[98] Whenever the volume of garbage increases, bulldozers are employed to compact it and then cover it with a layer of clay.

When the landfill is full to maximum capacity, it is often buried under a thick layer of soil, about two feet thick. Since decomposing garbage produces liquids and other hazardous gases, the guidelines propose that vents be made into the landfill to allow the gases to escape and prevent potential hazards. To limit the amount of gases released into the atmosphere from the landfill and to protect the environment from pollution, most industrialized nations have gas recovery wells throughout their landfills, which capture the gases for their energy value. After the landfill has been buried and its surface has been properly leveled, it can be turned into a recreational facility such as a golf course or a community park. It is important to ensure that these landfills are located at a safe distance from residential areas to avoid a repeat of what happened at the Fresh Kills landfill that was located on Staten Island, a borough of New York.

According to Schneider, the residents of Fresh Kill complained about a landfill close by and its threat to their health. Their complaints caught the attention of the Environmental Protection Agency (EPA).[99] Fresh Kills landfill had been open for use since 1948 and by 1996 13,000 tons of garbage were being deposited in it every day, making it the biggest garbage dump in the world. When public hysteria broke up about the potential health threat posed by the landfill, the mayor of the city had to propose to close the landfill.

Waste Management in Developing Nations

According to research by Zerbock, developing nations have unique types of waste management problems compared with developed or industrialized nations partly because of differences

The Perfect Prescription

in the composition of the waste they deal with.[100] The waste in developing nations is usually two or three times denser than that of developed nations and has a moisture content that is about three times more than that of industrialized nations. Garbage in developing nations is mostly composed of organic materials such as vegetable matter.

These differences in garbage content require that a unique and appropriate waste management system be designed to accommodate the unique composition of garbage from developing nations. The problem of waste management in developing nations is a palpable one, which is further compounded by the rapid urbanization that is currently taking place in many nations.

Zerbock observes that about 50% of the population in developing nations lives in urban areas or peri-urban areas. Peri-urban areas are residential areas that immediately adjoin an urban area. They are located between the suburbs and the countryside. Peri-urban areas are mostly found in the developing nations of English-speaking Africa and Asia. The rate of growth of urban areas in Africa is over 4%. But the revenues spent on waste management are unable to match this extraordinary growth and its associated garbage management demands and needs.

Some developing nations have solicited help from foreign bilateral and multilateral agencies and organizations in their effort to improve their waste management systems.[101] Sometimes collaborations between native governments and these foreign agencies have been established and waste management programs and systems have been implemented. Tragically, although some of the projects have succeeded for a while, most of them have failed to be sustained by the host governments after the foreign agencies have withdrawn their support. Most developing nations are beleaguered by unanticipated financial constraints that curtail the continuation of vital national programs such as waste management systems. Technological handicap is an added constraint that cripples most projects in these nations.

Collection and Transportation of Garbage

Governments in developing nations do not have adequate skilled human capital or resources to manage waste management processes or to match the rate at which urbanization is occurring. Lack of skilled manpower is compounded by the fact that most of the rapidly growing areas are areas in peripherals of existing cities and their sanitation systems are often an extension of the city center sanitation services. This places an added burden on already inadequate existing sanitary services and resources in city centers. Transporting garbage from sites of generation such as households and industrial locations to garbage dumps is a challenge.

To address the challenge, most cities have devised a system in which they have a neighborhood common collection point to which household owners are responsible to transport their garbage so that the municipal or private companies can pick it up from there and take it to its final destination. In cases where transportation is dependent on privately hired operational vehicles, it is not uncommon to experience automobile breakdowns due mostly to lack of parts or proper maintenance.

Where municipal or contracted private vehicle services are available to pick garbage straight from households, for a fee, usually the garbage is not properly packaged for lack of standardized garbage containers to allow for proper storage and pick up. Sometimes old oil drums or grocery bags are used as garbage storage facilities before pick up. Animals usually have access to these garbage bags and scatter the garbage around. Corrosion-resistant containers would be ideal for protecting the garbage from pets and wild animals. They would also prevent the garbage from being soaked by rain, making an unsightly mess and health problem. But they are not always available.

The springing up of shanty compounds close to landfills is another problem confronting developing nations. For example, in the Philippines, the Smoky Mountain garbage dump has approximately 10,000 families living adjacent to it in shacks exposing themselves to obvious health hazards.[102] It is not uncommon for individuals living close to these dumps to scavenge for "valuable" solid waste to sell and earn a living or to collect food stuffs for themselves and their families.

Johannessen reports that the Bisasar Road landfill of Durban, South Africa, at one time provided a living for about 200 families who earned an equivalent of $15,500 a month by selling "products" from the landfill; each family averaged a monthly income of $77.00.[103] Because the garbage is so dense, compaction becomes quite difficult and requires equipment not readily available in most parts of the developing world. In rural Africa, villagers are encouraged to bury their garbage by digging holes in the ground. They are also instructed to build latrines to take care of sewage issues. Government health officials provide guidelines and enforce adherence to prescribed standards for building these latrines. Periodically, public health professionals inspect villages to ensure that they all have latrines.

Human Health Risks

Although garbage collection is generally a risky business even in industrialized nations, the problem becomes more intense and widespread in developing nations. Sometimes fecal matter and hazardous industrial waste material is found in open garbage dumps. In areas where there are inadequate sanitary disposal systems, such as shanty compounds, the amount of fecal matter and other solid waste can be very high.

This is a health hazard for garbage workers and individuals who scavenge in these garbage dumps. Usually these dumps are characterized by foul smells emitted by decomposing solids. Soil and water contaminants are also produced by decomposition of garbage. While laws regulating the presence of toxic substances in solid waste are very stringent in industrialized nations, the problem remains acute in developing nations.

Environmental Problems and Garbage Disposal

Decomposing waste matter can trigger environmental pollution through the production of noxious gases. Methane is usually produced by bacteria present in landfills. If not properly captured and used, methane can seep into the soil, posing an explosion risk. Carbon dioxide is another gas produced by decomposing waste matter in landfills. A concentration of gases released from landfills can contribute to the greenhouse gases (GHGs) problem.

Liquid leachate management is another problem associated with waste management. In industrialized nations leachate management involves placing a layer of dense clay at the bottom and sides of the landfill and then covering that layer with plastic sheet to prevent liquids produced by the decomposition process from leaching into the soil and contaminating it and its ground water.

Usually leachate management plants are established not very far from landfills. These plants conduct leachate treatment processes using stipulated biological, chemical, and physical guidelines in order to prevent leachate from infiltrating the soil and causing pollution. Developing nations have very limited and sometimes no viable leachate management programs at all. Sometimes the leachate management system involves allowing the liquids from decomposed garbage to be discharged into municipal sewage systems or in surface water such as rivers or lakes, becoming a potential health threat.

Modern-day waste management has become a particularly expensive process, and reducing costs is a monumental task. Landfills continue to be an important component of waste management systems. Unlike in open dumps where waste is disposed of without proper covering, sanitary landfills have their waste compacted and covered with dirt each day. Open dumpsites have no controlled access regulations or stringent environmental controls.[104] Open dumpsites can easily contaminate ground water and surface water. Their presence can devalue surrounding properties and their open structure leaves them accessible to a myriad of disease-carrying agents.

The fact that open dumpsites have traditionally been in wetlands made them a significant source of ground water contamination. Because of the volume of garbage being produced in modern times, different methods of controlling waste production and management are being explored such as recycling the waste products so that they can be re-useable and reducing waste material production at the sources.

Recycling can dramatically reduce waste material production. A workable reduction of waste materials requires that customers refrain from demanding excessive and bulky packaging. Using biodegradable and reusable items such as reusable napkins, dishes, towels, and cups is another method of reducing the amount of waste being produced each day. Recycling bottles and cans reduces waste production by producing new products out of discarded ones.

However, ventures such as recycling demand time, labor, and financial resources in order to successfully process old products into new, usable ones. Manufacturers who conduct these processes need proper equipment and technology to be able to successfully recycle different types of materials. The benefits of recycling garbage include reduction of environmental pollution, conservation of natural resources, and creation of jobs. Composting is also another method that can be used to recycle organic household waste under aerobic conditions. The bacteria convert the waste into humus, which is an integral component for reclaiming fertility in the soil.

CHAPTER 9

INFECTIOUS DISEASES

For he will deliver you from the snare of the fowler and from the deadly pestilence.

(Psalm 91:3_

Infectious diseases have plagued mankind from time immemorial. Although health professionals have discovered means to prevent and control some infectious diseases, there has not been a single generation of humanity that has been completely free from the scourge of infectious diseases.

General life expectancy has improved and deaths from infectious diseases have been reduced drastically in most parts of the world, but this planet is far from being free of all infectious diseases. God instructed the nation of Israel to have individuals who had bodily discharges bathe in running water.

> "Say to the people of Israel, When any man has a discharge from his body, his discharge is unclean. And this is the law of his uncleanness for a discharge: whether his body runs with his discharge, or his body is stopped from discharge, it is uncleanness in him. And when he who has a discharge is cleansed of his discharge, then he shall count for himself

seven days for his cleansing, and wash his clothes; and he shall bathe his body in running water, and shall be clean."

(Leviticus 15: 2, 3, 13)

It is important to understand that this law did not say that the person who had a discharge was sinful but rather that they were unclean, giving us a hygienic perspective. Pathogens that are disease-carrying agents that include viruses and bacteria can be found in human body fluids such as blood and semen. Vaginal fluids, nasal discharges, and other secretions can also carry pathogens.[105]

Anyone who comes into contact with them can be in danger of being infected by whatever disease they are carrying. This is the reason why Scripture said that the individual who touched a person with a bodily discharge was also deemed unclean: "And whoever touches the body of him who has the discharge shall wash his clothes, and bathe himself in water, and be unclean until the evening" (Leviticus 15: 7). Even touching the property of the individual who had a discharge rendered one unclean: "And anyone who touches his bed shall wash his clothes, and bathe himself in water, and be unclean until the evening,"(Leviticus 15:5).

Anyone who came into contact with a dead body was unclean too. All open vessels that were in the same house with a dead body were deemed defiled. This was to protect any individual who would have wanted to touch or use these items just in case they had been contaminated by the same disease-carrying organisms of the deceased individual: "This is the law when a man dies in a tent: everyone who comes into the tent, and everyone who is in the tent, shall be unclean seven days. And every open vessel, which has no cover fastened upon it, is unclean. Whoever in the open field touches one who is slain with a sword, or a dead body, or a bone of a man, or a grave, shall be unclean seven days" (Numbers 19: 14-16).

The Perfect Prescription

It was possible for the people who came into contact with a dead body through the process of preparing for burial to have been exposed to the pathogens that had killed the individual. As such, they were to be kept separate from everybody else until it was proved that they had not contracted the dead person's disease. The practice of separating those who have come into contact with a dead body until they have thoroughly been disinfected is a standard modern-day public health procedure.

Any articles recovered after wars or taken as spoil were to be purged by fire or cleansed in water. This spoil was collected from diverse individuals coming from foreign backgrounds and cultures. Not knowing the health status of the previous owners of these items required that the items themselves be treated as if they were contaminated. The clothing and other personal items could have been reservoirs for deadly pathogens.

To prevent potential disease outbreak and to safeguard the health of the nation of Israel, the spoil had to be purged and made safe for use. It is a common modern health procedure to require that used items such as clothing, cooking utensils, flatware, and non-disposable drinking utensils should be disinfected and washed to make them safe for the next user. Here is what the Bible says about purifying booty from battlefields:

> And Elea'zar the priest said to the men of war who had gone to battle: "This is the statute of the law which the Lord has commanded Moses: only the gold, the silver, the bronze, the iron, the tin, and the lead, everything that can stand the fire, you shall pass through the fire, and it shall be clean. Nevertheless it shall also be purified with the water of impurity; and whatever cannot stand the fire, you shall pass through the water."
>
> (Numbers 31:21–23)

HAND WASHING AND HEALTH

Recently, modern medicine discovered the benefits of washing hands in running water. Early in the 19th century, physicians merely wiped their hands on cloths as they moved from one patient to another even after performing a postmortem—transmitting undetectable pathogens that clung to their hands to their next patient. Transmission of disease can take place in an environment where an infectious agent has access to a vulnerable host.

Oliver Morgan of the London School of Hygiene and Tropical Medicine, Public and Environmental Health Research Unit confirms that the human body is home to an array of organisms.[106] Some of these organisms are harmless, but others are pathogenic and can spread from one individual to another with catastrophic consequences.

In endeavoring to promote the health of the general public, one of the main duties of public health professionals is to protect susceptible individuals from noxious and infectious agents. Infection can happen in any setting, including healthcare institutions. Infection that takes place in healthcare institutions such as hospitals is called nosocomial infection. Webster's New World Medical Dictionary defines nosocomial infection as "an infection acquired in a hospital. Specifically an infection that was not present or incubating prior to the patient being admitted to the hospital but occurred within seventy-two hours after admittance to the hospital."[107] In the United States, studies on nosocomial infections in the medical intensive care units reveal an alarming situation.

Research conducted by Richards and associates in 1999 on the epidemiology of nosocomial infection in medical intensive care units in the United States revealed a grim picture.[108] The findings demonstrated that the most frequent nosocomial infections were urinary tract infections (31%), pneumonia (27%), and primary bloodstream infections (19%). The problem of nosocomial infections is not a new phenomenon.

In Vienna during the 17th century, a Hungarian physician named Ignaz Semmelweis who worked for the First Obstetrical Clinic at the Vienna General Hospital, which was established to train physicians to deliver babies, was confronted by incredible cases of nosocomial infection.[109] The fatalities from these infections were also incredibly high. In Semmelweis's time, the medical community did not have the knowledge that diseases can easily be transmitted from one person to another. In the hospital where he worked, Semmelweis noticed that mortality rates among women attended to by interns who also delivered babies was alarmingly high, particularly after delivering babies. About one in eight women died from pueperal fever. However, in the wards where deliveries were administered by midwives, the death rate was significantly lower. The only difference between the interns and midwives as far as performing their responsibilities was concerned was that interns performed autopsies while the midwives did not.

During this time, it was standard procedure for physicians to perform autopsies with their bare hands without surgical gloves. After the autopsies, the students would wipe their hands on rags to remove the blood. Then the young interns would head straight to the maternity wards to internally examine women in labor and deliver babies.

Semmelweis noticed a pattern in which the participation of interns in performing autopsies and their subsequent delivery of babies was often followed by onset of fatal pueperal fever among mothers. Commenting on the work of Semmelweis, Julie Cwikel indicates that the frequent presence and participation of medical trainees at autopsies implied to Semmelweis that "the transfer of cadaverous material might be the source of the rampant childbed fever, which killed the women" (Cwikel, 2008).[110]

Semmelweis's theory was that the pathogens were sticking to the hands of the interns during autopsies and were being inadvertently transmitted to the women in the delivery wards through the unsterilized hands of these interns. Sterilizing hands after each medical procedure was an unknown, unobserved procedure in the medical community then. Semmelweis decided to test his hypothesis by instituting a rule requiring thorough hand-washing procedures by interns after each autopsy and before performing examinations on women in labor using chlorinated water. Within six months of instituting the hand-washing practice, the death rate among the women fell significantly.

Cwikel further observes that in modern times maternal morbidity and mortality still remains a main indicator of the unfortunate gap existing between the rich and the poor, who still do not have proper physician care during and after delivery. In today's world, the largest burden of maternal morbidity and mortality is borne by developing nations. Of the 600,000 maternal deaths that occur each year from pregnancy and delivery complications, about 99% of them take place in developing nations. Pueperal or sepsis fever remains one of the leading causes of death among mothers in these nations.

Semmelweis's contribution to the control of nosocomial infection by frequent hand washing practices among healthcare providers has become the foundation for modern-day health tools as an effective response to high maternal morbidity and mortality. It continues to be of great interest to public health professionals and is being taught across cultures. Semmelweis tapped into effective biblical wisdom about prevention of infection by washing hands after touching a dead body instituted thousands of years earlier. He understood the biblical principle of separating the dead from the living.

The Lord God commanded Israel that those who touched dead bodies had to sever all contact with the rest of the living, including their own families, for seven days. Unfortunately, the medical authorities of Semmelweis's time were still blinded by ignorance and denied that not washing hands by physicians was a causative factor for the high prevalence of deaths from pueperal fever at the hospital.

The Centers for Disease Control and Prevention (CDC) designed a Hand Hygiene Guidelines Fact Sheet that stipulates how health workers should wash their hands. The CDC observe that hand washing is "the single most effective way to prevent the transmission of disease."[111] In the United States, approximately 2 million nosocomial infections take place annually, and an estimated 90,000 people die from those infections because of poor hygiene practices of nurses, physicians, technologists, and others in the health care profession who come into contact with many patients.[112]

According to a report by Delaney and Gunderman, an Australian research study conducted to review hand-washing practices among physicians at the Royal Children's Hospital in Melbourne, although the self-report input by physicians indicated that they washed their hand between 50% and 95% of the time when hand washing was assessed among them without their knowledge, it was discovered that only about 9% of them actually washed their hands according to the recommended protocol.[113]

A similar study was conducted by Albert and Condie at the University of Washington Veterans Administration Medical Center in Seattle, Washington, among intensive care unit physicians, interns, and nurses to assess hand washing patterns in medical intensive care units.[114] The findings of the study demonstrated that physicians washed their hands 28% of the time, while nurses did so 48% of the time. The same study observed hand-washing practices among physicians and nurses working at a different private hospital locations. The findings were even more dismal. Physicians washed their hands only 14% of the time and nurses only 28% of the time in spite of having admitted earlier that they were aware of the strong correlation between inadequate hand washing and high transmission rates of infectious diseases.

Pathogenic organisms can easily be transferred from a dead body to a living individual by touching the body. The diseases that are likely to be contracted from a dead body include tuberculosis, gastrointestinal disease, streptococcus organisms, hepatitis B and C, and HIV, among others.

God, the omniscient Creator of the human body, knew that individuals who were given the responsibility of taking care of the dead needed to observe stringent hygiene standards to protect them and everybody else they came in contact with from deadly diseases. The Lord God commanded Israel to purify all people who came into contact with a dead body by washing themselves and their clothes in clean water. The same law applied to an individual who touched a dead person's bone or grave or one who entered a tent or house where a person had died.

Open containers found in the tent or house were to be destroyed, (see Numbers 19:14-16). Affected individuals who refused to adhere to this requirement were cut off from the rest of the community to prevent the spread of disease to the rest of the people.

In Numbers chapter 19, the Bible introduces us to a mysterious sacrifice of the red heifer, which obviously had spiritual significance for the nation of Israel. Nevertheless, physicians like Drs. McMillen and Stern (2000) now help us understand that the water of purification described in the biblical text of Numbers 19 also had the ability to destroy germs and infection among the people.

God instructed Israel to sacrifice a red heifer by burning it with cedar wood, hyssop, and scarlet. The product of this burning would be gathered and would be mixed with fresh water to form a purification solution. At face value, this solution sounds like a superstitious potion without any medicinal benefits. However, Butt asserts that this is a brilliant antibacterial solution.[115]

Drs. Mcmillen and Stern further enlighten us that hyssop contains an antiseptic called thymol, which is an ingredient found in some brands of mouthwash. The oil of hyssop leaves contains about 50% carvacrol, which is both an antifungal and antibacterial agent. Other items used in formulating the water of purification included cedar wood, which is used in storage cabinets to repel insects likely to start the process of decay. In oil form, cedar has antiseptic and antifungal properties. Scarlet, a third ingredient of the solution was probably scarlet wool. Adding it to the solution would have made it the ancient equivalent of Lava soap with an abrasive quality.

In modern developed nations, pathologists, mortuary or professional funeral staff are entrusted with the responsibility of handling and preparing cadavers using special equipment and antibacterial materials, at a fee of course. Even burials are conducted by professional funeral home personnel. The only thing relatives have to do is pay for the work done and attend the funeral. This is not always the case in certain countries. There are still societies where family members prepare the body of their deceased for burial. They even place the body in the coffin and deliver it to the cemetery where other family members dig the grave and bury their dead. This intimate management of cadavers by individuals who may not be professionally trained to handle dead bodies exposes them to infections agents. It is only logical that these individuals wash their hands after performing these tasks. They might not necessarily have to wash their entire bodies and clothes, but hand washing is critical in such cases. The World Health Organization (WHO) urges individuals who handle corpses to "Ensure hand-washing with soap after handling bodies and before eating." This is for their protection and for the protection of other people, from infectious diseases. The World Health Organization does not make any exception concerning who should wash hands after handling corpses; whether professionally trained or not, the WHO insists that anyone who handles a dead body must thoroughly wash their hands with soap.

God also commanded the nation of Israel that a woman who had just given birth was "unclean" for seven days. In other words, she was off limits. This restriction would continue for the next thirty-three days if she had given birth to a baby boy. If she gave birth to a baby girl she would be "unclean" for two weeks, after which she would continue to be separated from the rest of the community for another sixty-six days.

> The LORD said to Moses, "Say to the people of Israel, If a woman conceives, and bears a male child, then she shall be unclean seven days; as at the time of her menstruation, she shall be unclean. And on the eighth day the flesh of his foreskin shall be circumcised. Then she shall continue for thirty-three days in the blood of her purifying; she shall not touch any hallowed thing, nor come into the sanctuary, until the days of her purifying are completed. But if she bears a female child, then she shall be unclean two weeks, as in her menstruation; and she shall continue in the blood of her purifying for sixty-six days.
>
> (Leviticus 12: 1-5)

The seclusion period following the birth of a baby girl was double that of a baby boy. God did not give the Israelites reasons for this distinction, although many theories have been advanced to explain it. Dr. Steven P. Shelov and Dr. Tanya R. Altmann claim that male infants tend to weigh slightly more and to be larger at birth than girls.[116]

The findings of a study conducted by the Harvard School of Public Health titled "Baby Boys 'Boost Appetite'" reported in a BBC News Report claimed that pregnant women carrying baby boys ate more than their counterparts carrying girls. The reason for this was that male fetuses tend to grow bigger than their female counterparts in the womb.

Professor Dimitrios Trichopoulos was quoted as having said about the findings that "Sad to say, but there is discrimination in nature. For evolutionary reasons–such as having to compete among themselves to gain the favours of women—males have to be bigger than females and this phenomenon has its origins in the womb."[117] A study by Del Bono and Ermisch has confirmed the same.[118]

Obviously, the biblical directive was necessary so that the mother could nurse and nurture the female baby a little longer, in seclusion, to allow her to gain the strength and resilience she needed before being released into the mainstream community. It was also necessary for neonatals to spend this time with their mother to bond with her. Health professionals inform us that the first week after the birth of a child is crucial for emotional bonding with the mother and that it provides indispensable emotional stability and security necessary for the infant.[119] This security and stability becomes the foundation for the early development of the child and for establishing relationships in its childhood and beyond.

Since the entrance of sin in this world, mankind has lived in a hostile environment replete with pathogens and other life-threatening agents. God gave commandments to augment the spiritual wellbeing of the nation of Israel and to avert potential physical health threats. Concerning the commands given in Leviticus chapter 12, verses 1-5, some have suggested that because God perfectly understood the susceptibility of new mothers and their infants to prevailing infectious diseases, he gave them these directives to protect them.

Although it may not be feasible to make it mandatory for new mothers of female infants to spend more time with them than those of male infants, as was the case with ancient Israel, due to a convergence of different deeply-embedded values and cultural perspectives that have evolved over time, women can still learn from the guidelines found in the Bible and make their own individual decisions regarding nurturing their infants based on those guidelines.

There are scientifically proven facts about the health benefits the infant obtains when the mother spends quality time with it, and the relationship between them is the foundation upon which all future human relationships are built.[120] The contact between the infant and its mother starting with the few hours of its life have long-term implications. A special bonding and strong mother-infant relationship occurs during this time, which must continue to be reinforced and nurtured by the mother as she spends quality time with the infant. There is often gentle touching, eye contact and soothing speech, which are necessary for healthy emotional development of the infant. A secure attachment bond, which is a unique, nonverbal relationship between the infant and its mother is an emotional exchange which makes the infant feel safe and secure. This is critical for optimal physical development and neurodevelopment of the infant. The bond is a significant "factor in the way your infant's brain organizes itself and influences your child's social, emotional, intellectual, and physical development"[121] so that the baby can grow into a healthy, responsible and productive adult. The mother also plays a significant role in ensuring that the baby is protected from disease including infectious ones by practicing good hygiene. That is why the Lord God gave instructions for the mother to spend time with her baby.

In recognition of the importance of the need for the mother to spend quality time with her infant some countries have made this easier for the mother by designating a significant amount of time as maternity leave. For example, countries who are members of the European Union give women fourteen weeks maternity leave during which the woman is paid either her salary or adequate allowance, and whatever benefits she qualifies for.[122] In Australia a new mother is entitled to fifty-two weeks maternity leave. In Canada maternity leave is administered on provincial level.

However, almost all of Canada's jurisdictions guarantee women seventeen weeks of maternity leave. Britain guarantees fifty-two weeks maternity leave with thirty-nine of them being paid leave.

As it was in Semmelweis' day so it is today. The post-partum health of a mother is of uttermost importance. It must be guarded so that she can be free of any type of disease that would impede her from nurturing her infant into a healthy, productive member of the community. In case of employed women, maternity leave helps their bodies recuperate and regain resilience to disease. It also helps them spend time nurturing the infant during that critical formative period of its life on earth.

MORE BENEFITS OF HAND-WASHING PRACTICES

Although hand washing is supposed to be a spontaneous process mostly among adults after using the bathroom and before handling food, the reality is that people are not as vigilant about hand-washing as they should be. The public health sector continues to release reminders about the importance of consistent hand-washing practices to prevent disease. In its 2010 *Fall Newsletter*, the American Public Health Association (APHA) featured the following article:

> To encourage healthy habits and keep families safe this flu season, the APHA's *Get Ready* campaign is launching a new initiative today aimed at promoting proper hand-washing. APHA is providing free hand-washing timers that when activated play a 20-second tune reminding everyone how long it takes to thoroughly wash your hands. This effort is in collaboration with the National Association of Child Care Professionals and funded by Colgate-Palmolive Company.
>
> (Get Read Newsletter, American Public Health Association, 2010)[123]

The health of young children and infants mainly depends on the caregivers' and mothers' hygiene and sanitation practices. If the caregiver or mother has lax hygiene practices, the infant will easily contract infectious and other diseases. In Southern Africa, in isolated villages, there are still some tribes who practice isolation of new mothers and their infants for about one month, similar to the biblical injunction.

Various reasons are given for this isolation, including shielding the infant and the vulnerable mother from diseases and evil. Only an elderly midwife, usually a very close relative of the new mother, has access to the infant and the mother for up to one month after delivery. She also provides guidance for the new mother on how to nurse her baby. She teaches her how to bathe the baby. She also supervises the diet of the mother, which is usually composed of cow or goat milk and millet porridge to help her secrete milk for the nursing infant.

The new mother and the baby are secluded in a separate hut from the husband's, away from the general community and even the nuclear family for about four weeks. The new mother is not allowed to cook or carry any heavy burdens during this time. Other people have to draw water for her from the river or from the well so that she and the baby can have their daily bath. From a health perspective, it is obvious that an unbridled interaction with the mainstream community at this time can easily expose the new mother and her infant to any type of pathogens. Visitors are warned in advance to stay clear of the nursing hut. After about a month, the infant is released to the nuclear family members. They are allowed to hold it. After another two weeks, the general community members can have access to the baby.

The time of a woman's impurity or seclusion after giving birth stipulated in the Bible should not be interpreted to mean that God has a negative attitude toward birth or childbearing. He is the One who commanded humans to be fruitful and to multiply: "And God blessed them, and God said to them, "Be fruitful and multiply, and fill the earth and subdue it; and have dominion over the fish of the sea and over the birds of the air and over every living thing that moves upon the earth," (Genesis 1:28), and Scripture further says that children are a gift from God: "Lo, sons are a heritage from the LORD, the fruit of the womb a reward," (Psalm 127:3).

The period of impurity marked by seclusion obviously gave the new mother time to recuperate from the physical challenge of carrying a baby for nine months as well as the rigors of the childbirth process. This was particularly necessary in Bible times when women did rigorous manual work characteristic of the agrarian communities to which they belonged. A period of recuperation is still given to new mothers in modern day, although its duration has been reduced.

Myers-Smith claims that after giving birth, women are advised to wait until after the six-week medical checkup before they can have sex again to allow the bleeding to stop and their bodies to heal properly.[124] Most women suffer from postpartum fatigue. Postpartum fatigue or new-mom fatigue is a condition caused by physical and psychological changes that inevitably take place during and after childbirth. This is a process in which the mother learns to breastfeed the infant and to change its diapers and clothing. These responsibilities result in fragmented and short spells of sleep, which can undermine the immune system of the mother.

Hobson states that sleep deprivation can compromise the immune system, making a person susceptible to infectious diseases.[125] Therefore, this time of seclusion and recuperation serves to protect the mother from exposure to infectious diseases and allows for rebuilding the immune system. It also protects the infant from exposure to infectious diseases.

The National Institute of Neurological Disorders and Stroke confirms that "Sleep may help the body conserve energy and other resources that the immune system needs to mount an attack" against pathogens (National Institute of Neurological Disorders and Stroke, 2007).[126] Sleep deprivation can depress the immune system. A body that has a strong immune system is resilient to disease including infectious diseases.

Disease avoidance is a central focus of public health. Throughout the history of mankind different methods and efforts have been made to control disease. No single community embraces disease. On the contrary, different communities have adopted different practices and strategies to combat disease, and to maximize the health of individuals and the general public. Although some of the disease-preventive methods have been modified over the years to a certain extent, they can still be traced to biblical teachings. By studying these methods, public health professionals have succeeded in reducing the burden of disease. This is how important our health and well-being are to God, and they should be to us, too. Regular hand washing after exposure to pathogens continues to be advocated as a sure way of disease prevention. The private time of a new mother with her infant promotes much needed rest and helps strengthen her immune system so that her body can be more resilient to disease. The mother's time with the infant is also beneficial for the infant's health.

CHAPTER 10

DEADLY INFECTIOUS DISEASES

And when he who has a discharge is cleansed of his discharge, then he shall count for himself seven days for his cleansing, and wash his clothes; and he shall bathe his body in running water, and shall be clean.

(Leviticus 15:13)

Infectious diseases have always been among the most feared diseases throughout the history of mankind. Their etiology and rapid spread was mainly enhanced by population growth and shifts facilitated by wars, poor sanitation, poor hygiene practices, crowding, unprecedented changes in ecologic, and climatic conditions and poverty.[127] There have been many deadly infectious diseases throughout history. Here we sample only seven of them. This planet is not yet completely free from emerging and re-emerging infectious diseases. According to the World Health Organization (WHO), "An infectious disease crisis of global proportions is today threatening hard-won gains in health and life expectancy."[128] The WHO also claims that infectious diseases have now become the main killer of little children and youth, worldwide. This means a threat to the future of the planet.

The WHO further claims that infectious diseases account for the deaths of 13 million people each year. In developing nations one in two deaths is caused by an infectious disease. Emerging and re-emerging infectious diseases have become a threat to all countries.

The five main agents of infectious diseases include "bacteria, viruses, fungi, protozoa, and helminths. In addition, a new class of infectious agents, the prions..."[129] These agents are still around today and they still have the potency and capacity to cause disease again. Most of the diseases listed in this chapter were caused by some of these agents. Although some of these diseases have been eradicated such as the bubonic plague, smallpox and Spanish Influenza, it is still appropriate to study them in order to further understand their microbial composition and their transmission modes in case of emergence or re-emergence. If we fail to remember our history we are doomed to repeat it.[130] The effects of the Bubonic Plague, Smallpox and Spanish Influenza were catastrophic. They adversely altered the demographic composition of the societies they attacked by decimating almost entire generations and damaging economies of those societies. To be complacently satisfied about having eradicated these microbial enemies of ours is to leave ourselves startlingly vulnerable to them. The Surgeon General, William Stewart, testified before Congress in 1969, two years after the global campaign to eradicate smallpox began, that the world could now "close the book on infectious disease" because of the discovery of efficacious antibiotics and vaccines.[131] The medical community and other health professionals thought the war against infectious diseases was over. But, today, we are still contending with emerging and re-emerging alarmingly virulent infectious diseases, forty-four years after the Surgeon General's testimony. The World Health Organization has collaborated with the Centers for Disease Control and Prevention in an intensified surveillance effort of infectious diseases, both emerging and re-emerging ones. What is more disconcerting is the fact that these diseases can easily change in virulence due to genome mutations. Global changes in temperatures, seasonal patterns, and ecological patterns are some of the risk factors for the emergence and re-emergence of these diseases. Studying these diseases gives public health professionals the impetus to mobilize resources and to conduct relevant community educational campaigns in case of a re-emergence of any of these diseases.[132] Being aware of the characteristics of these diseases further legitimizes the engagement of health professionals in the development of new innovative solutions as well as in the development of public health policy aimed at planning for prevention of these diseases. In a nutshell, to study them is to be ready for them whenever and wherever they may appear.

Some of the diseases listed in this chapter such as tuberculosis, malaria and cholera are still endemic in some countries around the world and they continue to devastate communities. In these areas clinicians continue to provide therapeutic services while public health professionals are engaged in community education to mitigate the impact and spread of these diseases. Research studies are also being conducted to find means of eradicating them.

BUBONIC PLAGUE

The bubonic plague was a disease that infected the lymph nodes. Its symptoms appeared between two to five days after infection. These symptoms included chills, high fever, severe headache, and muscle pain. The bubonic plague was also known as the black plague or Black Death. It ravaged medieval Europe at different times. The worst outbreaks were between 1347 and 1350. This disease killed approximately 25 million people during this time. It also weakened the economy of fourteenth century Europe. This caused a significant economic recession that continued into the 16th century.[133] The bubonic plague was caused by a bacterium or bacillus called *Yersinia Pestis*. It was transmitted to humans by fleas or through direct contact with tissues of an infected animal.

SMALL POX

Small pox was another deadly infectious disease that is reported to have killed more human beings than any other infectious disease in history.[134] In the 18th century, small pox killed 400,000 people in Europe. Most of the people who survived were left blind. The fatality rate among adults was between 20% and 60%. Among infants it was 80% in the city of London and 98% in Berlin. Significant financial costs were incurred by governments in conducting research for a smallpox vaccine. After the discovery of the smallpox vaccine by Jenner, millions of lives were saved, especially in developed countries where rigorous population vaccination programs were designed and implemented almost immediately after discovering the vaccine. But the developing world lagged behind in this area and the disease continued to claim lives until the introduction of the smallpox eradication global immunization program spearheaded by the World Health Organization and the United Nations Children's Fund (UNICEF) from 1967 to 1977.[135] The program required routine immunization of children in developing nations. As a result hundreds of millions of lives have been saved from the scourge of smallpox. The World Health Organization claims that smallpox has been totally eradicated worldwide.

SPANISH INFLUENZA

The Spanish influenza was also a deadly infectious disease that lasted from 1918 until 1919. This disease is reported to have killed about 40 million people worldwide.[136] The devastation and virulence of this pandemic was so severe that life expectancy was reduced by 10 years in the United States. The impact of the 1918 influenza epidemic is still reverberating in the public health arena because all cases of influenza worldwide, apart from those caused by avian viruses, have their roots in the 1918 flu virus, including the H1N1, H2N2 and H3N2 viruses. In the United States, public health professionals have attempted to estimate the economic impact of a potential influenza epidemic as a way of designing related interventions as indicated in the following quote.

> We estimated the possible effects of the next influenza pandemic in the United States and analyzed the economic impact of vaccine-based interventions. Using death rates, hospitalization data, and outpatient visits, we estimated 89,000 to 207,000 deaths; 314,000 to 734,000 hospitalizations; 18 to 42 million outpatient visits; and 20 to 47 million additional illnesses. Patients at high risk (15% of the population) would account for approximately 84% of all deaths. The estimated economic impact would be US$71.3 to $166.5 billion, excluding disruptions to commerce and society.
>
> (Meltzer, Cox & Fukuda, 1999)[137]

TUBERCULOSIS (TB)

Tuberculosis is yet another infectious disease that has ravaged humanity for millennia. It escalated into an epidemic in North America and Europe during the 18th and 19th centuries.[138] This disease has been known by other names such as phthisis, inflammation of the lungs, scrofula, gastric fever, and tabes, as well as consumption. Before a cure was discovered, many methods were prescribed for treatment of tuberculosis, including continuous rest, drinking large amounts of goat or cow milk, and milk from pregnant women.[139] Sometimes drastic measures were applied such as bloodletting, a procedure used to drain infected blood from the lungs of the patient.

In 1882, Koch identified infectious agents known as *tubercle bacilli* as the causative agents for tuberculosis. In 1889, the National Tuberculosis Association in the United States came to understand that tuberculosis was not hereditary but an infectious disease that was preventable.[140] Large-scale campaigns were implemented to educate communities about the modes of the transmission of tuberculosis from one person to another.

With the discovery of the antibiotic streptomycin in 1944, many individuals were cured of the disease, and by the 1960s most sanatoriums were closed as the battle against the disease was being won. For over three decades the incidence of tuberculosis (TB) significantly declined. After that, this age old disease began to make a global re-emergence. Tragically, the same medication used for tuberculosis treatment had become a catalyst for the development of a new wave of TB resistance.[141] Patients given TB medication had been allowed to take their medication at home without supervision by a health care professional.

In such cases, if the patient fails to complete the prescribed course of treatment, the disease can become drug resistant. In 1993, the World Health Organization (WHO) declared TB a "global emergency."[142] Currently, tuberculosis is one of the leading killers among infectious diseases worldwide. In developing nations, TB causes 26% of preventable deaths. The receding tide of TB in developed nations is being reversed, with Canada experiencing 2,000 cases of TB annually. Delahanty and Johnson list the contributing factors to the re-emergence of tuberculosis as follows:

1. An unprecedented increase in migration and international travel. Tourists traveling to countries where TB is endemic are likely to be infected. Also, infected travelers are likely to infect fellow passengers or residents of the host country. For example, in 1994, a Korean woman infected with TB was reported to have infected some of her fellow passengers on a flight

from Chicago to Honolulu. In Canada about 58% of TB cases were diagnosed in immigrants;

2. Increase in the prevalence and incidence of HIV/AIDS is another contributing factor. People with a compromised immune system are vulnerable to tuberculosis infection; Tuberculosis is now the leading cause of death among individuals living with HIV/AIDS;

3. Weak and unprepared healthcare systems. For instance, in New York the number of individuals with TB increased by 300% between 1978 and 1992. Proper treatment choices for multi drug resistant TB (MDRTB) have been hampered by "lengthy delays in the availability of drug susceptibility results by conventional methods," (Cooksey, et al., 1997).[143]

4. Research findings indicate that "The main causes of MDRTB are poor patient management, non-adherence to the prescribed regimen, a poor national programme or some combination of these three," (Beale, 2001).[144] Tuberculosis is also a disease of poverty. The increase in TB prevalence and incidence especially in developing nations is exacerbated by the growth of urban slums without proper sanitation or clean water. Multi-drug resistant TB usually found in previously treated patients is resistant to the most effective TB treatment drugs such as isoniazid and rifampicin.

(Delahanty & Johnson, 1998)[145]

According to the National Institute on Drug Abuse (NIDA), the Centers for Disease Control and Prevention (CDC) report indicates that about $617 million was spent on tuberculosis-related inpatient and outpatient services in 1991.[146] Research conducted by the CDC and the National Institute of Allergy and Infectious Diseases (NIAID) on tuberculosis cost $50 million. The annual treatment regimen for each individual suffering from MDRTB has been estimated to be $250,000, especially if there is need to hospitalize the patient or if the patient has a concurrence of MDRTB, HIV, and AIDS. The Centers for Disease Control and Prevention and the National Institute of Allergy and Infectious Diseases are both concerned that these figures could escalate as the cases of MDRTB increase.

Malaria

Yet another dreaded infectious disease is malaria. Malaria has been eradicated in wealthy and industrialized nations. However, it remains endemic in Africa, where it continues to kill at least one million people per year.[147] Malaria kills more than 3,000 African children each day. That means a child dies every 30 seconds from malaria in Africa. Malaria is also one of the greatest threats to the health of pregnant women in Africa. The World Health Organization claims that "Malaria causes more than three hundred million acute illnesses... Ninety percent of deaths due to malaria occur in Africa, south of the Sahara, and most deaths occur in children under the age of five," (WHO, 2012).[148] Malaria is caused by parasites that are transmitted form one individual to another through the bite of infected *Anopheles* mosquitoes.

Efforts to control malaria should first of all control populations of *Anopheles* mosquitoes. Congenital malaria is being reported increasingly among infants born in malaria endemic areas. Approximately 7% to 10% of newborns are reported to have been found with malaria parasites in their placental blood. Malaria parasites from the mother can infect the baby in utero.[149] Blood transfusions from infected individuals can cause infection of malaria too. Mosquitoes that transmit malaria from one person to another breed in stagnant water sites. Therefore, an effective way to reduce or eradicate populations of mosquitoes around the home is to eliminate any form of stagnant water sites. Clogged up rain gutters can serve as a breeding ground for mosquitoes. Any stagnant water resulting from malfunctioning rain gutters should be drained out. Proper hygiene and cleanliness around the home are critical for prevention of mosquito breeding grounds.

ECONOMIC COST OF MALARIA

The World Health Organization's new global strategy for eradicating malaria called Roll Back Malaria (RBM) founded in 1998 to reduce the human and economic costs incurred due to the scourge of malaria claims that malaria has been significantly linked to major economic constraints and stagnation in affected countries.[150] In 2009, the Catholic Relief Services working with the Roll Back Malaria program claimed that "providing access to malaria prevention and treatment to every person at risk will cost between $5 and $6 billion per year over the next 12 years, which is more than four times the annual funding that was available for malaria in 2007," (World Malaria Day, 2010).[151] The war against malaria, especially in Africa, continues to rage.

CHOLERA

Up to the 19th century, cholera has mostly been confined to the Indian sub-continent where cholera outbreaks are seasonal.[152] After the 19th century, however, cholera spread from the Indian sub-continent to other continents and countries, including Indonesia, Latin America, and Africa. Cholera is an extremely virulent waterborne disease that is accompanied by severe, watery diarrhea, which quickly dehydrates the victim, causing imminent death.

Cholera epidemics are usually caused by contaminated water and food supplies, reinforced by poor hygiene and sanitation. In 1855, a fearful wave of cholera devastated the city of London. Thousands of lives were lost before John Snow identified the Broad Street water pump as the source of the disease. Cholera remains a significant health threat to people living mainly in developing nations. Peri-urban slums and refugee camps with inadequate social amenities such as safer water and toilet facilities are at increased risk of contracting cholera. The incidence of cholera continues to rise in endemic areas. The WHO reports that:

> From 2004 to 2008, cases increased by 24% compared with the period from 2000 to 2004. For 2008 alone, a total of 190,130 cases were notified from 56 countries, including 5,143 deaths. Many more cases were unaccounted for due to limitations in surveillance systems and fear of trade and travel sanctions. The true burden of the disease is estimated to be 3–5 million cases and 100, 000–120, 000 deaths annually.
>
> (World Health Organization, 2010)[153]

EBOLA

The World Health Organization (WHO) classified the Ebola virus under the Filoviridae family of viruses.[154] The Ebola virus derives its name from a river in the Democratic Republic of the Congo (formerly Zaire) where the disease appeared first. There are five sub-types of the ebola virus: Ebola-Zaire, Ebola-Ivory Coast, Ebola-Sudan, Ebola-Bundibugyo, and Ebola-Reston.

Ebola-Reston is the only known filovirus of Asian origin. Its genetic traits are similar to those of Ebola-Zaire. According to the European Center for Disease Prevention and Control, Stockholm, infection with the Ebola-Reston virus (REBOV) was first recognized in pigs in the Philippines.[155] But infection with the same virus in human beings does not cause clinical illness. The REBOV first appeared in the United States in the quarantine facilities of Virginia in 1989 when monkeys imported from Calamba in the Philippines were taken ill and died.

The African Ebola species can be transmitted from one individual to another through the exchange of or direct contact with blood, organs, and other body secretions of infected individuals. Direct contact with the body of a person who has died from Ebola virus can transmit the virus. Human beings handling dead or living infected animals can be infected with the virus. Healthcare professionals coming into direct contact with people infected with ebola without proper infection control precautions are at a high risk of infection.

The symptoms of infection with the Ebola virus include a sudden onset of high fever, sore throat, muscle aches, headache, and weakness followed by vomiting, development of rash, diarrhea, and both internal and external bleeding. Other symptoms include impaired kidney and liver functions. To control the spread of the disease, it is necessary to quarantine infected individuals and to observe stringent hygiene and sanitary measures. The WHO report claims that in 1976, in the Sudan, the Ebola virus killed 151 people between June and November.[156] In the same year, 280 people died in the Democratic Republic of the Congo (then Zaire). In 1979, 33 people died from a second Ebola outbreak in the Sudan. Another outbreak killed 250 people in Zaire in Kikwit in 1995. In Gabon, an estimated 75 people died from Ebola virus infection and in Uganda 224 deaths were reported. A second and third wave left 254 people dead between 2001 and 2003 in Gabon and Zaire.

Most of the infectious diseases cited above can be mitigated or completely prevented by applying simple practices of regular hand washing, especially before handling or preparing food and after using the toilet. Other ways of preventing the spread of such diseases include maintaining proper sanitation systems so that the community is not exposed to sewage. Other preventive measures include providing health education at community level to address the technicalities of disease transmission and prevention among local people to educate people about maintaining stringent health promoting measures in the food service establishments that cater for a lot of people. There is also a need for strict observation of infection control and hygiene measures in healthcare institutions.

In the Bible, we are told that the Israelites always washed their hands before eating. This was a tradition that had been handed down by their forbears: "Then Pharisees and scribes came to Jesus from Jerusalem and said, "Why do your disciples transgress the tradition of the elders? For they do not wash their hands when they eat," (Matthew 15: 1-2). In modern day, public health officials struggle to enforce the practice of hand washing and yet, if strictly applied, this practice can significantly improve the health profile of multitudes of people, as was the case during the time of Dr. Ignaz Semmelweiss.

During the 14th century, as the Black Death wreaked havoc in Europe, the Jewish people, led by Balavignus who was both a physician and a student of the Old Testament and was familiar with biblical health laws which he applied, observed stringent hygiene practices in their residential areas.[157] All refuse was either burned or buried. As a result, the mortality rate from the Black Death among the Jewish communities was only five percent of what it was among the rest of the population.

The adoption of biblical laws regarding disease prevention are not outdated. God's Word remains viable to the end of time. Biblical hand hygiene (see Leviticus 15: 11), a codification of biblical law is one of the strategies advocated by public health officials because it has great potential for prevention and control of infectious diseases. Additionally proper sanitation as indicated in Scripture (see Deuteronomy 23:9–14) is another effective method for preventing the occurrence and spread of infectious diseases and for reduction chances of recurrence of some of them. Eradication of vectors such as mosquitoes and rodents is also an effective method for disease prevention. These practices, which can be adopted at personal and community levels have the potential to break the life cycle, spread and multiplication of infectious agents. Besides, they are less expensive than treating and containing the disease in the community after it has broken out. Although the threat of the re-emergence of some infectious diseases is increasing, having and knowing the proper methods of combating them can allay our apprehension.

Chapter 11

Quarantine

He shall remain unclean as long as he has the disease; he is unclean; he shall dwell alone in a habitation outside the camp.

(Leviticus 13:46)

The biblical health laws mandated quarantining individuals who were afflicted by certain types of contagious and infectious diseases. One such disease was leprosy. Leprosy was a dreaded disease that traumatized not only the patients but their families as well as entire communities. Individuals who suffered from those diseases were commanded to live or dwell in isolation outside the camp, away from the mainstream community:

> The LORD said to Moses and Aaron, "When a man has on the skin of his body a swelling or an eruption or a spot, and it turns into a leprous disease on the skin of his body, then he shall be brought to Aaron the priest or to one of his sons the priests, and the priest shall examine the diseased spot on the skin of his body; and if the hair in the diseased spot has turned white and the disease appears to be deeper than the skin of his body, it is a leprous disease; when the priest has examined him he shall pronounce him unclean.

> He shall remain unclean as long as he has the disease; he is unclean; he shall dwell alone in a habitation outside the camp.
>
> (Leviticus 13: 1-3, 46)

One specific narrative of an incident involving the isolation of an individual who had leprosy is found in 2 Chronicles:

> Then Uzzi'ah was angry. Now he had a censer in his hand to burn incense, and when he became angry with the priests leprosy broke out on his forehead, in the presence of the priests in the house of the LORD, by the altar of incense. And Azari'ah the chief priest, and all the priests, looked at him, and behold, he was leprous in his forehead! And they thrust him out quickly, and he himself hastened to go out, because the LORD had smitten him. And King Uzzi'ah was a leper to the day of his death, and being a leper dwelt in a separate house, for he was excluded from the house of the LORD. And Jotham his son was over the king's household, governing the people of the land.
>
> (2 Chronicles 26:19-21)

Whenever the diseased person (who lived in isolation, particularly one who had leprosy) came into close proximity with the rest of the community who did not have the disease, he was required to cover his moustache or mouth and shout "unclean, unclean" to warn them to avoid contact with him:

> "The leper who has the disease shall wear torn clothes and let the hair of his head hang loose, and he shall cover his upper lip and cry, 'Unclean, unclean.' He shall remain unclean as long as he has the disease; he is unclean; he shall dwell alone in a habitation outside the camp."
>
> (Leviticus 13: 45-46)

By covering his mouth, the afflicted individual was preventing saliva from spraying and spreading from his mouth through the air to other people who did not have the disease. Similarly, the Centers for Disease Control and Prevention (CDC) instructs the general public to cover their mouths whenever they cough as a measure of infection control.

Some have argued that what was termed as leprosy in Bible times was not always Hansen's disease as we know it today. They assert that, in some cases, the disease was actually any type of infectious skin condition characterized by lesions or pustules. Nevertheless, the infectious nature of the disease, whatever it was, legitimized the isolation of the afflicted individual. This practice has been adopted by modern public health professionals. In the *Encyclopedia of Medical History,* McGrew asserts that "the idea of contagion was foreign to the classic medical tradition and found no place in the voluminous Hippocratic writings. The Old Testament, however, is a rich source for contagionist sentiment, especially in regard to leprosy and venereal disease" (McGrew, 1985).[158]

Leprosy mercilessly ravaged Europe in the 13th and 14th centuries. Norway, England, Sweden, and Iceland suffered alarming high percentages of leprosy cases. According to Drs. McMillen and Stern, authors of the book, *None of These Diseases,* the profile of the disease changed when in 1873 Dr. Armauer Hansen, a physician in Norway who had been conducting research on the causes of leprosy, looked into his microscope on a slide at a sample culture taken from a leprosy patient.[159]

There he saw what looked like tiny red dots, which he identified as leprosy bacteria. This opened the way for the understanding that leprosy was actually an infectious disease caused by bacteria found in the nose. This is the reason why leprosy is also known as Hansen's disease. Droplets emitted by an infected person when sneezing could easily transmit the disease to the next individual.

During this same period, it was also discovered that the leprosy bacteria had the ability to survive in a dry environment for several days, so if an uninfected person came into contact with the leprosy bacteria several days later, he would still be infected. Norway caught on to what Hansen had discovered—the high infectivity rate of the disease—and passed the Norwegian Leprosy Act, which enforced quarantining of infected individuals.

Leprosy mainly damages the peripheral nerves. This can range from mild to severe. Leprosy-related morbidity can have a negative social and psychological impact on the patient. The affected areas become numb as bumps and rashes begin to attack them. If they do not receive timely treatment, people with leprosy become disfigured, as they tend to lose their fingers, noses, and toes. They become significantly disabled and are usually feared and shunned. The *Merck Manual Handbook* indicates that in 2006, 137 new cases of leprosy were reported in the United States.

Over 50% of them were reported in "California, Florida, Louisiana, Massachusetts, New York, and Texas," (Merck Manual Handbook, 2010).[160] Almost all of them involved individuals who had emigrated from developing nations. The Handbook further informs us that in 2007, 250,000 new cases of leprosy were reported worldwide. An estimated 90% of these occurred in the nations of "India, Brazil, Indonesia, Congo, Bangladesh, Nigeria, Nepal, and Ethiopia."

Following Norway's quarantine law, other countries soon introduced stringent isolation laws to separate individuals who had leprosy from those who did not and the incidence of the disease began to reduce soon after that. Commenting on this achievement, Dr. Atkinson says that

"It is most singular that a description of leprosy, as found in the thirteenth chapter of Leviticus, could have been written so long before our time. It is to be noticed that such an accurate description of this dread malady as it appears in the biblical narrative is not to be found in the literature of any nation for the next seventeen hundred years," (Atkinson, 1950).[161]

Dr. Atkinson further comments that "Moses ordered that cases of leprosy should be segregated, that dwellings from which infected Jews had gone should be inspected before again being occupied, and that persons recovering from contagious disease were not to be allowed to go abroad until examined. The modern quarantine harks back to these sanitary regulations of the Old Testament."

Modern medicine and public health practice acknowledges the benefits of the practice of quarantine as a critical method of stemming the spread of communicable diseases. Other official campaigns of quarantine practices took place in 1485 when Venice established a forty-day quarantine practice, which required that any arriving ship that was suspected of having a plague aboard was to anchor in an isolated place for forty days without communicating with anyone from the mainland. Then in 1626 Marseille established the first quarantine station, which was followed by the introduction of a bill of health. The bill of health certified that ships coming into the harbor were free from disease.

In the United States, the first quarantine practice took place in Massachusetts Bay Colony, followed by the Philadelphia quarantine after the outbreak of yellow fever.[162] [163] In 1848 the National Quarantine Act was passed. This Act transferred quarantine powers from individual states to the federal government. Finally, in 1944, the Public Health Service Act was passed, which became the foundation of the current federal quarantine practices.

Quarantine is the separation and restriction of the movement of people who are well but are presumed to have been exposed to some contagion. It is also the separation and restricted movement of people who have contracted a contagious disease in hospitals or other enclosures. Quarantine is applied mainly at individual level, but population groups can also be quarantined depending on the magnitude of the disease outbreak. Quarantine can be voluntary or mandatory depending on the virulence and infectivity of the disease in question.

Following the outbreak of the Severe Acute Respiratory Syndrome (SARS), individuals who exhibited symptoms of the disease were isolated from the rest of the community until they were no longer infectious. But no large-scale quarantine measures were deemed necessary. By isolating them, the patients were given time to receive the care they need. According to the World Health Organization (WHO), the Severe Acute Respiratory Syndrome (SARS) emerged in Southern China in late 2002 and early 2003. Before long it had spread to 30 countries of Asia, North America, as well as Europe. The World Health Organization acknowledges that the disease was halted "through strict implementation of quarantine and isolation procedures," (WHO, 2010).[164]

In addressing the benefits of quarantining infected individuals as prescribed by biblical health laws, Gwilt elaborates on the severity of the Black Plague that ravaged Europe in the 14th century and how efforts to contain it were futile until "the city leaders of Venice decided to adopt the 40-day segregation practices employed by the Jewish ghettos at the time," (Gwilt, 1987).[165]

After observing a significant reduction of disease rates due to the practice of isolating infected individuals, the city leaders began to view the practice favorably and encouraged other cities to adopt it. The term quarantine (quaranta meaning 40) was adopted to refer to the number of days that were required to be spent in isolation. In the document of the *Epidemic Alert and Response to SARS* by the World Health Organization (WHO), Angus Nicoll, a WHO spokesperson, states that: "The evidence presented at the Global Meeting on the Epidemiology of SARS and published data have confirmed the efficacy of traditional public health measures, which include early case detection and isolation, vigorous contact tracing, voluntary home quarantine of close contacts for the duration of the incubation period, and public information and education to encourage prompt reporting of symptoms," (Nicoll, 2003).[166]

Biblical health laws continue to prove their efficacy as health-promoting guidelines millennia after they were first given.

CHAPTER 12

INCEST

None of you shall approach any one near of kin to him to uncover nakedness. I am the Lord.

(Leviticus 18:6)

Incest is the sexual abuse of another human being by a close family member or relative. Incest can also take place between related as well as quasi-related individuals. Author and researcher Dr. Christine A. Courtois observes that when the perpetrator of an incestuous relationship is older and much bigger or stronger or has the advantage of power differential—such as a parent with a child, a grandparent with a grandchild, an aunt with a nephew, or an uncle with a niece—then that incestuous expression becomes child abuse too.[167] Data on sexual offenses that take place in the family is difficult to obtain because there is usually a wall of silence, which makes the discussion of such issues taboo. Most of the time family members who may be aware of a nonconsensual incestuous relationship taking place between an adult and a minor in the family may be unwilling to discuss the matter because of the upheaval such a discussion might incite in the family. Incest is regarded as a deeply "private and sensitive matter, the exposure of which can shroud the family in feelings of shame, guilt, and embarrassment."[168] However, studies have been conducted which have pin-pointed the personalities of individuals who are perpetrators of incest. Although perpetrators of incest can be grandparents, aunts, uncles and siblings, researchers have discovered that most incest offenses are more likely to occur between father and daughter.[169] Most of the fathers who commit incest have a symbiotic personality characteristic of a person whose emotional needs such as affection were never met in their childhood. Such people do not know how to have a close relationship with anyone in a non-physical and non-sexual manner.

Incest is one of the toxic stressors whose traumatic consequences can be both short-term and long-term, particularly for the victim. The effects of incestuous relationships on the victim can last a lifetime. Victims of incest tend to have emotional, relational, and sexual scars that outlast the physical scars. What makes incest virulent is that is rarely occurs alone. It is often accompanied and reinforced by other types of family problems such as spousal abuse, child negligence and ill-treatment as well as abandonment of the child. The convergence of these other problems makes incest even more damaging to the victim. Whenever incest occurs between an adult and a minor, the burden of guilt is placed on the adult and not on the minor. The consequences resulting from incestuous relationships between an adult and a child are more serious if it starts when the child is still very young or when the child is in early puberty. Additionally, great damage is incurred by the child if the perpetrator is forceful and violent or if the child is blamed for the occurrence of the incestuous relationship. Physical penetration and continuous recurrence of incest by a person living under the same roof with the child further exacerbates the adverse effects of incest. Apart from being traumatized by incest the victim can also suffer from secondary trauma from family members, particularly if the perpetrator denies the accusation and convinces the family of his or her innocence. This can cause the family to blame the victim and to withdraw any form of social support, making the victim feel emotionally abandoned. With such a hostile environment the family might become reluctant to obtain therapeutic services for the victim. Sometimes the hostility in the family can cause the victim to recant the exposure of incestuous relationship with the perpetrator just to keep the peace in the family and to comply with the rules obtaining in the family while the perpetrator continues with the incestuous practice, wounding the victim even more.

Incest offenders usually prey on the trust of their victim and use it to manipulate them into submission, particularly when the victim is young. Perpetrators of incest are astute in selecting the vulnerabilities of their target, particularly children.[170] They can easily identify the weaknesses in the personality of their victim. These personality weaknesses are sometimes compounded by the child's life circumstances such as loneliness and passiveness. Additionally, children who seek attention or have no siblings living with them at home or are quiet and have low self-esteem seem to be regular targets of incest predators.

The findings of a study by Bushnell and associates conducted among women aged 18-44 in New Zealand to assess potential long-term effects of intra-familial sexual abuse during their childhood years demonstrated that incestuous sexual abuse during childhood was significantly associated with increased mental problems including depression, bulimia, and anxiety. The study found a significant prevalence of intra-familial incest practices in the target population group.[171] By destabilizing the mental faculties of its victims, incest undermines their ability to be productive members of society and to fulfill their calling. This is not only a loss to the victim, it is also a loss to the broader community of mankind. As such, incest is an affront to all of us.

The New York City Alliance Against Sexual Assault Fact Sheet states that in the United States, 46% of children who are subjected to sexual abuse are victims of their own family members in acts of incest and about 61% of them are subjected to this abuse before they are 18.[172] Twenty-nine percent of these sexual abuses take place when the victims are below 11 years old. About 11% of victims are sexually abused by their own fathers or stepfathers. Posttraumatic stress disorder is a prevalent health condition among individuals who are incest survivors.

Societal taboo against incest forces the victims to carry and keep to themselves this violation for many years. A child who has been sexually victimized in an act of incest by a close relative living away from home can turn home to the loved ones for safety and support, but a child who is sexually abused by a person at home, in the same family, has nowhere to run to for security.

As such, victims usually do not report the abuse because they fear that no one in the family will believe them or that they will be blamed for it. They also fear that they will endanger their stay in the family. Sometimes they do not report it because they are not aware that it is a crime against them. In most cases, the victims of incestuous sexual abuse carry feelings of betrayal, especially toward the perpetrator who did not honor the trust they had in him or her.

Later in life, these individuals might find it difficult to develop relationships in which trust is the fundamental ingredient. They also feel betrayed by their mother (if the perpetrator was any other family member other than the mother) who should have protected them but did not.

Sexual abuse by a father is one of the deepest betrayals a child can experience, because in the balance of power in the family, the father is a symbol of authority and security. Fathers betray their roles as protectors of their families when they rape their children. The father in the family is supposed to protect everybody who comes under his roof from such violations. He is the head of the family, and power and authority differentials are skewed in his favor. Therefore, when the father becomes the perpetrator, the children feel trapped. Incestuous relationships between mother and son can be equally traumatic to the victim.

An abused child has very little knowledge about therapeutic resources that might exist outside the family. As a consequence, recovery from the violation becomes very difficult. Although in all cases of incest, the survivors of incest know that there was nothing they could have done to prevent it, they still experience a sense of guilt and shame because of their involvement. A young child does not always understand that it is the responsibility of the perpetrator, if he or she is an adult, to set the standard for appropriate behavioral patterns that prevent perverted sexual expressions from taking place.

Another research study conducted by Read and Argyle among psychiatric in-patients who were survivors of childhood physical and sexual abuse in New Zealand revealed that hallucinations were more frequent among patients who had experienced incest than among those who had been physically abused.[173] According to researchers Lubin and associates, early childhood incestuous experience and abuse have been implicated in the etiology of an array of psychopathological conditions in adult survivors.[174] These conditions include multiple personality disorders, depression, substance abuse, and somatoform disorders. The American Academy of Family Physicians defines somatoform disorder as:

> "The somatoform disorders are a group of psychiatric disorders that cause unexplained physical symptoms. They include somatization disorder (involving multisystem physical symptoms), undifferentiated somatoform disorder (fewer symptoms than somatization disorder), conversion disorder (voluntary motor or sensory function symptoms), pain disorder (pain with strong psychological involvement), hypochondriasis (fear of having a life-threatening illness or condition), body dysmorphic disorder (preoccupation with a real or imagined physical defect), and somatoform

> disorder not otherwise specified (used when criteria are not clearly met for one of the other somatoform disorders).
>
> (Oyama, Paltoo & Greengold, 2007)[175]

The negative effects of incest become more virulent particularly if it starts very early in childhood or if it is prolonged or accompanied by violence or coercion. Incest can also have adverse effects if it is blamed on the victim or if it involves penetration by more than one perpetrator. When incest is protracted without any prospect of intervention, the victim feels trapped and may resort to dissociating from reality in order to cope with what is happening to her or him. Victims of childhood incestuous relationships tend to be prone to suicidal behavior, self-harm, sexual dysfunction, substance abuse, and cognitive distortion. Researcher Gelinas reports that survivors of incest usually manifest disorders that include self-mutilation and sleep disorders that include nightmares.[176]

Modern-day medicine has intervention strategies designed to bring healing to both incest victims and their perpetrators. Therapy for victims is aimed at helping them realize that the occurrence of incest was not their fault and that they are not to blame. The victims are encouraged to understand that the perpetrator was the only person who could have prevented it from happening. This is intended to help the victim have a sense of self-worth and cease from blaming herself or himself about the abuse.

Linda S. Coker introduces us to a three-phase treatment model that serves as a therapeutic approach for the adult female victim of incest.[177] The model enumerates the issues and tasks that each survivor must deal with before they can achieve the ascribed therapeutic goals. The first phase is conducted in group settings. The second phase involves individual sessions between the therapist and each member of the victim's family, and the third phase is a hybrid of individual and group sessions.

Concerning therapy for perpetrators, Coker informs us that there are treatment options that include offender-oriented cognitive/behavioral therapy (CBT). There are also family-focused multimodal systems of therapy for the families of the perpetrator. The cognitive/behavioral therapy model was designed by merging behavioral therapy with cognitive therapy. It focuses on personal counseling of the offender by a psychotherapist. The cognitive/behavioral therapy (CBT) model has been reported to reduce recidivism by between 20% and 30%. Although they are effective, these therapies are curative not preventive. This means that they are conducted after the violations have already been committed. The ideal would be to find means that would prevent the occurrence of the violation altogether.

According to a report in *Psychology Today*, incestuous relationships have a biological cost.[178] Apart from the emotional and psychological damage, adverse effects of incest to the victim and the perpetrator, children that are born of incestuous acts have a high rate of birth defect. In a study conducted among Czechoslovakian children who were sired by very close relatives of their mothers it was discovered that 42% of the offspring had severe birth defects and 11% had moderate mental impairment. The study included a control group constituting "offspring of the same mothers but whose fathers were not the mothers' relatives." When the same women had children from other men who were not their close relatives, only 7% of the children born from these relationships had birth defects.

God's methods of maximizing the health of his people is through prevention of the health threat. We have seen the destructive effects of incestuous relationships in our day, both forced and consensual. God desires for his people to prosper and be in good health (3 John 1:2), physically and spiritually. Incest hinders this prosperity. The Bible does not condone forcing anyone into a sexual relationship of any type (see Deuteronomy 22: 28-29), let alone abusing a young child in any manner (Matthew

18: 1-6). Concerning incest the Lord God commanded Israel that "None of you shall approach any one near of kin to him to uncover nakedness. I am the LORD" (Leviticus 18:6). Although marrying an individual who was near of kin immediately after the fall of man and prior to the giving of this law was lawful, the Lord forbade the practice later probably because the genetic mutation had started having a cumulative effect on the human race. In their Apologetics Press article, Thompson and Major had the following to say:

> There was no need for strict laws on marriage partners in the early Patriarchal Age (apart from the divine "one man, one woman, for life" institution), and for at least one good reason: during this time, man was in a relatively pure state, at least physically, having left not long before the perfect condition in which he was created and the Garden that had sustained his life... No harmful genetic traits had emerged at this point that could have been expressed in the children of closely related partners. However, after many generations, and especially after the Noahic Flood (Genesis 6-9), solar and cosmic radiation, chemical and viral mutagens, and DNA replication errors, led to the multiplication of genetic disorders. God protected His people by instituting strict laws against incestuous marriages in the eighteenth chapter of Leviticus.
>
> (Thompson & Major, 1987)[179]

Although Cain could safely have married his sister because the genetic pool was still pristine from the Creator's hand, by Moses's day the genetic error had augmented considerably and incest was out of question.

This chapter has depicted the grim picture of the effects of incest. Therefore, it is only logical to conclude that ways must be found to protect those who are vulnerable to incest perpetrators from being exposed to such an atrocity by finding ways to prevent it from happening and identifying it when it is happening so that the victim can be admitted to services and resources, which can bring healing. Stiffer sentences should also be meted out to those who perpetrate incest against little children. Parents, guardians, clinicians and public health professionals as well as other allied health professionals should make a concerted effort to watch out for any signs of rape or incest and identify them. They should also listen attentively to the victims and encourage them to expose the perpetrators so that the scourge can be reduced or completely eliminated.

CHAPTER 13

RAPE

But if in the open country a man meets a young woman who is betrothed, and the man seizes her and lies with her, then only the man who lay with her shall die.

(Deuteronomy 22: 25)

Rape is unwanted or forced sexual intercourse. It is sexual contact with an individual that takes place without the consent of the victim. Sexual intercourse is a very personal and private experience that should never be forced on anyone. Rape or forced sexual intercourse negatively impacts the psychological, emotional, and physical wellbeing of the victim.[180] It violates the privacy and human rights of the victim. It also humiliates the victim irreparably. No victim of rape can ever forget the violation.

What is stolen by the perpetrator can never be returned back to the victim. No attempted remedial action can completely wipe out the experience or restore the victim to the state they were before the rape took place. However, it is possible for some amount of healing to take place with the passage of time and with proper treatment, counseling, and therapy.

According to the World Health Organization (WHO), rape is a universal problem. It cuts across race, gender, class, ethnicity, sexual orientation, geographical, and religious boundaries.[181] The risk factors for rape include authority and power differentials based on gender and age. Some societies still view women and young girls as disposable sexual objects to be experimented with and discarded at will.

Other risk factors for rape include war, poverty, alcohol, and drug abuse. Often the documentation of every rape occurrence during times of war is scarce because perpetrators are usually never persecuted. Prior to the Nuremberg and Tokyo tribunals established in 1945 and 1946, respectively, and the prohibition stipulated in the Fourth Geneva Convention of 1949 as well as the Additional Protocols of 1977 aimed at punishing perpetrators of rape during times of war, rape was perceived as a reward for the victors of war.[182]

A research study conducted by Lilly found out that American GIs raped more than 17,000 women in Germany, United Kingdom, and France during World War II between 1942 and 1945. German soldiers also used rape as a war tactic.[183] The soldiers would invade villages and have their way with the women and young girls. It is estimated that over 50,000 women were locked up in enclosures during the war for the sexual pleasure of the German soldiers in the villages and towns they invaded.

Beevor, a historian, estimates that Russian soldiers raped about two million German women during the final days of the war.[184] Similarly, according to reports by Wood, when the Japanese soldiers overran the city of Nanking in December of 1937, they raped up to 80,000 women and then executed them afterwards.[185] Hu, writing for the Chinese American Forum, 1992, presents the following eyewitness report given to him by a missionary at Nanking Drum Tower Hospital who witnessed the rapes:

> Never have I heard or read of such brutality. Rape! Rape! Rape! We estimate at least 1,000 cases a night, and many by day. In case of resistance or anything that seems like

The Perfect Prescription

disapproval there is a bayonet stab or a bullet... People are hysterical... Women are being carried off every morning and evening. The whole Japanese army seems to be free to go and come anywhere it pleases, and to do what it pleases.

(Hu, 1992)[186]

Researcher and author Inger Skjelsbæk claims that rape was a tactic used by state forces against insurgents in Guatemala during the civil war that took place between 1960 and 1996.[187] A similar strategy was used in El Salvador, Nicaragua, and Cambodia, although the actual quantification of the atrocities is unavailable. In Khmer Rouge, rape was particularly used against women who were captured during the war. Skjelsbæk further claims that in Mozambique during the brutal civil war between the political parties, Frelimo and Renamo, which lasted from 1977 to 1992, women and girls as young as 8 years old were raped in front of their own families while fathers were forced to commit incest with their own daughters or nieces or daughters-in-law.

In Uganda, about 70% of women in Luwero District were raped by soldiers in 1991, and about 200,000 Somali women refugees were raped in their camps in Kenya. In Bosnia and Herzegovina from 1992 to 1995, mass rape was used as a weapon of war, and between 10,000 and 60,000 women were raped there. In Rwanda, the world witnessed one of the most heinous genocides of the 20th century in 1994. The Rwandan civil war was characterized by the most extreme and senseless violence imaginable, particularly against vulnerable population groups such as women and children and the elderly.

The absence of international intervention during the 100-day genocide intensified incredible anarchy. It has been estimated that between 250,000 and 500,000 women were raped or subjected to other despicable forms of sexual violence during this period. The rapes were motivated by an intention to humiliate and then to kill the victims.

In Kosovo during the war, large-scale rape took place in women's homes and in detention facilities. The Kosovo Liberation Army soldiers committed rape against Serbian, Albanian, and Roma women in Kosovo. Recently, the armed forces of the government of Sudan launched horrible attacks on the non-Arab people of Darfur in the Sudan, particularly women and children.

The *Janjaweed* or armed gunmen of Darfur collaborated with the armed forces of the Government of the Sudan and embarked on a massive campaign of rape as a deliberate strategy of their military assault against their victims. Reporting on the atrocities, the Genocide Intervention Fund observed that:

> The fight for women's lives is being lost in Darfur. While the violence in Darfur is a human rights atrocity for all Darfurians, the situation on the ground is especially dangerous for women because the Janjaweed militiamen are employing rape and other acts of sexual violence as systematic weapons of genocide and ethnic cleansing. Women—from young girls to grandmothers—are raped and brutally assaulted during attacks on their villages, as they attempt to flee, and in refugee camps. It is difficult to gauge the true extent of abuse against women in Darfur due to social stigmas surrounding sexual abuse that keep women silent about the issue, but survivors' testimonies reveal that violence against women is widespread.
>
> (Genocide Intervention Fund, n.d)[188]

Gender-based inequality often creates a conducive environment for rape.[189] Rapists, in such cases, tend to have the mistaken belief that women are somewhat inferior to men. They hold deeply embedded beliefs that men should exhibit sexual prowess and women should be at their disposal to satisfy their sexual hunger with or without the women's consent.

In such communities, rape is perceived to be the fault of the woman involved. The victims are usually in denial of the deleteriousness of the crime on their general health. Commonly held beliefs among societies that promote gender inequality are that the man should have sex in order to prove his masculinity and that when women say no to sex, they actually mean yes and so their protests should not be taken seriously. Other negative beliefs stipulate that if the woman consents to kissing or any kind of petting, she is obligated to have sexual intercourse. In these societies, rapists are rarely punished and male entitlement denies the women the right to refuse sex. The victims do not report rapes in these cases for fear of being punished themselves by the existing so-called criminal justice system.

Holly Burkhalter, vice president of Governmental Relations for International Justice Mission, was quoted by the World Bank Group as follows: "I think that it is not going too far to say the world will never successfully confront the global AIDS pandemic if it does not simultaneously confront the epidemic of sexual violence in the world today, because sexual violence is behind women and girls' vulnerability to the disease."[190]

Ban Ki-Moon, United Nations Secretary General, also underscored the insidiousness and repugnancy of violent crimes against women. Ban Ki-Moon was also quoted by the same World Bank Group that quoted Burkhalter when he said that "Violence against women and girls continues unabated in every continent, country and culture. It takes a devastating toll on women's lives, on their families, and on society as a whole. Most societies prohibit such violence—yet the reality is that too often, it is covered up or tacitly condoned."

In the United States, rape is one of the most under reported crimes.[191] In 1996, over two-thirds of rapes committed were not reported. The treatment of victims of rape by the criminal justice system in the United States has been questioned in the past. But since the establishment of the first rape crisis center in the 1970s, hundreds of laws have been passed aimed at protecting rape victims in courts. Medical protocols for rape victims have also been designed and implemented widely. Mental health professionals are being equipped with the necessary skills to understand and effectively deal with the mental impact of rape on the victim. However, gaps still exist in medical treatment and assistance of rape victims.

Sometimes the quantification of rape occurrences is often not an easy undertaking because the scale and nature of rape crimes is heavily dependent on how rape is defined and determined by different communities and societies. A report from the Federal Bureau of Investigations (FBI) indicated that there were 96,122 rapes committed in 1997 in the United States. Kilpatrick (2000), writing for National Violence against Women Prevention Research Center, claims that using a definition that describes rape as any forced vaginal, anal, and oral sex, the National Violence Against Women Survey discovered that 1 out of every six women and 1 in every 33 men in the United States have experienced a rape or an attempted rape at one time or other in their lives. An estimated 1.5 million women and 834,700 men have been raped or assaulted by someone who is intimate to them.

A survey conducted by the National Survey on Adolescents funded by the National Institute of Justice among 4,023 adolescents aged 12 to 17 revealed that about 8.1% of the participants had already experienced at least one sexual assault.[192] Kilpatrick further reports on the findings of a three-year prospective study funded by the National Institute of Drug Abuse conducted among 4,008 women aged 18 and above aimed at assessing the incidence of rape among the study participants that approximately "seven-tenths of one percent of all women surveyed had experienced a completed forcible rape in the past year."[193]

Overall 683,000 adult American women get raped each year. About twenty-two percent of rape victims are raped by strangers; nine percent are raped by husbands or former husbands, eleven percent by fathers and stepfathers, ten percent by boyfriends or ex-boyfriends, sixteen percent by extended family relatives, and twenty-nine percent by neighbors or friends. Apart from sustaining lifelong psychological wounds as a result of rape, the victims also sustain physical injuries.

In the HIV/AIDS era, the horror of rape has intensified for women and girls. To be raped by an individual who is HIV positive is to be infected with HIV. In areas where gender imbalances are endemic, this becomes a constantly threatening and looming nightmare. Some societies in which HIV/AIDS is endemic have adopted HIV infection strategies called "ABC," meaning Abstain, Be Faithful, and use a Condom.

However, women in societies where gender discrimination abounds are in no position to benefit from abstaining from sex, being faithful, or using condoms unless these imbalances are redressed. The United Nations Theme Group on HIV and AIDS reports that in Kenya, 46% of women reported at least one episode of sexual abuse in their childhood, and only 12% of them reported the incident to an individual in authority such as the police.[194] Twenty-five percent of the women lost their virginity through forced sex or rape.

It is not unusual for the Nairobi Women's Hospital to receive an average of 18 cases of rape or incest each day. The Human immunodeficiency virus (HIV) prevalence among women aged between 15 and 49 is about 8.7%, while the prevalence among men in the same age group is 4.6%. The ratio is almost 2:1. The Human immunodeficiency virus (HIV) prevalence among girls aged 15 to 19 is six times higher than in the boys of the same age group, and HIV prevalence among women aged 20 to 24 is about four times more than that of men in the same age bracket.

Women who have been raped are highly susceptible to infection with sexually transmitted diseases, including HIV since the violence that characterizes rape damages the membranes of the genital area leaving open sores and lesions through which pathogens can penetrate the body. There has been no law in

Kenya against domestic violence as such. However, there are signs that the Republic of Kenya is beginning to take significant steps to address this issue. The government and many NGOs have committed themselves to establishing a legal system that will protect Kenyan women's rights.

The issue of widow inheritance in some African countries is another risk factor for HIV infection. In these countries, it is mandatory for the widow to have sexual intercourse with the individual deemed to inherit her and her children. Often this individual is a close relative of the deceased. Sexual intercourse must take place even when the husband of the widow has died of a highly virulent and infectious disease such as AIDS. However, the high death rates from AIDS and the irreversible loss of human capital that has paralyzed economies of the countries where HIV/AIDS is endemic has compelled local governments to take steps to criminalize the dangerous practice of widow inheritance.

In Zambia, traditionally women are advised never to refuse their husbands' sexual advances. They are also advised never to insist that their sexual partner should use a condom, as this would indicate lack of trust on the part of the woman. In a country where power differentials are skewed toward the men, that kind of behavior is perceived as insubordination and deviant from the norm. The women are merely required to submit.

In a behavioral survey conducted among Zambian women by the Zambia Ministry of Health/National AIDS Council, about 15% of women reported forced sex, although this may not reflect an accurate percentage, as many women could not disclose this information for fear of reprisals if discovered. However, the Zambian government is one of the governments in the region that have taken steps to protect the women particularly from customs such as widow inheritance.

The Zambian government has officially condemned the practice of sexual cleansing and has urged its citizens to seek alternative methods that are less traumatic than the sexual cleansing practice. In Uganda, the practice is decreasing. In Tanzania, men are beginning to openly question the benefits of the practice. Aggressive education campaigns about the potential harm these practices can cause has been of some benefit, particularly in the fight against HIV infection in these countries.

Mike Earl-Taylor, a university researcher in South Africa, states that in 2002 there were between 4.2 and 4.7 million people infected and affected by the HIV/AIDS pandemic in South Africa.[195] South Africa has one of the highest incidences of rape in the world, including child rape. About five children are raped every hour. In 2001, about 21,000 child rapes were reported and another 37,000 adult rapes were reported in South Africa.

According to the South African police, only 1 in 35 cases are reported. Therefore, the actual statistics of rape incidents could be well above what was been reported then. The myth of virgin cure from AIDS implies that an individual with AIDS can be cured if they have sexual intercourse with a young virgin. Earl-Taylor claims that this myth is pervasive and not confined to the African continent only. India and Thailand have entrenched beliefs in this myth. This myth, according to Earl-Taylor:

> Has a rich and culturally diverse history stretching back to 16th century Europe, and more prominently to be found in 19th century Victorian England, where, in spite of the emphasis on morality, rectitude and family values, there existed a widespread belief, that sexual intercourse with a virgin was a cure for syphilis, gonorrhea, [and other STDs]. Syphilis, like HIV/AIDS, was fatal in its terminal stages. In the Eastern Cape of South Africa, when a significant outbreak of STD's was spread by troops returning home from overseas after WWII, the Virgin Cure was widely sought among the population.
>
> (Earl-Taylor, 20002)

The Global Coalition on Women and AIDS, a UNAIDS-initiative group has committed itself to mitigating the impact of the AIDS pandemic on women around the world by galvanizing AIDS-related programs that are aimed at improving the lives of women and girls. Some of its objectives include reduction of violence among women and girls, prevention of HIV infection among women and girls, protection of women's rights and ensuring that women and girls have equal access to healthcare resources and treatment.

In commenting on the impact of rape on the victim, Kilpatrick observes that Posttraumatic Stress Disorder (PTSD) is one of the consequences of rape. Approximately 31% of rape victims suffer PTSD at some time in their life. About 11% continue to carry this disorder most of their lives. Thirty-three percent of rape victims have contemplated committing suicide. About 13.4% of the victims have major alcohol addiction problems, and another 7.8% are likely to have major drug addiction problems.

Thus, rape is a significant problem for the public health system, the criminal justice system, the mental health system, as well as the medical care system. A concerted effort involving all these systems would be an effective approach for designing and implementing workable policies to alleviate suffering typical of rape, and to meet the needs of rape victims and their families.

Deuteronomy 22:25-27 says:

> "But if in the open country a man meets a young woman who is betrothed, and the man seizes her and lies with her, then only the man who lay with her shall die. But to the young woman you shall do nothing; in the young woman there is no offense punishable by death, for this case is like that of a man attacking and murdering his neighbor; because he came upon her in the open country, and though the betrothed young woman cried for help there was no one to rescue her."

The woman depicted in this text is being coerced into a sexual encounter. Her resentment toward the impending violation causes her to scream for help, but because this is happening in some isolated field where there is limited human traffic, no one hears her screams. The rape takes place regardless of her protests. The assailant has taken advantage of his strength and has overpowered the woman. This man, therefore, is deserving of death, according to the Bible. The death penalty is a deterrent measure against such morally perverse practices so that they do not become commonplace in the nation.

In Deuteronomy 22:28-29, the Bible says, "If a man meets a virgin who is not betrothed, and seizes her and lies with her, and they are found, then the man who lay with her shall give to the father of the young woman fifty shekels of silver, and she shall be his wife, because he has violated her; he may not put her away all his days."

According to author McIntosh, if the above Scripture is to be interpreted as another form of rape, the occurrence still required disciplinary measures and restitution.[196] The perpetrator, in this case, was given two types of punishments. The first one was to marry his victim. The second one was to pay the father of his victim fifty shekels of silver. Viewed from the perspective of modern-day life, this seems like a horrific directive: the rape victim marrying her assailant! However, McIntosh further asserts that it is important for us to understand that there were no federal welfare systems then to take care of the economically disadvantaged. Being a virgin was a valued evidence of chastity and a source of pride in ancient Israel, while premarital unchastity was so abhorrent that if a bride was not found to be a virgin, she was condemned to death as stipulated in Deuteronomy 22:20-21 that "if the thing is true, that the tokens of virginity were not found in the young woman, then they shall bring out the young woman to the door of her father's house, and the men of her city shall stone her to death with stones, because she has wrought folly in Israel by playing the harlot in her father's house; so you shall purge the evil from the midst of you."

From the above Scripture it is evident that the woman whose virginity was stolen by a rapist was made unmarriageable by the occurrence. No other man would have her as a wife. No one married a non-virgin unless she was a widow. Marriage and children were indicative of a fulfilled life, then. The rape victim would have to live with her parents all her life, and if they died before her, she would have no source of support at all. Possibly, she would sell herself into slavery to earn a living.

Therefore, the directive given in Deuteronomy 22:28-29 for the assailant to marry his victim and never to divorce her was meant to ensure the violated woman was taken care of and not discarded to live a life of poverty, ostracism, and shame. Other men had the option of divorcing their wives if they no longer found favor in their sight (Deuteronomy 24:1), but not the man who had married someone he had violated.

He had to live with her and support her all her life. Divorce was out of question for him. Although the directive to marry the assailant was a difficult position for the victim to find herself in, especially when perceived from modern society, the alternative would have been even worse for her. The very fact that the men were punished for committing any type of rape in Israel suggests that crimes against women were not inconsequential or that they could just be dismissed without accountability by the perpetrator.

McIntosh further claims that instituting a law to punish rapists at all in ancient Israel was a revolutionary concept during that period of time. No other ancient legal system punished the crime of rape particularly to the degree outlined in Deuteronomy 22:22-29. This law serves as a foundation for modern-day penalties against rapists.

Some Bible commentators view the text in Deuteronomy 22:28-29 from a different perspective than that of McIntosh. They believe that the text does not address rape but a form of

The Perfect Prescription

seduction leading to consensual premarital sexual intercourse separate from the text in Deuteronomy 22:25-27. For example, James Jordan from the Institute for Christian Economics made this comment about the same text:

> "At first sight, this seems to allow for rape of an unbetrothed girl. In Hebrew, however, the verb 'seize' is a weaker verb than the verb for 'force' used in the same passage (v.25) to describe rape. This stronger verb is also used for the rape of Tamar (2 Sam. 13:11). Implied here is a notion of catching the girl, but not a notion that she fought back with anything more than a token resistance."
>
> (Jordan, 1984)[197]

Sam Shamoun, another Bible commentator, affirms Jordan's position when he indicates that the Hebrew text does not present the text found in Deuteronomy 22:28-29 as a rape case but rather a seduction of an unbetrothed virgin by a man. He links this text to the one found in Exodus 22:16-17: "If a man seduces a virgin who is not betrothed, and lies with her, he shall give the marriage present for her, and make her his wife. If her father utterly refuses to give her to him, he shall pay money equivalent to the marriage present for virgins," and concludes that in both these texts there is no forcible rape at all.

Shamoun further observes that the woman in Deuteronomy 22:28-29 is unlike the woman in Deuteronomy 22:25-27 who is said to be not guilty. The father of the victim portrayed in Exodus 22:16-17 had the option of refusing to allow his daughter to marry her violator, in which case he would take it upon himself to be responsible for the long-term welfare of his daughter whose chances of marriage had been dashed by the assault.

However, the principle still standards: no one has the right to forcefully have sex with another human being or to beguile or manipulate them into having sex. Both occurrences demanded restitution and punishment to stem the evil of having forced intercourse with women from the community. The punishment was also a way of protecting people from spreading sexually transmitted diseases through having indiscriminate sexual intercourse. Although a death sentence was imposed against convicted rapists, rape was not completely eradicated in Israel, as we read later in 2 Samuel 13:10-15 in which a prince, Amnon, raped his half-sister Tamar, and like most rapists, cruelly despised his victim after humiliating her.

> Then Amnon said to Tamar, "Bring the food into the chamber that I may eat from your hand." And Tamar took the cakes she had made, and brought them into the chamber to Amnon her brother. But when she brought them near him to eat, he took hold of her, and said to her, "Come, lie with me, my sister." She answered him, "No, my brother, do not force me; for such a thing is not done in Israel; do not do this wanton folly. As for me, where could I carry my shame? And as for you, you would be as one of the wanton fools in Israel. Now therefore, I pray you, speak to the king; for he will not withhold me from you." But he would not listen to her; and being stronger than she, he forced her, and lay with her. Then Amnon hated her with very great hatred; so that the hatred with which he hated her was greater than the love with which he had loved her. And Amnon said to her, "Arise, be gone."

Severe consequences followed this rape case. Amnon ended up losing his own life in Absalom's carefully planned murder plot as restitution for the rape of Tamar, his sister. Probably because King David did not punish Amnon for the rape of Tamar, Absalom felt betrayed by his own father and took matters in his own hands to avenge the evil done to his sister.

As a result, Absalom carefully organized an insurrection, which attempted to depose his father as king of Israel so that he could become king instead. King David had to flee hastily from Jerusalem to save his life. In an unprecedented act of treason and outrageous treachery, Absalom pitched a tent on a rooftop and lay with his father's concubines in broad daylight and in total view of the people of Israel.

Sleeping with the king's wife or concubine could only be done by the successor to the throne in the event of the death of the king not while he was still alive. Absalom himself died later in a bloody civil war at the hands of Joab, the commander of the army of Israel. One rape case had spiraled into a murderous rebellion and deadly civil war that adversely affected an entire kingdom and caused the death of hundreds of people. David lost two sons and almost lost his kingdom.

God gave mankind guidelines to deal with sinful and health-threatening occurrences such as rape. If we modify or defy his guidelines and counsel, the aftermath should never be blamed on him. Every human being has been endowed with the power of choice. Philip Yancey, a prolific and inspiring Christian author of our time, has this to say about our power to choose. "Our heavenly Father, it seems, 'errs' on the side of human freedom, subjecting himself to our choices and working from within his creation rather than acting on it from the outside" (Yancey, 2002).[198] The Lord Jesus Christ, working in tandem with his Father, also honors our power of choice, as Yancey further observes: "I see the same gentleness and refusal to coerce in the life of God's Son. In dealing with people, he states the consequences of a choice, then hands the decision back to the other party." Every choice has a consequence.

Although rape is rarely if at all punishable by death in modern societies even when it happens to a betrothed woman, it is still treated as a crime against humanity in corroboration with biblical health laws. Public health professionals and some other organizations within the World Health Organization such as the Sexual Violence Research Initiative (SVRI) as well as other different community-based organizations around the world are spearheading a global awareness by holding dialogues with governments about the societal disruptiveness and destructiveness of the crime of rape. They are demanding that perpetrators be persecuted and penalized for these crimes.

Biblical health laws provide the groundwork that galvanizes these organizations to zealously fight the evils of rape around the world and to restore dignity to those who have been violated by it, although these organizations may not consciously be aware of the biblical origin or abhorrence of rape. In his word, God has plainly revealed how he feels about the health and well-being of the marginalized, ostracized, and vulnerable.

An array of organizations, including legal systems, committed to alleviating the plight of the economically and financially disadvantaged and those who have no access to health care services and resources have picked up on it, unawares, and are fiercely defending the cause of "these, the least of my brethren;" providing them with a voice to seek redress where possible and to reduce suffering at the hands of other human beings. The echoes of God's statutes continue to stimulate the establishment of many more such campaigns.

Chapter 14

Stress

Thou dost keep him in perfect peace, whose mind is stayed on thee, because he trusts in thee.

(Isaiah 26:3)

Stress-related health problems are a major public health concern in developed nations. The incidence of stress-induced health disorders is expected to rise in the coming decades, and the global impact of stress-related health conditions is expected to rise significantly so that by 2020, stress-related depression and anxiety might be second only to ischemic heart disease in their prevalence.[199] This rise in these health conditions is likely to negatively affect the economy by disrupting work hours and productivity in general. Job stress is a threat to production.[200]

The Hungarian scientist, Hans Selye, discovered what we now know as stress in 1936.[201] But he called it the General Adaptation Syndrome (GAS). The GAS was the process by which the human body confronted what he called noxious agents. Selye's definition of stress is "the non-specific response of the body to any demand for change" (The American Institute of Stress, 1979).

Selye explained that any event that threatened an organism's well-being (a stressor) yielded three types of response: Alarm, Resistance, and Exhaustion.[202] In the alarm stage, the body reacts with either flight or fight response. In the resistance mode, the blood glucose becomes high, and adrenalin and cortisol continue to circulate at elevated levels.

The heart rate and blood pressure increase as well. In the exhaustion state, the organism exhausts all its resources and becomes susceptible to disease and even death. Selye understood that this could be a risk factor for disease. The General Adaptation Syndrome, which we now know as stress, can cause the blood to become thicker than is good for general health.

Thick blood hampers the proper circulation of oxygen, nutrients, and hormones to various tissues of the body, resulting in significant nutritional impairment as well as hormonal deficiency. This condition can lead to hypoxia, a condition in which oxygen levels fall below normal. A further decrease in oxygen levels can cause anoxia. Anoxia is a condition in which there is such an acute decrease in oxygen levels of the body so that the organism experiences impairment of cognitive skills and other psychological and physical functions.

Stress has been implicated as a risk factor for a number of other health disorders, including insomnia. A considerable number of research studies have been conducted to explore the relationship between stress and the etiology of insomnia. Some studies have demonstrated a positive association between stress generated by familial conflict and insomnia in little children, young adults, and adults.

Exposure to chronic stressful events in early life can also contribute to long-term sleep disorders. A retrospective study conducted by Healey and associates demonstrated that the participants who manifested chronic insomnia reported having experienced negative life events in the form of personal losses and illness and difficulties with parents in the year preceding the onset of insomnia.[203]

Studies such as that of Healey and associates have also indicated that although exposure to major life events can elicit insomnia, minor life events can also be a major contributor to sleep disorders and insomnia. Kim and associates conducted a population-based study in Japan among the general population to assess the prevalence of insomnia.[204]

The findings revealed that there was a correlation between the occurrence of stressful events as well as the lifestyle of the participants and onset of sleep disorders. The sleep disorders in this study included difficulty initiating sleep, difficulty maintaining sleep, and poor quality of sleep. Dr. Ruth Benca, professor in the Departments of Psychology and Psychiatry at the University of Wisconsin-Madison, claims that:

> Individuals in stressful situations commonly experience difficulty sleeping, and transient insomnia can occur in almost anyone in response to acute stressors, such as illness, personal conflict, work-related stress, environmental factors, and sudden schedule changes. In most cases of transient insomnia, the cause is obvious and sleep improves once the stressor is eliminated. Stress also appears to play a role in chronic insomnia, with severity and frequency of stressors as well as the individual's response to them contributing to the development of persistent difficulties with sleep.
>
> (Benca, n.d.)[205]

An epidemiologic study to evaluate the prevalence and correlates of sleep disorders in adolescents studying at 15 secondary schools in France was conducted by Vignau and associates.[206] The results of the results demonstrated that approximately 40.8% of the student participants reported at least one type of sleep disorder, including difficulties falling asleep or staying asleep, a need for more sleep, chronic use of sleeping pills, and early awakenings. Almost all of these disorders were highly correlated with high rates of divorce in their families, poor familial relationships, and death of parents.

Other studies have focused on the development of sleep disorders due to work-related stress. A survey study was conducted in 1999 by the National Sleep Foundation in conjunction with the Gallup Organization using telephone interviews among 1,000 Americans to assess the prevalence and nature of sleep disorders among the sample.[207] Approximately one-third of the sample reported at least one type of sleep disorder, and twenty-five percent reported insomnia; another nine percent reported regular sleep difficulties. The participants who reported insomnia complained that they woke up every morning feeling tired and drowsy due to waking up and staying awake in the middle of the night.

A myriad of job-induced stressful factors were implicated in the onset of these sleep disorders, including shift work and frequent traveling across multiple time zones. Job-induced stress has also been linked to anxiety, nervousness, and depression. Additionally, this type of stress can be exacerbated by little or lack of support from management, supervisors, and colleagues in the workplace.

Stress is a major risk factor for heart disease because it raises the blood pressure in the body, which is a risk factor for heart disease.[208] It also raises insulin, cholesterol, and sugar levels, which can work in concert or individually to facilitate onset of heart disease. Elevated insulin levels can cause sodium retention in the body, which can lead to fluid retention. Fluid retention can, in turn, lead invariably to high blood pressure and finally congestive heart failure.

The physical changes triggered by stress can instigate a host of negative health outcomes, including the development and acceleration of arteriosclerosis. Additionally, unbridled stress levels induced by real-life cataclysmic events such as natural disasters in the form of hurricanes, tsunamis, and earthquakes can raise the rates of heart attacks and sudden deaths. Heart disease has been reported to be more common in individuals who have been subjected to constant stressful experiences in their lives. Serum cholesterol levels in any individual at any given time are dependent on the interaction between environmental and biological factors. Stress is reported to be one of the factors that induce cholesterol elevation.

A study supported by Research Grant H-1891, National Heart Institute, and in part by the Tobacco Industry Research Committee assessed the effect of stress on cholesterol levels among Johns-Hopkins medical students.[209] The investigators conducted serum cholesterol assessments among 52 male medical students studying at Johns-Hopkins during three academic events: first, during admission to medical school (Test I); second, during final anatomy examination (Test II); and third, during a period of regular school work (Test III).

The assessments demonstrated that during the period of admission to medical school (Test I) and during the final anatomy examination (Test II), mean cholesterol levels were remarkably higher than when the students were doing regular academic work (Test III). These findings affirmed the prevailing hypothesis that significant stress levels among students facing admissions to medical school and critical final examinations is accompanied by a remarkable rise in cholesterol level.

In Pakistan, scientists Wattoo and associates conducted a quantitative analysis to measure the association between stress and cholesterol levels among local university teachers and housewives.[210] The researchers recruited 40 university teachers and 40 housewives from middle socioeconomic groups for the study. The participants were aged between 30 and 45 years. The researchers utilized the Likert Scale type of questionnaire to measure environmental, psychological, and physiological stress levels among the participants.

Total cholesterol, namely, LDL, cholesterol, and HDL cholesterol was measured using the CHOD-PAP method, and triglyceride levels were measured by glycerol-3-phosphate oxidase (GPO) method. The results of the study demonstrated that housewives had high levels of LDL cholesterol and triglycerides but low levels of HDL cholesterol compared to university teachers. Low-density lipoprotein (LDL) cholesterol is what is known as the "bad" cholesterol and high-density lipoprotein (HDL) protein is what is known as the "good" cholesterol.

Psychological, physiological, and environmental stress levels were much higher among housewives than among university teachers. Housework in Pakistan is perceived as of low status marked by societal isolation and limited interaction with the mainstream society. This perception can trigger stress, depression, and unhappiness in housewives. In traditional Pakistan, teaching is held in high esteem, making teachers develop and harbor a healthier sense of self-worth and security compared to their counterparts, the housewives. In addition, university teachers experience financial autonomy that housewives do not. A low level of HDL is a risk factor for heart disease.

Another research study was conducted among accountants to assess changes in their serum cholesterol and blood clotting time when subjected to occupational stress.[211] The reason for selecting this occupational group was that their routine work schedule is, seasonally, interrupted by urgent tax deadlines usually marked with high levels of stress. The researchers took blood samples from the participants every fortnight for serum cholesterol. Blood samples were also taken every month to assess blood-clotting time for a period of six months—that is, from January to June. The results of the study demonstrated that "severe occupational stress…was associated with a sudden and often significant rise on serum cholesterol. Results also showed a remarkable acceleration of blood coagulation time" (Friedman, et al. 1958).

According to researcher Kivimäki and associates, there is an increasing interest and concern about the relationship between job-induced strain and stress and associated negative health outcomes, particularly the risk of heart disease.[212] These researchers posit that two models have been used to identify "stressful components of the psychosocial work environment" (Kivimäki et al., 2002). One is the job strain model and the other is the effort-reward imbalance model.

According to the job strain model, high job demands coupled with low job control in work environments can be a threat to the health of employees. To validate this claim, researchers Altman, Shekelle, and Burau conducted a 25-year prospective study among 1,683 men aged between 38 and 56 in the Chicago Western Electric Study between 1957 and 1983.[213] Scores were given to the participants based on their job title at baseline to indicate decision latitude and psychological demand.

The results of this study revealed "a moderate prospective association between job strain and fatal cardiovascular disease" (Alteman, Shekelle & Burau, 1994). The second model, the effort-reward imbalance model, relates to the effect the labor market conditions can exert on health. A study by Bosma and associates examined the relationship between effort-reward imbalance model and the job-strain model and the risk of coronary heart disease among male and female British civil servants.[214]

The results of the assessment of the correlation between the effort-reward imbalance model and onset of coronary heart disease revealed that an imbalance between personal efforts and rewards at work such as not being promoted had a 2.15 high risk of new coronary heart disease. Similarly, a case-control study conducted by Xu and associates among a Chinese population assessed the relationship between job stress and coronary heart disease. The results of the study revealed that the combination of high effort-reward imbalance (ERI) and overcommitment to work had the highest risk for coronary heart disease.[215] High rewards reduced the incidence of coronary heart disease. The findings of the study confirmed that job-induced stress is a risk factor for coronary heart disease.

On October 25, 2008, a news article written by Roger Dobson in The Telegraph claimed that "Treating ill health caused by the stress of bad debts costs the NHS millions of pounds a year."[216] Twenty-one percent of the 5,000 adults surveyed in England and Wales reported having suffered from stress-related physical illness as a result of debt. Debt-related stress plagues both developed and developing nations. One of the main sources of stress is credit card debt.[217] This is the case because such debt is usually accompanied by high interest rates, which place a financial burden on the debtor. The obligation to pay the principal amount and interest can lead to high levels of stress, particularly in times of economic instability.

Recently, we have witnessed a significant home mortgage crisis in the United States and around the world. With an alarming rate of home foreclosures, "lenders are tightening mortgage lending standards, making it harder for families to maintain their consumption in the face of weakening income growth" (Westrich & Weller, 2008).[218] Although banks have restricted access to mortgages, they still continue to offer credit cards. Most credit cards come not only with high interest rates but with complicated repayment terms as well. These terms could easily lead to increased failure to pay in the long run. Acting out of desperation, consumers have begun to use their credit cards to purchase daily essentials, including groceries and gasoline. Individuals who have not been unable to meet their monthly mortgage payments use their credit cards to get by.

A report of a survey conducted by Ohio State University's Consumer Finance Monthly (CFM) in 2007, which appeared in the 2008 issue of *Filene Research Institute*, portrayed a bleak picture of the debt problem in the United States.[219] The findings of the survey demonstrated that about eight million households in the United States worry constantly about the amount of debt they have. About 7% are worried that they might not be able to pay off their debt, and another 6% report that their debt elicits in them "a great deal of stress."

Approximately 16% of consumers surveyed reported that they had at least one credit card account that has been submitted to a collection agency in the previous six months, which was another source of stress due to the constant telephone calls made by collection agencies demanding payment. One in ten respondents reported having filed for bankruptcy at one time in their lives. Respondents who had filed for bankruptcy reported having experienced an increased level of debt stress.

ECONOMIC COST OF STRESS DISORDERS

The World Health Organization (WHO) Global Burden of Disease claims that stress-related health problems will be one of the major causes of disabilities by the year 2020.[220] A report from Medibank Private in Australia indicates that job-related stress costs the economy $14.81 billion, annually, and employers are losing $10.11 billion a year due to employee absenteeism.[221] Further, each worker loses about 3.2 days each year due to job stress. In the United States, a survey of 300 businesses revealed that the rate of employee absenteeism has escalated alarmingly in the last few decades.[222]

About one million employees are absent from work every day because of stress. Approximately $602.00 is lost every week by American companies to employee absenteeism. Statistics from the American Institute of Stress indicate that 40% of job turnover is a result of stress; between 60%-80% of job-related accidents are due to stress, and "in California, the number of Workers' compensation claims for mental stress increased by almost 700 percent over eight years and ninety percent were successful with an average award of $15,000 compared to a national average of $3,420" (American Institute of Stress, 2011). In addition, employee stress costs American business approximately $50-$150 billion in health and productivity expenses each year.[223]

Although the actual term *stress* does not appear in Scripture, the Bible still addresses conditions we term as stressful. In modern times, almost everybody has some level of stress. This is one of the reasons for the booming market of self-help books, time-management seminars, therapists and massage businesses. Most people are desperately looking for ways to reduce stress levels in their lives. Most of the time we work ourselves almost to exhaustion to satiate our craving for a comfortable lifestyle, but that comfort continues to elude us and the craving continues.

Life seems meaningless, particularly if we have not discovered our purpose in life. Some of the stress that we experience stems from not knowing who we really are or why we were created. Each one of us is likely to face stressful events at one time or other. But the most important thing is how we react to those stressful events. Our reaction can either stimulate character growth or undermine it altogether. The Bible cautions us against excessive worrying because of the negative effects it has on spiritual growth and on physical health and well-being. The apostle Paul, writing from a Roman jail, exhorts us thus: "Have no anxiety about anything, but in everything by prayer and supplication with thanksgiving let your requests be made known to God. And the peace of God, which passes all understanding, will keep your hearts and your minds in Christ Jesus" (Philippians 4: 6-7). This scripture is a warning against entertaining and harboring toxic thoughts of worry and anxiety, which can distort our outlook to life and set us on a dangerous road to disease. It also cautions us against being driven by anxiety or being fearful of life.

The apostle Paul urges his audience to confidently let God know about their specific needs in every area of their lives. That is not to say God does not already know what we need. It means that we must be in a position to recognize and evaluate what is happening to us and then communicate it to him with gratitude for his promises and blessings, which builds and strengthens the relationship between us and him. It causes us to think within the parameters that acknowledge him as the center or our existence. The result of such a state of mind is mental tranquility and a much-needed relief from stress. The apostle's exhortation is similar to the Lord Jesus' counsel found in Matthew 6:25-34. Our future is a landscape that has been carefully marked by our loving heavenly Father, and we can confidently trust it to him.

The Bible does not condemn the borrower or label debt as sin. Instead, it warns us against the inevitable consequences of misusing it. Proverbs 22:7 tells us that "the borrower is the slave of the lender." When we borrow, we enter into an agreement with the lender. The agreement binds us until the debt is repaid. Borrowing can lead to a kind of enslavement because the borrower has to repay the debt on the lender's terms. Failure to pay on time is usually penalized by late fee charges and interest, making the burden of debt even more acute.

As such, we need to be careful to avoid acquiring debt, indiscriminately. However, there are occasions when emergencies arise that require significant expenditure such as illnesses in the family or any similar emergencies. In such circumstances, restoring the afflicted back to health might be, understandably, a primary reason for entering into debt should health insurance carriers refuse to pay for the medical services any longer. This is where we need to bear each other's burdens, and often there are Christian counselors and church organizations that provide services that can mitigate the negative consequences of debt such as foreclosures, broken homes and bankruptcies, and reduce stress levels.

CHAPTER 15

MENTAL ILLNESS

> *Have no anxiety about anything, but in everything by prayer and supplication with thanksgiving let your requests be made known to God. And the peace of God, which passes all understanding, will keep your hearts and your minds in Christ Jesus.*
>
> (Philippians 4: 6, 7)

Although mental illness has been reported to be a significant source of morbidity worldwide, not much is known about its etiology or causative factors because its symptoms are varied and complicated.[224] With technological advancement and medical research, however, it has become clear that mental illness can be triggered by biological, environmental, and psychosocial factors interacting with each other.

Mental illness can adversely affect cognition, emotional, and behavioral control.[225] It can also impair the ability to learn new skills and disrupt the ability to function well at work and in the family. Sometimes mental illness starts early in life and keeps recurring throughout the life of the individual. Research has demonstrated that susceptibility to mental disorders such as schizophrenia, manic depression, and attention deficit hyperactivity disorder can be genetic.

However, sometimes the etiology of mental illness can be triggered by an interaction between an array of genetic factors and non-genetic factors interacting with each other. Gender also plays a significant role as a risk factor for mental illness. Females are mostly vulnerable to depression, anxiety, and eating disorders, while their male counterparts are usually more susceptible to other types of mental disorders, which include attention deficit hyperactivity disorders, substance abuse disorders, and autism. Trauma to the brain can also be a risk factor for mental disorder.

According to the National Alliance on Mental illness, out of all individuals diagnosed with mental illness, 29% abuse either alcohol or drugs. About 50% of individuals with severe mental illness have a substance abuse habit of one kind or another.[226] An estimated 37% of people with mental disorders abuse alcohol, and 57% of individuals who abuse drugs suffer from at least one type of mental illness. The National Institute of Mental Health (NIMH) describe some mental disorders in the manner that is stipulated below:[227]

SCHIZOPHRENIA

Schizophrenia is a mental disorder that interferes with an individual's ability to distinguish between reality and fantasy. Schizophrenia also interferes with the ability to make proper decisions and to manage emotions. It is a chronic disorder that is characterized by sporadic episodes of hallucinations. Schizophrenia can also impair the patient's social skills. The hallucinations experienced by the patient usually happen in the absence of stimuli.

Sometimes the patient hears voices. Other times the patient becomes delusional and holds on to false beliefs that are not part of their belief system. No reasonable explanation can be given to them to refute those beliefs. The Global Burden of Disease (GBD) study—which began in 1992 as a collaborative initiative of the World Health Organization, the Harvard School of Public Health, and the World Bank—have placed schizophrenia as one of the top ten most incapacitating diseases worldwide.[228] There is no specific symptom that can positively identify schizophrenia because its symptoms are present in other mental disorders as well. The onset of schizophrenia occurs usually in adolescence for males and in early adulthood for females.

Manic Depressive Disorder

This is a mental disorder that is sometimes referred to as bipolar disorder. It causes extreme mood changes. It also causes shifts in energy and general activity levels. Symptoms of manic-depressive disorder include mood swings such as being in an elated state at one moment and being agitated, angry, or irritable the next moment. An individual with manic depression has poor sleeping habits and behaves impulsively. Bipolar disorders can result in ruined relationships, poor performance at work, and suicidal behavior.

Depression

This is another phase of bipolar disorder. The National Alliance on Mental Illness describes the symptoms of this health condition as loss of energy, protracted sadness, reduced energy, irritability and restlessness, lack of concentration or focus, anxiety, thoughts of suicide, and feelings of hopelessness. Sometimes individuals with this phase of bipolar experience a shift in appetite marked by over-eating or reduced eating. They also experience sleep disorders marked by either sleeping a lot or sleeping less.

Anxiety Disorders

This mental disorder is ubiquitous and cuts across cultural boundaries. It is generally characterized by chronic anxiety, tension, and exaggerated and unprovoked worry.[229] Individuals with anxiety disorders experience a regular sense of foreboding and anticipate disasters and difficulties in their lives usually related to money or family. Approximately 6.8 million people have anxiety disorders in the United States.[230] The onset of this disorder is gradual. Anxiety disorder can also include panic disorders, social phobia, and obsessive-compulsive disorder.

The Office of the Surgeon General 1999 report defines panic disorders as periods of intense fear and discomfort. Panic disorders associated with anxiety disorders can manifest themselves through other somatic and cognitive symptoms. The symptoms of this disorder include heart palpitations, nausea, feelings of choking on something, gastrointestinal distress, and dizziness.

> "A person who experiences recurrent panic attacks, at least one of which leads to at least a month of increased anxiety or avoidant behavior, is said to have panic disorder. Panic disorder may also be indicated if a person experiences fewer than four panic episodes but has recurrent or constant fears of having another panic attack."
>
> (National Alliance on Mental Illness, 2012)[231]

Researchers, Hayman and associates observe that "Because of the combination of high prevalence, early onset, persistence, and impairment, mental disorders make a major contribution to total disease burden" (Hayman et al. 2006). However, the severity of the burden of disease has somewhat been mitigated by the discovery of efficacious treatment regimens for mental health. This is what Hayman and associates say about the discovery of treatment regimes:

The Perfect Prescription

> Beginning in the early 1950s, effective psychotropic drugs were discovered that treated the symptoms of schizophrenia, bipolar disorder, major depression, anxiety disorders, obsessive-compulsive disorder, attention deficit hyperactivity disorder, and others. The safety and efficacy of antipsychotic, mood-stabilizing, antidepressant, anxiolytic, and stimulant drugs have been established through a large number of randomized clinical trials. Psychosocial treatments have been developed and tested using modern methodologies. Brief, symptom-focused psychotherapies such as cognitive-behavioral therapies have been shown to be efficacious for panic disorder, phobias, obsessive compulsive disorder, and major depression.
>
> (Hayman et al., 2006)[232]

Although this is a significant medical achievement that will substantially reduce the burden of mental illness, its benefits are mostly limited to developed nations. Access to effective mental illness treatment methods has yet to be a reality in most parts of the developing world, although the prevalence of the condition is as significant in the developing nations as it is in developed nations. Speaking at a mental health awareness event in Beijing, then Director-General of the World Health Organization, Dr. Brundtland, revealed that there were 340 million global cases of mental illness at the time of the report in 1999.[233] In Africa, approximately 50% of the population afflicted by mental illness has no access to necessary mental health drugs, particularly in rural areas and villages where treatment drugs such as antidepressants, antipsychotic and anticonvulsants are unavailable. Dr. Brundtland added that there were more than 45 million cases of schizophrenia worldwide. Between 10-20 million individuals with mental illness attempt to commit suicide each year.

Dr. Brundtland further said that "five of the 10 leading causes of disability worldwide…are mental problems" (Brundtlan, 1999). She listed these mental problems as major depression, schizophrenia, bipolar disorders, alcohol abuse and obsessive-compulsive disorders. She also stated that "They are as relevant in poor countries as they are in rich ones, and all predictions are that there will be a dramatic increase in mental problems in the coming years" (Brundtland, 1999).

Disabilities caused by mental disorders have been increasing steadily from 10.5% in 1990 to 12% in 1998. A 15% increase has been predicted by the 2020. Where counseling and treatment regimens are available for individuals with mental disorders, they should be used as prescribed. Dr. Brundtland further stated that the current increase in mental illness worldwide has been exacerbated by many factors, including cultural issues.

> "Many societies and communities that customarily offered support to their needier members through family and social bonds now find it much harder to do so. Then there are the obvious cases of civil war and chaos, as well as more subtle threats...radical shifts in society towards technology, changes in family and societal supports and networks and the commercialization of existence which may account for the current epidemic of depression and other psychiatric disorders."
>
> (Brundtland, 2000)[234]

ENVIRONMENTAL FACTORS AND MENTAL ILLNESS

Scientists believe that a successful identification and validation of environmental risk factors for mental illness could be useful in unlocking effective preventive measures that could significantly lower the incidence of mental illness and the associated morbidity.[235] Although genetic research scientists have made fascinating headway in discovering genes that predispose an individual to mental disorders, scientists believe that "mental illness increasingly falls into the realm of environmental health.

And from that platform... new treatment advances could soon emerge" (Schmidt, 2007).

An array of environmental factors that have the potential to trigger mental health includes abuse of pharmaceutical and illicit drugs, trauma or injury to the brain, and nutritional deficiency. Other negative conditions such as sexual abuse, death of a close relative or spouse, divorce, disintegration of a close relationship, and being victimized by a criminal event can also be sources of stress. These occurrences can also trigger depression or anxiety or both. Psychosocial and physiological conditions can work in concert with genetic susceptibility to alter, distort or impair brain chemistry, which can lead to a disruption in the mental stability of an individual.

STIGMATIZATION MENTAL ILLNESS

Many individuals suffering from mental illness experience another worldwide problem: stigma. This is compounded by unfounded beliefs that mental illness afflicts people with tainted or weak characters. Mental illness invokes fear in some societies because it is viewed as a shameful disease and that it is hopeless and lifelong. About two-thirds of all individuals who have been diagnosed with mental illness do not seek treatment because of fear of disclosure, fear of being rejected by friends, and lack of knowledge about available treatment options. This problem is usually exacerbated by some healthcare professionals who exhibit negative attitudes toward patients with mental illness.

To investigate the levels of stigma among healthcare professionals against people with mental illness, Bell and colleagues conducted an international research study among 649 pharmacy students from Australia, Finland, Belgium, India, Finland, Estonia and Latvia.[236] The pharmacy students' attitude toward people with mental illness was measured using the Social Distance Scale (SDS). The results of the study revealed that, generally, the students had stigmatizing attitudes toward people with mental illness. These attitudes were similar in each country.

In Nigeria, Gureje and associates used a multistage, clustered sample of household respondents to determine the knowledge and attitudes of the participants toward people with mental illness.[237] To collect information from the participants about their knowledge and attitude toward schizophrenia, a questionnaire in the format of the World Psychiatric Association Programme to Reduce Stigma and Discrimination Because of Schizophrenia was distributed. The World Psychiatric Association Programme to Reduce Stigma and Discrimination Because of Schizophrenia was launched in 1996.

It has since established projects to fight stigma in 20 countries using social marketing techniques to enhance effectiveness. The study found that the participants attributed the cause of mental illness mostly to demon possession. Trauma, stress, and heredity were also mentioned as secondary probable causes. Nine percent of the respondents believed that mental illness was a punishment from God, and another 6 percent thought poverty was the cause. The results explained, to some extent, the reason why negative attitudes toward the mentally ill are widespread in the society. This makes it difficult to socially integrate them into the mainstream society even after their situation has improved.

Researchers Kapungwe and associates conducted a research study to "explore the possible presence, likely causes, and potential means of addressing stigma and discrimination against the mentally ill in Zambia" using fifty semi-structured interviews and six focus group discussions to obtain the information they needed.[238] Their participants were recruited from three different provinces in the country. The results of their research study revealed widespread stigma against people with mental illness among the general public, among healthcare providers, among family members of those suffering from mental illness, as well as among some individuals at government level. The attitudes exhibited by the participants included fear of contagion, fear of potential violent behavior from the mentally ill, and a lack of understanding about the cause of mental illness. This study highlighted the dire need for aggressive community education campaigns and an urgent need to review and re-evaluate the existing legislation on mental health.

There is a lot that remains to be done at the global level to educate the general public about the etiology of mental illness. Aggressive education campaigns might reduce the unnecessary burden and stress caused by stigma among people with mental illness. Individuals with mental disorders need medication to control the symptoms of the disease, but most of all they need supportive counseling, some form of rehabilitative services, financial assistance to achieve recovery, and a strong spiritual family to provide support for them and their families during difficult times.

Economic Cost of Mental Illness

Mental illness accounts for more than 15% of the overall burden of disease from all causes.[239] Failure to provide the needed and timely treatment can have drastic consequences, such as degeneration of the condition and disruption of families. Untreated mental illness is reported to be the leading cause of morbidity and suicide, imposing significant costs at federal, state, and local government levels.

Untreated individuals who have mental problems lose their ability to be independent and productive members of their communities. Sometimes they become homeless and end up in correctional institutions. Young children who are left untreated lose the ability to learn or to participate in any productive school programs to develop and hone their skills.

While economic costs incurred by mental illness form approximately 6.2% of United States total expenditure on health care, these costs are difficult to analyze and quantify because some of them are indirect while others are direct.[240] Indirect costs take the form of reduced labor, drawing support from public funds, disrupted educational attainment, unemployment, suicide, and other costs related to mental illness such as homelessness. Direct costs take the form of doctors' office visits, hospital admissions, and prescription medication costs. Some mentally ill individuals do not have the motivation to seek treatment or any related resources at all.

According to the National Alliance on Mental Illness, untreated mental illness has staggering consequences. The total cost of untreated mental illness in the United States is more than $100 billion per year.[241] In 1992, mental illness accounted for 32,400 deaths in the United States. The economic cost for premature death from mental illness was about $10.6 billion in 1992. The economic cost associated with severe and persistent mental illness in the same year was about $10.5 billion with a death toll of 28,200.

Impaired productivity associated with mental illness cost $83 billion as lost productivity. Direct health care costs for mental illness, which included prevention interventions cost $63 billion in 1992. Severely and persistently mentally ill people exert a significant burden on the criminal justice system through arrests associated with offenses of public disorder and vagrancy resulting in police arrests, court procedures and correctional incarceration. The economic cost for these behaviors was about $723 million in 1992.

In developing nations, quantification of the precise economic cost of mental illness is quite scarce, since about 50% of this population group has no access to counseling services or any other related treatment options, and most of them live in remote rural areas far from urban health care services. In some developing nations, only about 1% of healthcare expenditure is allotted to mental illness services.

Pastoral Counseling and Mental Health

The person of faith who has a mental disorder should not hesitate to seek help from both the minister of religion and the healthcare provider. JCecil3 writing for *Progressive Catholic Reflections* states that:

> Psychiatrists are medical doctors best suited for those with chronic neurobiological disorders. Psychologists have doctoral degrees in psychology, and use various personality testing methods and talk therapy, though they are trained to identify serious mental disorders, and in some states can write prescriptions. Social workers and marriage or family therapists are highly trained master's level counselors who use the techniques of psychotherapy. Pastoral counselors integrate a faith perspective with a specialization in one of the fields of general psychotherapy.
>
> (JCecil3, 2003)[242]

Pastoral counselors are ministers or individuals who are endorsed by a religious faith and are also mental health professionals.[243] Pastoral counseling constitutes a significant and necessary resource for community mental health services, both therapeutic and preventive. This is because religious communities provide principal gateways for individuals and families seeking relief from issues associated with human suffering such as mental and emotional illness, alcohol and drug abuse, suicide, depression, family problems, juvenile delinquency, and child and spouse abuse.

Pastoral counseling has become a major mental health provider in the United States, offering individual, group, and family therapy. Pastoral counseling is a vital resource for people seeking spiritual modalities of treatment. The Gallup poll of 1992 revealed that 66% of the people surveyed preferred a professional counselor who also represented spiritual values and beliefs.[244] The American Association of Pastoral Counselors (AAPC) is a member of the national mental health community and is actively involved in a number of health as well as mental health coalitions.

Pastoral counselors certified by the American Association of Pastoral Counselors are highly educated individuals who have studied both theology and psychology. This means that they are trained in two disciplines necessary for addressing mental health issues. Because they are often willing to work for modest salaries compared to other mental health professionals, pastoral counselors provide one of the most cost-effective and accessible modalities of treatment in the field of mental health.

The Bible tells us to "Bear one another's burdens"(Galatians 6:2) and to be compassionate toward each other in all circumstances. There are many burdens that afflict people, such as emotional problems, physical illnesses or disabilities due to illness or old age or accidents, and financial calamities brought by retrenchments or medical conditions. The church, the Body of Christ, has a responsibility to lighten these burdens by developing programs aimed at identifying those who are going through a difficult time among its parishioners and in the general community in order to meet their needs as best as it can.

When people with mental disorders are given social support, fellowship, and encouragement from their church family, they usually develop the fortitude and resolve needed to work through their problems. This is one way of restoring their physical and mental well-being. Their outlook to life becomes optimistic and hopeful once again. A hopeful attitude can make a big, positive difference in their entire mental state.

Dr. Archibald Hart, in his book, *The Anxiety Cure*, asserts that a positive attitude toward life "is known to improve recovery from surgery and the immune system's ability to fight off disease as well as aid in cancer recovery, to reduce the fight-or-flight response and hence stress disease [and can]…restore our tranquility and turn our unhappy, anxiety-producing hormones into happy ones."[245]

The Perfect Prescription

In Philippians 4:8, Scripture tells us that "Finally, brothers, whatever is true, whatever is honorable, whatever is just, whatever is pure, whatever is lovely, whatever is gracious, if there is any excellence, if there is anything worthy of praise, think about these things."

A research finding published by the Mayo Clinic claims that optimism and pessimism can significantly affect one's life.[246] Optimists believe positive things will happen in their lives, which is an important ingredient for reducing stress. However, having a positive attitude does not mean being oblivious to the fact that unpleasant things can also happen in life. It means approaching life's irritants in a more productive and positive manner. Thinking takes place in a self-talk manner and self-talk is persistently endless.

Dr. McMillen enlightens us that the brain is able to affect every organ in the body through its intricate network of nerves. Whenever an abnormal chemistry is present in the brain, triggered by one event or another, the entire body is affected. Human beings are complex organisms because they are spiritual beings. "We are spiritual at our very nature. Our spirituality is what the Bible calls the "image of God," (Dr. McMillen, 2000).[247] This divine endowment is what distinguishes humanity from all other animate and inanimate forms of life.

If the spirit (*pneuma*) becomes agitated, upset, or restless, the mind (*psyche*) becomes perturbed as well. Then the physical body becomes equally, negatively affected (*soma*). Therefore, a distressed spirit can have a domino effect of ill health to the mind and the body. Worrying or being in a state of continual anxiety or agitation or distress, can trigger an adrenaline rush into the body, which can progress into serious physical or mental disorders.

Scientists have discovered that faith is significantly beneficial to prevention and treatment of many illnesses including mental illness. In his book *Modern Man in Search of His Soul*, Carl Jung observed that "there has not been one [of my patients] whose problem in the last resort was not that of finding a religious outlook on life...None of them has been really healed who did not regain his religious outlook" (Jung, 1934).[248] Carl Jung was a scientist, an influential thinker who founded analytical psychology. But he acknowledged the important role religion played in the health of his patients. Other modern studies have verified the positive effect of faith on mental and physical health. For example, the results of a study conducted by Williams and associates indicate that "religion may be a potent coping strategy that facilitates adjustment to the stress of life" (Williams et al.1991).[249] Similarly, a research study conducted by Harris and associates on *The Role of Religion in Heart-Transplant Recipients' Long-Term Health and Well Being* "found empirical evidence that recipients with strong beliefs who participated in religious activities had better physical and emotional well-being, fewer health worries, and better medical compliance by the final 12-month assessment."[250]

Dr. Harold G. Koenig, Director of the Duke University Center for the Study of Religion, Spirituality and Health and Associate Professor of Psychiatry and Behavioral Sciences, and Assistant Professor of Medicine at Duke, in his book *The Healing Power of Faith: Science Explores Medicine's Last Great Frontier*, gives a report of the findings of his study on the role of religion on health and well-being.[251]

The findings confirmed that the faith of religious individuals directly motivates them to adopt health-promoting behavioral choices and gives them the impetus to avoid unhealthy habits that could lead to physical and mental health disorders. These choices lead to lower rates of divorce, crime, and general stress. In addition, people of faith experience lower rates of liver disease caused by alcohol consumption because they refrain from abusing alcohol.

They also have lower rates of abuse of other mind-altering substances that usually cause mental disorders. "The deeper a person's religious faith, the less likely he or she is to be crippled by depression" (Koenig, 1999) in the face of traumatic experiences. Active faith, therefore, enhances both physical and mental health by bringing tranquility to the mind. Dr. Koenig encourages his colleagues to try and integrate their patients' personal faith with modern science and to endeavor to find out how these two can work in tandem to restore the patients to health. The idea is not to force the patients to adopt a religious belief if they are not so inclined but rather to encourage those who already believe.

In their efforts to prevent acute rates of morbidity from mental health, public health professionals focus on providing social support for the mentally ill.[252] They develop, implement, and foster befriending programs that provide networks of friends to help reduce loneliness by increasing opportunities for meeting new people and making new friends. This is an echo of the Scripture in Galatians 6:2 quoted above, which exhorts us to "Bear one another's burdens."

Any church that practices the scriptural counsel to bear each other's burdens can help reduce the severity and incidence of mental illness by providing spiritual nurturing and other services mentioned above. Secular mental health self-help groups and psychosocial clubhouses for individuals suffering from mental illness can work in partnership with the church to help people with mental disorders access social, vocational, and educational opportunities and resources.

Chapter 16

Mold and Fungus in Buildings

Then the priest shall command that they empty the house before the priest goes to examine the disease, lest all that is in the house be declared unclean; and afterward the priest shall go in to see the house. And he shall examine the disease; and if the disease is in the walls of the house with greenish or reddish spots, and if it appears to be deeper than the surface, then the priest shall go out of the house to the door of the house, and shut up the house seven days.

(Leviticus 14: 36-38)

Mold is a type of fungus that includes mildew yeasts and mushrooms. Fungi are ubiquitous eukaryotic organisms that constitute a variety of species.[253] They can be transported into a building via the surface of new materials or on clothing. Sometimes they access a building through passive (desiccant) or active (dehumidifier) ventilation systems. A desiccant ventilation system removes moisture from air using absorption so that the air is much drier when it leaves the desiccant than when it entered.[254]

Dehumidifier ventilating systems are believed to be one of the best methods of controlling humidity levels, although they are thought to be too expensive for normal residential buildings.[255] As a result, they are often used in commercial buildings. Fungi thrive in damp, dark areas of the building. Dampness in the building can be caused by rainwater or groundwater leaking through the roofs and walls. Plumbing leaks and spills can also be another cause of dampness in the building.

Yet another cause is by infiltration of warm, moist indoor air blowing through cracks in the wall. Once they are brought into the home, fungi can grow exponentially, particularly in a moist environment. They derive their nutrients from materials such as wallpaper, paint, glue and wood, dust or soil, books, and many other sources. To detect the presence of mold, it is necessary to carefully observe discoloration or leaching from plaster.

According to the Institute of Medicine, mold and other microbial organisms thrive in excessively damp, indoor environments.[256] The Institute of Medicine further claims that there is a significant association between damp indoor environments and upper respiratory tract health problems such as asthma, coughing, and wheezing.[257] Shenessa and associates conducted a survey study in eight European cities to evaluate a previously reported association between residing in a damp and moldy environment and the risk of depression.[258] The researchers created "a dampness and mold score...from resident- and inspector-reported data"(Shenessa et al.2007). They assessed depression in the participants using a validated index of depressive symptoms. Their findings demonstrated that dampness and mold were significantly associated with depressive symptoms.

Another study was conducted by Dales, Burnett, and Zwanenburg in six regions of Canada to measure the association between indoor dampness and mold, and health.[259] The findings indicated that the presence of dampness and mold in the home environment was associated with a significant prevalence of lower respiratory symptoms. This association persisted even after adjusting for sociodemographic variables that included gender, age, and region. The association still persisted when adjustments were made for exposure variables such as passive cigarette smoking, natural gas heating system, and wood stoves.

In their quantitative meta-analysis focused on the assessment of the effect of residential dampness on risk of respiratory problems, Fisk and associates received and evaluated research studies that were available to them so far.[260] The findings of the meta-analysis indicated that "building dampness and mould are associated with approximately 30–50% increases in a variety of respiratory and asthma-related health outcomes" (Fisk, Lei-Gomez & Mendell, 2007).

Stachybotrys chartarum, a greenish-black fungus, is usually found outdoors, but it can also be found in damp or flooded homes. Dr. Berlin D. Nelson, a mycologist, claims that for over fifteen years in the United States evidence has mounted implicating Stachybotrys chartarum as a severe problem in homes and buildings.[261] Mycotoxin is a potentially harmful chemical compound that is produced by fungi. It can be harmful to the health of humans and animals. It has also been implicated as a causative factor for "sick building syndrome." Dr. Nelson also reports that in the 1930s, in the Ukraine, a new disease was detected in horses and other animals, with symptoms of irritation of the mouth, throat and nose, dermal necrosis, hemorrhage, and a decreased level of leukocytes. In 1938, Russian scientists discovered that the disease was associated with *S. chartarum* then known as *S. alternans*, which was growing on the straw and grain that was being fed to the animals.[262] Intensive research studies followed this discovery in which horses were fed cultures of *S. chartarum*. Altogether about 30 petri dishes of the fungus were fed to the horses, and the result was death of the animals.

In 1986, an outbreak of trichothecene toxicosis was reported in a Chicago residence.[263] For five years, the occupants complained of headaches, sore throat, diarrhea, flu symptoms, dermatitis, and general malaise. When the air of the home was sampled, it was discovered the there were spores of *S. chartarum*. The fungus was growing on an uninsulated cold air duct and on some wooden ceiling material. The chronic moisture in the home favored the growth of mold. Extracts of samples from the contaminated duct debris proved toxic to the animals on which it was tested. The health problems of the occupants disappeared after the mold problem was rectified.

The overall problem of mold and its adverse effects on health finally managed to catch the attention of the World Health Organization (WHO). As a result, the WHO embarked on a process of reviewing and evaluating epidemiological evidence presented by previous published research studies conducted by various scientists. The WHO also reviewed the report by the Institute of Medicine on the topic of mold and health. Consistent with the findings by the Institute of Medicine, the WHO confirmed that there was sufficient evidence from the studies to indicate that occupants of moldy buildings are at increased risk of developing respiratory symptoms, respiratory infection, allergic rhinitis, and exacerbation of asthma.[264]

There was also evidence from the findings of the studies that being exposed to mold and other microbial agents in damp environments can increase the risk of rare conditions such as hypersensitivity pneumonitis, allergic alveolitis, allergic fungal sinusitis, and chronic rhinosinusitis. Additionally, the World Health Organization (WHO) acknowledged that microbial pollution in the form of bacteria and fungi, particularly filamentous fungi (also known as mold), which grows indoors where there is dampness or moisture, can be detrimental to health.

In the light of the above findings, therefore, the WHO designed and issued worldwide guidelines to protect the health of the general public living in varied socioeconomic and general environments. Local governments are cautioned to select guidelines that are viewed as appropriate for the local environment and the prevailing circumstances to help achieve their goals for optimal public health. The guidelines are intended to help public health professionals and also the general public to identify potential hazards and reduce risks. The following are some of the WHO health-promoting guidelines (World Health Organization, 2009).

1. Continuous indoor dampness and moisture-related microbial growth should be prevented or minimized because they can lead to poor health outcomes;
2. Whenever indoor microbial growth is suspected, thorough inspection should be conducted by experts and appropriate assessments should be used either to confirm the suspicion or to dismiss it;
3. When dampness and mold-related problems recur, they need to be properly corrected to eradicate any potential recurrence and future hazardous exposure to microbes and deleterious chemicals;
4. Building codes should be established in a way that ensures that building envelopes are well maintained and well constructed to prevent and control excess moisture and microbial growth. The building envelopes, which are the physical separators between the interior and exterior environments of the buildings, should be able to prevent thermal bridges and entry of vapor-phase water;
5. Ventilation should be distributed properly around the building and stagnant air zones should be avoided;
6. Individuals who own buildings should provide a healthy environment for their tenants by ensuring that the buildings are properly constructed and maintained. The tenants should utilize water, ventilation, and heating in such a way as not to promote dampness and growth of mould spores;
7. Local recommendations for various geographical areas should be updated and modified to suite the prevailing climatic conditions in order to effectively

control dampness and mould growth in buildings. Indoor air quality should be always desirable and safe and;

8. Remediation of conditions that can lead to exposure to mold should be enforced to prevent poor public health outcomes.

Writing about managing mold and lawsuits in an article in *The New York Times Archives* in 2003, Romano claimed that at that time the Insurance Information Institute, a New York-based organization, reported that there were more than 10,000 mold-related lawsuits in state courts all over the United States.[265] Most of these lawsuits are in Florida, California, and Texas, where the weather conditions are conducive for indoor mold growth. Multimillion-dollar awards to tenants have inspired an increase in the number of mold-related claims. This has motivated property managers, their lawyers, and the lawyers representing corporations, condominiums, and other rental property to ensure that the buildings are built as mold-proof as possible so that they do not end up among those facing mold-related litigation.

Researchers Mudarri and Fisk claim that out of 21.8 million individuals reported to be suffering from asthma in the United States, an estimated 4.6 million cases have been reported to be a consequence of exposure to mold and dampness.[266] Mudarri and Fisk further claim that "the national annual cost of asthma that is attributable to dampness and mold exposure in the home is estimated to be $3.5 billion" (Mudarri & Fisk, 2007).

In 2001, in Texas alone, insurance companies paid about $1.2 billion in mold-related claims.[267] In 2007, an employee sued his employer, a software company, for irreversible damages to his vestibular system due to occupational exposure to mold at the company's facility, according to a report from BLR=Business & Legal Resources.[268] The plaintiff contended that the building had a musty smell due to water leakages and damage. Fellow employees also complained about the leakages and reportedly suffered from increased upper respiratory problems. An environmental testing procedure was conducted, which confirmed the presence of mold. The plaintiff was awarded $1.6 million and his wife was awarded $ 200,000 for loss of consortium claim.

God foresaw the public health problems associated with the presence of mold and fungus in His people's homes and established guidelines to counter them and to promote public health. A blog entry dated March 11, 2011, by Nathan Albright explained in detail how the process of mold removal from homes in ancient Israel was treated and who was responsible for the remediation process.[269] In Leviticus 14:33-48, God gave specific instructions about mold remediation. These instructions were to be followed step by step as they are presented below in order to effectively deal with the threat of mold or with the actual presence of mold in the home so that the health of the community could be protected.

> Step No. 1. When you come into the land of Canaan, which I give you for a possession, and I put a leprous disease in a house in the land of your possession, then he who owns the house shall come and tell the priest, 'There seems to me to be some sort of disease in my house.' Then the priest shall command that they empty the house before the priest goes to examine the disease, lest all that is in the house be declared unclean; and afterward the priest shall go in to see the house.
>
> (Leviticus 14: 34-36)

As is indicated in the above passage, the Lord God commanded the nation of ancient Israel that dwelling places that had developed mold and mildew on the interior walls were to be evacuated even before the priest went inside the home to find out what the problem was. This same principle is still being applied in modern times. Families living in homes that are suspected of having developed mold and mildew are often required to evacuate the premises while experts access the premises to investigate the suspected mold problem.

> Step No. 2. And he (the priest) shall examine the disease; and if the disease is in the walls of the house with greenish or reddish spots, and if it appears to be deeper than the surface, then the priest shall go out of the house to the door of the house, and shut up the house seven days.
>
> (Leviticus 14: 37-38)

Because the people of ancient Israel did not have the technological methods we have in modern day to conduct a sophisticated mold-testing procedure, the priest among them was endowed with the visual acuity, which was honed by years of experience to help him inspect and verify the threat or presence of mold in a home. He mainly looked for evidence of green or red mold, which is usually a dangerous and toxic type of mold. Although it is not as common as green mold, red mold can appear on walls, in carpeting, and even in air conditioning coils. It can also attack clothing. If the presence of mold was confirmed, the priest was required to seal the home and declare it off limits so that no one could have access to it and be exposed to the mold and endanger their health. The building was quarantined for seven days.

> Step No. 3. And the priest shall come again on the seventh day, and look; and if the disease has spread in the walls of the house, then the priest shall command that they take out the stones in which is the disease and throw them into an unclean place outside the city; and he shall cause the inside of the house to be scraped round about, and the plaster that they scrape off they shall pour into an unclean place outside the city; then they shall take other stones and put them in the place of those stones, and he shall take other plaster and plaster the house.
>
> (Leviticus 14:39-42)

The Perfect Prescription

The priest was required to come back after seven days had elapsed to inspect the house again and to find out whether the mold was still present. If the mold had spread farther across the wall of the house, he ordered the removal of all the stones that were affected by the mold. This is a similar procedure to that which is applied in modern-day mold remediation processes.

The material that is affected by mold has to be removed from the building and be replaced with newer, safer material. In Bible times, the moldy materials that were taken out of the affected house were carefully removed and dumped in an isolated place away from the community residential area to ensure that no one else was exposed to the mold spores. In ancient Israel, new stones replaced the molded ones in the wall and the house was plastered afresh.

> Step No. 4. If the disease breaks out again in the house, after he has taken out the stones and scraped the house and plastered it, then the priest shall go and look; and if the disease has spread in the house, it is a malignant leprosy in the house; it is unclean. And he shall break down the house, its stones and timber and all the plaster of the house; and he shall carry them forth out of the city to an unclean place.
>
> (Leviticus 14: 43-45)

The affected building was under observation for a while to make sure the mold problem had been effectively treated. As such, the priest was required to conduct another inspection on the house to make sure that the mold had not returned. If the mold returned, this time the entire house was condemned and demolished. It was no longer fit for human habitation. Whenever toxic mold is detected in a building in modern day and if for some reason it becomes difficult to completely remove it, the building is evacuated and then demolished.[270] The building materials of such a building are destroyed as a protective measure.

> Step No. 5. Moreover he who enters the house while it is shut up shall be unclean until the evening; and he who lies down in the house shall wash his clothes; and he who eats in the house shall wash his clothes.
>
> (Leviticus 14: 46-47)

The Lord God warned Israel that if any one went into the house that had developed mold while it was still sealed, they would be declared unclean. This was a method for protecting the people from inhaling the mold and being exposed to mold spores, which would have had adverse health effects.

> Step No.6. But if the priest comes and makes an examination, and the disease has not spread in the house after the house was plastered, then the priest shall pronounce the house clean, for the disease is healed. And for the cleansing of the house he shall take two small birds, with cedarwood and scarlet stuff and hyssop, and shall kill one of the birds in an earthen vessel over running water, and shall take the cedarwood and the hyssop and the scarlet stuff, along with the living bird, and dip them in the blood of the bird that was killed and in the running water, and sprinkle the house seven times.
>
> (Leviticus 14:48-51)

This chapter depicts the seriousness with which God views mold in the home because of its harmful nature to the health of the occupants. When God stresses a point there is always a significant reason for it. It may not be necessary for us living in modern day to follow the steps enumerated above to eliminate mold from our homes, but the rigorousness and thoroughness of the process portrayed in the Bible underscores the seriousness of mold as a health threat. It also means we should not trivialize it either. The other point is that mold should be completely remediated for all homes where it may appear. The step by step process indicated in the verses ensured that the mold was completely taken care of and that the health of the owners of the home was protected. Shortly after they opened the tomb of King Tutankhamun of Egypt, Lord Carnarvon and his 26 colleagues died from a mysterious disease.[271] At first the deaths were attributed to Egyptian curses. Only later was it established that the tomb of King Tutankhamun had been heavily infested with dangerously toxic mold spores when it was opened. There is no difference between the biochemical composition of ancient Israelites to whom this law was given and ours as far as susceptibility to illness due to mold is concerned. Human beings of every age in the history of this planet are all vulnerable to the harmful nature of mold if exposed to it. Therefore, the counsel found in this Scripture continues to be relevant to all people. Whatever is written in the Bible is for our instruction, for us to learn from. Therefore, whenever we detect mold in our dwelling places we must, as a matter of urgency, contact certified experts who are able to identify the mold and prescribe the type of remediation procedure necessary to protect our health.

CHAPTER 17

SEXUALLY TRANSMITTED DISEASES

You were bought with a price. So glorify God in your body.
(1 Corinthians 6:20)

In most societies, social change occurs as a process that is often propelled by mechanical inventions and scientific discoveries.[272] These inventions and discoveries can instigate dramatic and evolutionary changes in a society's culture, values, and social norms. For example, the discovery of contraceptives revolutionized the overall structure of human sexual perceptions and practices. The origin of the unprecedented sexual revolution of the 1960s and 1970s has been attributed mainly to the discovery of contraceptives. In the 1900s, only an estimated 6% of unmarried teenage girls dared engage in premarital sex. By the beginning of the 21st century, however, that percentage had swelled to 75%.[273, 274] With the increase in the frequency of premarital sexual intercourse came an almost inevitable increase in the number of sexual partners per individual involved. The rise in premarital sex was buttressed by reduction in the risk of pregnancy due to the availability of contraceptives.

Another factor that led to the increase of premarital sex was the easy availability of abortion options for unintended pregnancies. The birth control movement originated with Margaret Sanger in 1914 when she wrote and published a pamphlet titled *Family Limitation*.[275] Although Sanger faced and experienced severe criticism and opposition from many circles, she had significant supporters for her work as well. The birth control movement took root, and its effects continue to reverberate in our societies today.

THE SEXUAL REVOLUTION

The sexual revolution of the mid-sixties and the seventies in the United States and other parts of the world not only changed young adults' perception of sex, it also changed their attitude and behavior regarding sex. Since the beginning of this period, the world has witnessed an unprecedented and continuous increase in the prevalence of sexual experimentation. Young people start experiencing sexual debut early in their teens as they become less and less inhibited about their sexual behavior.

In an article that appeared in the 2008 copy of the *Journal of American Physicians and Surgeons*, Sheetal Malhotra claimed that adolescents and young adults began to engage in risky sexual experimentation as a result of the sexual revolution.[276] That propensity toward engaging in risky sexual behavior has not changed much among adolescents and young adults with the passage of time. It has actually increased in intensity.

Malhotra further reports that approximately 50% of youth aged 15-19 have already had an experiment with vaginal sex; more than 50% of the same age group have tried oral sex, and 11% have had experiments with anal sex. Over one third of youth aged 15-19 have had more than one sexual partner already. These behavioral traits seem to be reinforced by age so that about 75% of young adults aged between 20-24 have already had sexual experiences with multiple partners; about 90% of this same age group has had vaginal sex; over 80% have engaged in oral sex at one time or other, and approximately 30% of them have had anal sex.

The strong inclination toward oral and anal sex is intensified by the belief that these practices do not result in pregnancy. These methods are regarded as safer and more appealing practices that outweigh the risk of contracting sexually transmitted diseases. However, Chlamydia, HIV, gonorrhea, and syphilis can easily be transmitted by engaging in oral as well as anal sexual intercourse.[277] The risk is especially great in anal sex because of the lacerations and tears that occur in the lower bowels during intercourse. These tears and lacerations create an environment that is conducive to infection with STDs.

THE MEDIA AND SEXUAL BEHAVIOR

The effect of the media has been implicated in fostering social behaviors that focus on sexual aggression, social attitudes, and stereotyping.[278] The media has the potential to educate young adults about responsible sexual behavior. This is one population group that is easily impressionable about romantic relationships, love, and sexuality. Portrayal of sex as something to be pursued and experimented with has steadily increased in music, television, and the movie industries in the past few decades.

Most of these portrayals depict intercourse between heterosexual, unmarried adults without any concern about STDs, including HIV/AIDS. Generally, female young adults depend heavily on magazines for information about STDs, sex, pregnancies, and birth control. The Internet is another source of information about sexual practices, STDs, and romantic relationships.

In 2008, the *Pediatrics Journal* reported a longitudinal survey study in which scientists assessed associations between exposure to television sexual content and the incidence of adolescent pregnancy.[279] Teens aged 12 and 17 were recruited for the study and were followed for the next three years. The results indicated that those adolescents or teens who were exposed to high levels of television sexual content had significantly higher rates of pregnancies compared with their counterparts who had relatively lower rates of exposure.

The reasons for the continuing engagement in risky sexual practices by young adults are numerous and varied, including peer pressure, alcohol consumption, illicit drug use, lack of proper parental guidance, and just plain curiosity about sex. Young adults who engage in experimental sexual intercourse early in their teens are usually at high risk for sexually transmitted diseases (STDs), unintended, nonmarital pregnancies, and poverty, which can lead to an assortment of physical and psychological problems such as contraction of an STD and depression.

There are two categories of STDs, namely viral and bacterial STDs. Viral STDs include genital herpes, which is a chronic infection that afflicts over 50 million individuals in the United States. Genital herpes is caused by the herpes simplex virus type 1 (HSV-1) or type 2 (HSV-2).[280] Most infected individuals manifest only minimal signs or herpes. Others do not have symptoms at all. But when the symptoms finally appear, they appear as one or more blisters on or around the genitals or the rectum. When these blisters break, they leave tender ulcers that may take about four weeks to heal after their first appearance. Another outbreak may take place some months after the first. Any person with genital herpes has a seven-fold risk of being infected with HIV.

In the United States, sexually transmitted diseases afflict about 19 million young adults under the age of 24 each year.[281] One of the most common STDs is human papillomavirus (HPV), which was recognized in 1986. The HPV frequently manifests itself in genital warts and can cause deadly cancers. Currently there are 100 types of HPV that are known by the medical community.[282] Of these, 40 types can cause genital tract and anus infection. The most common among the types that infect the anogenital tract are HPV types 6, 11, 16, and 18. These are high-risk HPV types that are associated with approximately 99% of cervical cancers. About 11,000 women are diagnosed with cervical cancer each year. The HPV afflicts 20 million people in the United States. It also kills a lot of women each year. In 1991, about 4,600 women succumbed to the HPV.[283]

Chlamydia is the most common sexually transmitted disease in the United States.[284] Chlamydia is a bacterial STD that infects over 2.8 million people each year. Infection with chlamydia can develop into pelvic inflammatory disease (PID). About 20% of women who get acute infection with PID become infertile, while 18% suffer chronic pelvic pain. Over 1 million cases of PID are diagnosed each year.

Gonorrhea is also a highly common sexually transmitted disease among women aged 15-19 and men aged 20-24.[285] Because gonorrhea is usually asymptomatic especially in men, it can spread quietly and ravage the body causing damage to the heart, joints, and brain if not treated on time. *Neisseria gonorrhoeae* is the second most commonly reported STD after chlamydia. In women, infection with gonorrhea can progress into cervicitis and PID. If left untreated, infection with gonorrhea can increase chances of infection with HIV.

Gonorrhea is an extremely common sexually transmitted disease in the United States. It infects about 700,000 new people each year.[286] Gonorrhea is caused by the bacterium *Neisseria gonorrhoeae*. It can be spread by oral, vaginal, or anal sexual intercourse. It can also be passed from a mother to her child during normal delivery. Perinatal transmission of gonorrhea to infants can cause severe cases of conjunctivitis that can progress to blindness if left untreated. Sometimes severe perinatal infection can result in sepsis with associated meningitis and arthritis.

Trichomoniasis is an STD caused by protozoa and is asymptomatic in 85% of men and in 50% to 80% of women. In pregnant women, this disease can be passed on to the infant. Infection with trichomoniasis increases the risk of being infected with HIV threefold. Most of the above STDs can be transmitted through oral and anal intercourse.

Condom use has been vigorously advocated as a way of reducing the risk of STD infection. Condoms may reduce the risk of infection, but they do not eliminate it. The National Institute of Health (NIH), in collaboration with the Centers for Disease Control and Prevention (CDC), the Food and Drug Administration (FDA), and the United States Agency for International Development (USAID) convened a workshop in 2000 to review the published evidence about the effectiveness of the male condom in preventing STDs and HIV infection. After the workshop, a Fact Sheet for public health personnel was produced. The following is a statement found in the opening pages of the Fact Sheet:

> The surest way to avoid transmission of sexually transmitted diseases is to abstain from sexual intercourse, or to be in a long-term mutually monogamous relationship with a partner who has been tested and you know is uninfected.... no protective method is 100 percent effective, and condom use cannot guarantee absolute protection against any STD.
>
> (Williams College Health Center, 2012)[287]

These institutions confirmed that abstinence and mutual fidelity in a monogamous lifetime relationship were the most effective safeguards against being infected with sexually transmitted disease. Condom use can only be protective to a limited extent.

ORAL CANCER

The rise in the incidence of oral cancer is causing concern in the United States. Scientists conducted a case-control research study nested within a longitudinal cohort of 100 patients who had recently been diagnosed with oropharyngeal cancer from 2000 to 2005.[288] The control group of the research study was composed of 200 eligible patients who did not have oropharyngeal cancer. Oropharyngeal cancer is cancer of the throat. The findings provided "support for the association between HPV and a subgroup of oropharyngeal cancers. The strength of the evidence is underscored by the associations of high-risk sexual behaviors, oral HPV infection, and HPV-16 exposure…with oropharyngeal cancer" (D'Souza, et al. 2007).

An analysis of throat swabs revealed that the oropharyngeal cancer patients were 12 times more likely to have infection of active HPV. Oral genital contact was significantly associated with oropharyngeal cancer. Other scientists affirm the above findings and indicate that "Both oral and oropharyngeal HPV infection and oral and oropharyngeal squamous cell carcinoma (SCC) are associated with the practice of orogenital sex" (Feller et al. 2010).[289]

Teen Pregnancies

Adolescents are prone to engaging in risky sexual behavior usually because of personal vulnerability and a focus on immediate rather than long-term consequences of their behavior.[290] Engaging in risky sexual behaviors can result in unintended negative health outcomes. Over the past few decades, there has been an alarming increase in teen pregnancies worldwide. Scientists and researchers claim that about 750,000 teen pregnancies occur every year in the United States alone. Most of them happen out of wedlock.[291] Some teens who get pregnant drop out of school and ultimately end up with no proper jobs and subsist on government public support program.

Alarming figures have been published about sexually transmitted diseases and their adverse effects. For example, as of December 2000, about 774,467 known AIDS cases were reported to the federal CDC. Over two-thirds of them were sexually transmitted or acquired. The human immunodeficiency virus (HIV) is perceived as a sexually transmitted disease because 75% of infections are acquired through sexual intercourse.[292, 293]

The 2001 *Surgeon General's Call to Promote Sexual Health and Responsible Sexual Behavior* emphasized the public health implications of sexual behavior. In this same report, the Surgeon General's office unveiled the following most important facts about sexual trends and the impact they have had in the United States. If studied carefully, these facts can be of uttermost help to teenagers and young adults in making decisions related to sexual relationships.

1. As of the year 2001, an estimated 800,000-900,000 persons are living with HIV in the United States. Although an estimated one-third of those living with HIV are aware of their status and are in treatment, another one-third are aware but not in treatment, and one-third have not been tested and are not aware. About 40,000 new HIV infections occur each year.

2. An estimated 1,366,000 induced abortions occurred in 1996. Commenting on the alarming rates of abortion and in an effort to promote sexual health and responsible sexual behavior, the *Surgeon General's Report* suggested that "The underpinning of the public health approach to this issue is to apply a variety of interventions at key points to prevent unintended pregnancy from occurring, and thus, ensure that all pregnancies are welcomed."

3. Nearly one-half of pregnancies among young adults are unintended or unplanned.

4. An estimated 22 percent of women and 2 percent of men have been victims of a forced sexual act at one time or other in their lives.

5. An estimated 104,000 children are victims of sexual abuse each year.

> (Office of the Surgeon General (US);
> Office of Population Affairs (US) 2001)[294]

Following biblical directives about sexual practices is a sure and effective way of preventing STD infections, unintended pregnancies, unfortunate occurrences such as abortions, forced sex as well as child sexual abuse. The effects of the above statistics are not limited to the individuals concerned, but they also adversely affect families, communities, and entire nations as well. Most often these problems and their ensuing consequences are skewed toward minority racial and ethnic groups.

The *Surgeon General Report* claims that Chlamydia infection rates for women from minority groups are significantly higher than the rates for white women and that the rates of gonorrhea are particularly high among individuals 15-19 years. These population groups also constitute the majority of individuals who are economically disadvantaged and do not have comprehensive access to the services and resources that could help mitigate the negative consequences of the problems listed above. This means that they are sometimes forced to rely on public programs for some time.

Sexual intercourse, which is a uniquely profound and intimate relationship and one that is supposed to be a source of indescribable joy, has become a source of public health concern in some cases. Health professionals now conduct workshops and seminars to educate people about responsible sexual conduct. Women and girls usually face sexual violence such as rape and incest in some communities, fueling susceptibility and vulnerability to HIV infection. The entire global community is faced with challenges associated with risky sexual behaviors. Some of these problems include infertility resulting from infection by some STDs. Other challenges are associated with the spread of the human immunodeficiency virus (HIV) and acquired immunodeficiency syndrome (AIDS), sexual abuse, unintended pregnancies, and abortion. The *Surgeon General's Report* further claims that "five of the ten most commonly reported diseases in the United States are STDs" (Office of the Surgeon General [US]; Office of Population Affairs [US] 2001).

God's approach in caring for his people is to prevent disease to curtail morbidity and mortality rates. That is why he allows certain activities to be performed only within prescribed parameters. For example, he allows and blesses sexual relationship when it takes place within the confines of a marriage relationship. He also commands that the marriage relationship be based on mutual fidelity and trust. Marriage in the Bible is treated as a sacred institution established by God himself when he presented Eve to Adam in the garden of Eden:

> So the LORD God caused a deep sleep to fall upon the man, and while he slept took one of his ribs and closed up its place with flesh; and the rib which the LORD God had taken from the man he made into a woman and brought her to the man. Then the man said, "This at last is bone of my bones and flesh of my flesh; she shall be called Woman, because she was taken out of Man." Therefore a man leaves his father and his mother and cleaves to his wife, and they become one flesh.
>
> (Genesis 2: 21-24)

The Scriptures also prescribe responsibilities for husbands and wives toward each other within the marriage relationship. The husband is commanded to love his wife as he loves his own body. The wife is also commanded to exhibit submissive devotion and commitment to her husband:

> Wives, be subject to your husbands, as to the Lord. For the husband is the head of the wife as Christ is the head

of the church, his body, and is himself its Savior. As the church is subject to Christ, so let wives also be subject in everything to their husbands. Even so husbands should love their wives as their own bodies. He who loves his wife loves himself. For no man ever hates his own flesh, but nourishes and cherishes it, as Christ does the church.

(Ephesians 5:22-24, 28, 29)

Marriages that are *truly* undergirded by biblical laws do not have to worry much about HIV infection or genital herpes infection or infection with any other sexually transmitted diseases resulting from promiscuity. These Scriptural directives about sexual behavior were aimed at preventing sexually transmitted diseases among the Israelites and for moral purity. God gave other commands to safeguard the sexual health of his people such as those prohibiting practices that include adultery (Exodus 20:10-12), homosexual practices (Leviticus 20:13), bestiality or sexual relationships with animals (Lev. 20:15-16). Other commands were given against incest (Leviticus 20:17, 19-20), prostitution (Leviticus 19:29), and rape (Deuteronomy 22:25-28). Marriages founded on a deep commitment to God and His health laws experience less divorce rates than their counterparts, which are not. According to the Bible, the marriage bed is a sacred place that ought to be respected: "Let marriage be held in honor among all, and let the marriage bed be undefiled; for God will judge the immoral and adulterous" (Hebrews 13:4).

The Bible takes an uncompromising stand against sexual promiscuity. In Leviticus 20:10-13, the Bible warns us that any sexual intercourse outside marriage is sinful. In Bible times sometimes promiscuity was punishable by death. Adherence to the commands about sexual behavior was enforced by religious leaders. These commands were not given to punish the people or to deny them sexual pleasure. On the contrary, they were given to promote optimum pleasure in secure and safe sexual relationships as well as to promote health in the community by preventing outbreaks of different diseases resulting from promiscuous behavior.

In modern times, those who are at the forefront in fighting HIV/AIDS and other debilitating sexually transmitted diseases are advocating observance of sexual laws similar to those found in Scripture. For example, they expressly advocate avoidance of multiple sexual partners. They also advocate abstinence. In his book *What the Bible Says About Healthy Living*, Dr. Russell gives us a graphic medical explanation as one reason why God prohibited the practice of homosexuality. Listen to how he explains it.

> The lining of the vagina is very tough and is designed to withstand the severe trauma during childbirth. Neither viruses, bacteria nor sperm can penetrate the lining of the vagina, and it is difficult for viruses to penetrate the vaginal wall. Healthy sperm, however, can easily swim through the birth canal and into the uterus or oviduct to penetrate an ovum, starting a new life. In contrast, the lining of the rectum is very fragile. Sperm placed in the rectum easily penetrate the mucosa and temporarily shut down the immune system, making the victim susceptible to infections. Thus, having a compromised immune system, any infection or latent cancer cells are poorly controlled. The consequences are often fatal.
>
> (Russell, R. 1996)[295]

The Creator God who designed the human body knows the conditions under which its health can thrive. Homosexuality is no more wrong than committing adultery, stealing, or lying. They are all sins that can separate us from the love of God. In the Book of Proverbs, the Bible gives us a list of other behavioral traits that are labeled as abomination to the Lord.

> There are six things which the LORD hates, seven which are an abomination to him: haughty eyes, a lying tongue, and hands that shed innocent blood, a heart that devises

wicked plans, feet that make haste to run to evil, a false witness who breathes out lies, and a man who sows discord among brothers.

(Proverbs 6:16-19)

In the same book, we are also told that "Lying lips are an abomination to the Lord, but those who act faithfully are his delight" (Proverbs 12:22).

The Bible, authoritatively and unequivocally, labels all of the above practices and many more as sins and God's word is immutable. Only he can change what is written in his word, not human beings, regardless of how much we may wish to do so. No amount of effort aimed at trying to justify our arguments against God's word can alter its stand about sin. However, no one is called to hate the sinner or to berate them.

As we remember our own vices and the mercy and grace God has given us, we must view each other with empathetic humility and pray for one another. God does not hate his children even when they disobey him. There is nothing anyone of us can do to make him love us any more or any less than he already does. He hates the wrongdoing because of what it does to us and to the relationship between him and us. His love is unconditional although the blessings are conditional. Those of us who claim to be his children should emulate him in our dealings with each other. Compassion is what undergirded the ministry of the Lord Jesus in the days of his flesh. The woman caught in the act of adultery found compassion in the Lord Jesus, although he did not condone the sin she had committed (John 8:1-11). Therefore, compassion for each other should be the bedrock of our ministry to each other. Our rebuke and warnings about the consequences of sin should be tempered with compassion and empathy, remembering that we, too, are sinners and are no better than anyone else.

We all need God's grace. When we accuse and berate and denigrate sinners of a different stripe, we begin to sound more like the devil and less like our Father. When we encounter individuals who are totally convinced that they cannot help doing wrong, it is not time to get into an argument about how wrong they are. It is time to intercede for them, to get on our knees and claim them for the kingdom of God by asking the Lord to shine his light into their hearts and show them the path of life. If we engage in arguments to try to prove how right we are, we might win the argument but lose the soul.

Wherever biblical health laws have been strictly observed and applied, the health outcomes have been impressive.[296] It is no wonder, therefore, that most of the interventions designed to prevent and stem epidemics echo biblical health principles.

CHAPTER 18

HIV/AIDS

In him was life, and the life was the light of men. The light shines in the darkness, and the darkness has not overcome it.

(John 1:4)

Since 75% of HIV infection occurs via sexual intercourse, it is important to address the incidence and prevalence of the disease and the extent of the devastation it has caused due to sexual behavioral choices. It is imperative to discuss the risk factors associated with the transmission of this disease and how this transmission can be mitigated. It is also necessary to find out what the Bible says about high-risk behaviors that can predispose people to infection with HIV and discover methods of avoiding those behaviors in order to reduce the incidence of this disease.[297]

Controversy continues to rage over to the origins of the human immunodeficiency virus (HIV). Researchers hold different viewpoints and opinions about this disease. For example, in his 2001 article from the *Philosophical Transactions of the Royal Society*, Julian Cribb called for an international multidisciplinary investigation into the origins of HIV/AIDS for the purpose of preventing similar pandemics.

Cribb made this interesting observation: "that AIDS may have started with an experimental polio vaccine used in central Africa is one of a number of possible explanations," (Cribb, 2001).[298] He further revealed that a growing number of authors have pointed out that this observation is backed by more scientific evidence than other competing theories. Other researchers such as Dr. Wolfe of Johns Hopkins Bloomberg School of Public Health have claimed that after examining and screening the blood sample of 1099 research participants from Cameroon for simian foamy virus (SFV) antibodies, the antibodies were detected in 10 participants of the sample.[299]

The ten individuals were reportedly infected with viruses from three different primate species. Ankomah, reporting for *New Africa*, contends that Nigel Hawkes, editor of *Times Science* speculated that the AIDS virus was first found in a "man from Central Africa" (Ankomah, 1998).[300] However, says Ankomah, Hawkes does not mention the man's name nor identify his race or ethnicity. The unspoken assumption is that because the person was from Central Africa, he must be a black African.

Similarly, Dr. Schneider claims that "*the most likely hypothesis is that HIV is a mutation of a monkey or ape virus that somehow spread to humans, probably in Africa*" (Schneider, 2004).[301] She does not explain why this is the most likely hypothesis. Dr. Schneider further indicates that "*Scientists conjecture* that the virus may have existed in isolated pockets of Africa" (italics mine).

The late Dr. Alan Cantwell Jr. scoffed at the theory that HIV originated from a green monkey. He was convinced that the virus was created by the Special Virus Cancer Program (SVCP), which began in 1964 and was funded by the National Cancer Institute.[302] Dr. Cantwell further claimed that at the National Cancer Institute—Bethesda, Maryland, the military's biological warfare researchers merged with the SVCP and that after this merger, the SVCP was transformed into a joint effort between the National Cancer Institute and the army's bio-warfare laboratories at nearby Fort Frederick, Maryland, where it became officially known as the National Cancer Institute-Frederick Cancer Research Center.

"To this facility," Dr. Cantwell claimed, "healthy animals such as monkeys, chimpanzees, mice and cats were shipped in from various parts of the world for breeding purposes and experimentation, and virus-infected animals were shipped out again to various labs" (Cantwell Jr., 2000).[303] Dr. Cantwell believed that these activities set the foundation for the creation of the HIV virus, which has infected and killed millions around the world.

Another individual who was convinced that HIV/AIDS is a manmade disease and attempted to prove it was the late Dr. Boyd E. Graves, who was an attorney and a graduate from the Naval Academy in Annapolis, Maryland. Graves demanded that the United States president and the government make a public apology for the development of the AIDS virus in the laboratories of the United States.[304] He drew up a time line depicting what he believed to be the activities that led to the development of the HIV virus, which he dubbed as "an ethnic cancer."

It is not the purpose of this book to conduct an investigation or a meta-analysis of different research studies on whether HIV/AIDS is manmade or not, much as that subject is an important one. That responsibility has been left in the capable hands of those who have been specifically called to do so. This book attempts to establish the relevance of biblical health principles to general health even as we witness the benefits of adopting them in some modern intervention strategies and health-promoting campaigns. HIV/AIDS is a monstrous disease that has brought incredible pain and suffering to those infected and affected by it.

The acquired immunodeficiency virus (HIV) was first noticed in Los Angeles in the United States in 1981 among gay individuals.[305] In the same year, the CDC issued a statement warning the public about a rare form of pneumonia that was manifesting itself among gay young men in Los Angeles.[306] This rare type of pneumonia was later identified as being AIDS-related.

By 1983, the causative agent for AIDS was identified as the human immunodeficiency virus (HIV).[307] Although some scientists believe that AIDS may have existed prior to 1981, the year 1981 has come to be recognized as the official beginning of the HIV/AIDS pandemic. Because the disease was first recognized among the gay community, a stereotype developed that associated HIV solely with the gay population groups. As a result, the heterosexual communities around the world became indifferent to it and were convinced that this was not their problem.

Another widespread belief accompanying the beginning of this disease was the misconception that it was mainly a disease targeting illicit drug injectors. Therefore, those who were not drug abusers somehow thought they were insulated from contracting the disease. When the disease crossed over to the heterosexual community, it became labeled as a disease for the poor and undernourished individuals, particularly from developing nations.

However, although AIDS is closely linked to nutrition, since malnutrition and undernourishment can speed the progression of the disease from HIV infection to AIDS in an infected person, it is not true that only the poor and undernourished can be infected with HIV. Anyone, regardless of gender, race, economic status or ethnicity, can be infected with HIV if they are exposed to it.

When HIV/AIDS was first recognized, many people felt confident that a cure would soon be discovered by the scientific community. But over a quarter of a century later, the disease is still raging, decimating almost entire generations in some parts of the world. Both the cure and vaccine continue to elude scientists and other health professionals. When the disease was first recognized among the gay community, it was labeled as a gay-related immune disease (GRID).

But this name was abandoned when the medical community discovered that the disease was no longer exclusive to the gay community. The stigma against HIV/AIDS is related, to some extent, to this initial labeling as a gay disease although there are also other factors that continue to intensify stigmatization against people living with HIV/AIDS. Some researchers claim that stigmatization against people living with HIV/AIDS stems from certain viewpoints. Some of these viewpoints are listed below.

1. HIV is usually associated with individuals known to engage in socially, culturally, and religiously deviant behaviors. These individuals constitute sex workers, injection drug users, individuals in concurrent multiple sexual relationships, and homosexuals;

2. Infection with HIV is believed to be a result of deliberate choices made by some individuals to engage in avoidable risky behaviors, which places the responsibility of infection on them. The infection is their fault.

3. There is still no cure for HIV/AIDS although advances in the medical field have produced therapies such as the highly active antiretroviral therapy (HAART), which slows the progression of the disease for many years, allowing the patients to live longer after infection. Nevertheless, the fact that there is still no complete cure for the disease still instills fear and dread in many people.

4. Because HIV infection is concealable, particularly during the incubation period before symptoms become apparent, no one can tell who has just been infected by the disease. The fact that the disease is infective even when it is asymptomatic makes it even more frightening, which encourages the stereotype that certain population groups such as sex workers and gay people are all HIV positive and should be ostracized.

(Swendeman, et al. 2006)[308]

Some researchers observe that HIV/AIDS is associated with symbolic stigma, which "involves a synergy between the stigma attached to AIDS as an illness and the stigma attached to the groups linked to AIDS in popular perceptions."[309] The human immunodeficiency virus is spread through activities that society usually finds difficult to discuss, to like, or to accept. Some societies compound these perceptions by harboring gender-based discrimination, often exalting the position of men above that of women. Male dominance and chauvinism is normative practice in certain societies. Speaking at the 16th International AIDS Conference in Toronto, Canada, in 2006, Melinda Gates recounted a moving scene she witnessed at an AIDS hospice in South India.

> The patients in the hospice were separated by gender. The long narrow trailer of the male ward was filled with families and flowers. Children came to spend precious last minutes with their fathers. Across a courtyard, we saw a very different scene. The female ward was a lonely, desolate place. There were no visitors—just women wasting away from AIDS. Some of them had managed to get themselves to the hospice, others had been abandoned there by a relative who no longer wanted anything to do with them. There was no love, no warmth, no comfort. Just wives and mothers, left alone to die.
>
> (Gates, 2006)[310]

Stigma is not limited to India. There are many other areas, societies, and communities where AIDS-related stigma of every type is rampant. In China, a research study conducted by Li and associates revealed that some health professionals harbored a more negative bias against AIDS patients than against hepatitis B patients.[311] The bias was underscored and reinforced by fear of contagion.

The Perfect Prescription

In Africa, where male dominance still abounds, untold stigma and ostracism against people living with AIDS is still widely prevalent, making it difficult for the patients, particularly women, to seek treatment and counseling services for fear of being identified. In South Africa, "HIV-positive persons are typically blamed for, or seen to be deserving of their status; they may be thought of as cursed or victims of witchcraft," (Forsyth et al. 2008).[312] Sometimes, these individuals are abandoned by their spouses or relatives.

Csete claims that, in some societies, individuals who are HIV-positive are denied entry into institutions of higher learning such as universities.[313] They are also forbidden to marry. Sometimes they are quarantined in prisons. Other times they are denied jobs and housing. Unfortunately, stigma makes the battle against AIDS difficult because it promotes secrecy and reluctance to disclose HIV statuses. People living with HIV/AIDS in these communities do not seek healthcare services or related resources due to fear of being discovered. Where stigma against HIV/AIDS prevails, open discussions about the disease are suppressed. This drives the disease underground, making it a clandestine and mysterious phenomenon. Where this state of affairs is prevalent, health professionals find it difficult to implement effective interventions.

HIV/AIDS is leaving, in its trail, millions of orphans, particularly in Africa. For example, Botswana has the second-highest rate of infection with HIV in the world after Swaziland.[314] Statistics indicate that one in three adults in the nation is infected with the disease. Approximately 12% of the children in Botswana have been orphaned by AIDS. According to USAID, about 16% of the population between the age of 15 and 49 in Zambia is HIV positive. Approximately two in five women living in urban areas aged 25-39 are HIV positive, and about 20,000 infants get infected with HIV annually.[315] USAID further reported that in the year 2007, there were 801,000 orphans in Zambia.

The United Nations Children's Fund (UNICEF) and UNAIDS have a lot to say about the devastation caused by AIDS around the world in their report. The report claimed that sub-Saharan Africa had 15 million children under the age of 18 who had lost at least one parent to AIDS and that by the end of the decade, there would be about 25 million children who will have been orphaned by AIDS.[316] In the United States, Drs. McMillen and Stern claim that "In America more children lose a parent to AIDS than to motor vehicle accidents" (McMillen & Stern, 2000).[317] In addition to losing their parents, some of these children have to deal with the harsh realities of stigma. Cruel cases of senseless stigma against AIDS orphans have been reported around the world.

In November of 2001, the United Nations General Assembly asked the Secretary-General to conduct research on violence against children.[318] The findings of this study were to be used to expose the extent of the problem of violence and to identify safeguards that would help ensure global protection of the children from violence. Because of its prevalence in some countries, stigma associated with HIV/AIDS is often referred to as the "the third epidemic" after HIV and AIDS.

The findings of the United Nations General Assembly research study revealed that often orphans whose parents died of AIDS were discriminated against in the homes of their guardians particularly in some African countries. In Uganda, orphans suffered discrimination both at home and at school. Some teachers tended to mistreat orphans whose parents had died of AIDS. There were reports of orphans being slapped and caned. Although hitting and caning children as punishment was, to a certain extent, culturally acceptable, the physical treatment of the orphans was described to be more violent and frequent than was acceptable, usually prompted by guardians' anger about having to care for extra children with meager resources.

The Perfect Prescription

The report from the Congressional Research Service reveals the findings of a survey conducted in India where 36% of the participants felt that people who were HIV-positive ought to kill themselves.[319] Another 34% said they would never associate with an individual who was HIV positive. To further highlight the stigma existing in this country, a story is recounted in the Congressional Research Service report about two HIV-positive orphans who were blocked every time they wanted to attend school for a period of two years. It was not until the children and their grandfather decided to protest in front of government offices that one school accepted them. However, the parents of the 100 students who were already enrolled in that school decided to withdraw them for fear that they would be infected with HIV by the two children. Finally, the government decided to hire a private tutor for the two orphans to teach them at home.

The same Congressional Research Service report claims that in Tobago and Trinidad some HIV positive children were also barred from attending school for about six months. Fortunately, one school decided to accept them. HIV/AIDS is our problem, each one of us. Although HIV is 100% preventable, any one of us can contract it. All it takes is a single mistake by a sexual partner or a single moment of contact with infected body fluids through a paper cut or a blood transfusion. Furthermore, people who are HIV negative can still suffer from the consequences of this dreadful disease by losing a loved one. We are all part of the human family, and the pain inflicted on one person touches each one of us in one way or another.

The agricultural industry, which is the bedrock of the agrarian economy for most developing nations, has been severely impaired by the HIV/AIDS pandemic, which has drastically reduced the workforce necessary to till the land resulting in what Mason and colleagues term as the "new variant famine."[320] This "new variant famine" is the negative outcome of the interactions between the effects of the HIV/AIDS pandemic and drought.[321]

HIV/AIDS has also depleted the current and future intellectual capital of the countries where it is terribly endemic; crippling innovation and economic progress, and undoing whatever development had taken place before the pandemic. Another negative impact caused by the scourge of HIV/AIDS is at microeconomic level where individual households have had to deal with numerous healthcare needs and funeral expenses of those who contracted HIV/AIDS in their families. Family trauma caused by these expenses is intensified by stigma and hostility from healthcare providers, neighbors, friends, and even some family members. Industries have also suffered terribly due to loss of productivity and growth associated with staff illnesses, deaths, and funerals. Industries have also had to pay higher insurance premiums.

The AIDS orphans living in societies replete with stigma have often exhibited low academic performance mainly because of being preoccupied with their own HIV-positive status as well as the loss of their parents. When these feelings are intensified by ostracism, the burden becomes too heavy for their young minds to continue focusing on school, particularly if they have no proper support from their guardians.

Further report from the Congressional Research Services claims that in Botswana, where the government has undertaken to provide support for the orphans, some caretakers are utilizing government orphan packages for personal gain while providing minimal care for the orphans. Some female orphans have reported terrible incidents of sexual abuse from people who are supposed to be their caretakers in their new homes.

Carol Bellamy, executive director of UNICEF, claims that although HIV/AIDS is a disease that is 100% preventable, it has become the leading cause of death in Africa and the fourth leading cause of death around the world. But the fight against HIV/AIDS starts at individual level. The sexual decisions taken at individual levels are critical in the war against HIV/AIDS.

In fact, they are more important than any government or community intervention program. People who are infected with HIV should be encouraged to understand that they have the power to protect other individuals from contracting the disease by disclosing their HIV status to their potential sexual partner. Knowing one's HIV status provides an opportunity to ensure that it is not spread to other people. HIV-positive individuals have the power to get involved in the process of stopping the spread of HIV. Those who are HIV negative should know how the disease is transmitted from one person to another and avoid taking risky behavioral choices to reduce their susceptibility to infection.

Currently, health professionals are forging various strategies to stem the spread of HIV, including mutual faithfulness to sexual partners, abstinence, and avoidance of sexual promiscuity, which is an echo of Scriptural counsel cautioning us against engaging in indiscriminate sexual unions. HIV/AIDS is also challenging the church worldwide to live what it preaches. Christians are being challenged to remember that since the fall of man, each human being has an ongoing struggle with one form of vice or another. This is why we need to exercise compassion toward each other.

The AIDS pandemic provides opportunities for the individual Christian and the church as a whole to exemplify the grace and love of God in its truest form by reaching out to alleviate HIV/AIDS-induced suffering. Some individuals, churches, and organizations are already working tirelessly to bring needed medication and other resources to areas where AIDS is endemic around the world. But the battle against HIV/AIDS is intense and a more concerted effort is required to stem its spread by teaching susceptible individuals and communities some health-enhancing principles, particularly those stipulated in Scripture.

Sexual socialization can been characterized by misinformation. This misinformation can easily corrupt the beauty of sexuality through misuse, abuse, fear and exploitation. The Bible has counsel and guidelines concerning our sexuality, how and when we should express this sexuality. God's ideal for us is to have monogamous relationships guarded by mutual faithfulness and fidelity toward each other: "You shall not commit adultery," (Exodus 20:14). Since 75% of HIV infection occurs via sexual intercourse, which means that a violation of the counsel concerning our sexuality has taken place. For example, some people may contract HIV through extra marital sexual relationships or through sex with strangers or rape or incest or through polygamous marriages with multiple sexual partners. All these situations depict the occurrence of a sexual anomaly, which endangered the health of the individuals involved. However, this scenario does not warrant placing blame on anyone. Rather, it serves to highlight the need for safe sex education in this area from both a health and biblical perspective. This is the reason why churches, public health professionals and other allied health professionals are making a concerted effort to conduct educational campaigns in various parts of the world to stem the spread of HIV. One of their main approaches is mutual faithfulness to sexual partners, abstinence, and avoidance of sexual promiscuity. In Matthew 15:19 the Bible says "For out of the heart come evil thoughts, murder, adultery, fornication, theft, false witness, slander." In Colossians 3:5 the Bible further says "Put to death therefore what is earthly in you: fornication, impurity, passion, evil desire, and covetousness, which is idolatry." Pointing people to scriptural and health counsel can help them make wise choices about their sexual conduct and reduce the spread of HIV.

Chapter 19

Child Sex Trafficking

See that you do not despise one of these little ones; for I tell you that in heaven their angels always behold the face of my Father who is in heaven.

(Matthew 18:10)

Since the Declaration of the Rights of the Child that was adopted in 1924 by the League of Nations stipulating the responsibility mankind has to give the best to every child, many efforts have been made at community, national, and international levels to protect the rights and interests of children.

For example, the special rights of the child were articulated in the Universal Declaration of Human Rights in 1948 when it was declared that "Motherhood and Childhood are entitled to special care and assistance" (Universal Declaration of Human Rights, n.d.).[322] The Declaration of the Rights of the Child, 1959 and the Convention of the Rights of the Child, 1989 of the United Nations, endorsed by most countries, have legal standards that grant social, health, economic, and cultural rights to children. Other legal instruments attempting to uphold the rights of children include the International Covenant on Civil and Political Rights and the Covenant of Economic, Social and Cultural Rights, 1966. The most recent is the comprehensive Children's Act, 2004. All these laws and Acts were instituted to make the life of a child much easier worldwide.

Children are the supreme and prized assets of every nation. They are one of humanity's greatest gifts. Although they are a vulnerable population group that relies on adults for their wellbeing, children are an indispensable human resource necessary for progress and survival of every nation.[323] United Nations Children's Fund (UNICEF) and other related organizations urge governments, worldwide, to ensure that their policies and efforts to serve the health and general wellbeing of children are continuous and consistent.

Unfortunately, children are sometimes subjected to crimes perpetrated by the very adults who should be protecting them. Some of these crimes include child trafficking and prostitution. Sexual promiscuity has become so prevalent that some individuals have resorted to taking advantage of children living in abject poverty by subjecting them to prostitution as a means of earning a livelihood. What constitutes the difference between child sex trafficking or prostitution and child molestation and incest is that child sex trafficking is perpetrated for commercial exploitation, while child molestation, which is an informal synonym for child sexual abuse, takes place when a child or a young person is pressurized or coerced or manipulated into participating in any form of sexual activity with an adult individual.[324] The sexual activity can include touching the young person's genitals, breasts, or having sexual intercourse.

The year 2009 witnessed the launching of a Training Manual to aide advocates for abolition of child trafficking for labor, sexual, and other forms of exploitation. The manual was compiled by the International Labor Organization, UNICEF and Global Initiative to Fight Human Trafficking (UN.GIFT).[325] This manual highlights the needs of governments and international agencies, non-governmental organizations (NGOs), and other similar organizations in responding to this complex human tragedy. According to UNICEF, sex is a highly personal, sensitive, and private matter. Usually people refrain from discussing it, let alone openly confronting an individual who may be suspected of sexually unbecoming behavior. The hesitancy places the victim in a more difficult situation and intensifies vulnerability, particularly if it is a child.

Child sex trafficking is as varied and diverse as the people who practice it. It can exist at international, national, regional, and inter-regional levels.[326] Children's psychological as well as other needs such as shelter and food are dependent upon the nature of their relationship with adults taking care of them. Therefore, acts of child trafficking and sexual prostitution by adults betray the trust children place in their parents and guardians and adults in general. Because of its criminal nature, sexual trafficking of children or any other population group is often a clandestine, sensitive practice that constantly changes its strategies, making it difficult to detect or address. In some societies, myths that include beliefs that HIV/AIDS can be cured by having sex with a virgin place female children at greater risk for sexual coercion and exploitation than their male counterparts.

Technological achievements such as the Internet, which are meant to enrich and enhance communication and to facilitate valuable information exchange at interpersonal and international levels, are sometimes abused and used as tools to encourage activities such as child pornography and child prostitution. In Mekong, South Asia, statistics indicate that 30% to 35% of sex workers are children aged between 12 and 17.[327] Dr. Sadig Rasheed, Regional Director of UNICEF was quoted by BBC News in 2004 as saying that the "trade in…children for sex is spiraling out of control in South Asia" (BBC News, 2004).[328]

In a special report on trafficking of persons that was published in the 2006 *International Journal of Gynecology and*

Obstetrics, Huda, then Special Rapporteur on Trafficking in Persons at the United Nations Office of the High Commission for Human Rights, revealed to us that "the continued existence of caste systems in some parts of Asia and other expressions of discrimination based on race, ethnicity, social origin or gender, exacerbates trafficking, as some people are assumed to be more exploitable and less worthy of protection than others" (Huda, 2006).[329]

In Lithuania, about 20-50% of prostitutes are reported to be minors.[330] Sometimes, children aged 10-12 are used to make pornographic movies. Others work as prostitutes. The report by UNICEF indicates that over one million children enter the sex trade worldwide each year.[331] Some of these children are under the age 10. In the last couple of decades, over 30 million children have lost their childhood due to sexual exploitation. Huda claims that Asia is one of the most vulnerable regions for this kind of trade due to a number of factors.

Often causal factors of child sex trafficking are poverty and illiteracy. Where these two prevail, job prospects are dreadfully bleak and unemployment is extremely high. This kind of situation can force people to resort to reprehensible practices such as child sex trafficking and exploitation in order to make a living. Sometimes children are sold as sex workers to make a living for their parents or guardians or whoever the predator is. Other times they are used to bring sexual pleasure even among members of their own families.

For example, in a 2001 UNICEF Report entitled *Profiting from Abuse,* a little girl called Marife from the Philippines revealed how she trembled at the sight of her stepfather during a confrontation inside a courtroom where she was required to testify against him for sexually abusing her.[332] Marife who had often remained at home with her unemployed stepfather, gave a moving account of how she was repeatedly raped by him and how he later sold her as a sex slave. In the Philippines, where a major government land development program has been launched, many people in rural areas are being displaced in order to make room for government projects. Young girls are fleeing to cities and other neighboring countries to look for employment where they sometimes end up in the hands of sexual predators. Approximately 40% of sex workers in cities in the Philippines are young girls who left their homes in rural areas.

A quantitative study undertaken by the United Nations Development Programme (UNDP) Regional HIV and Development Programme in conjunction with the Harvard School of Public Health explored the subject of sex trafficking and STD/ HIV infection in Southeast Asia.[333] The findings revealed that sex trafficking was highly associated with a high risk of STDs/HIV infection among the victims. Predators often hide their victims in deplorable and unsanitary locations where they are unlikely to be discovered. This increases not only their risk of contracting STD/HIV infection but other diseases as well. In addition, the above study found out that most sex trafficking victims were also subjected to physical and sexual abuse and ill-treatment in the context of their sex work. The study highlighted the high cost of sex trafficking on the victim in terms of loss of personal dignity, human rights, health, and general well-being. But what was most disconcerting about the findings of the study was that sex trafficking was found to be a major component of the persistence of the HIV pandemic, not only in Asia, but in most other societies where sex trafficking is endemic.

In post-war Bosnia-Herzegovina, the squalid conditions most people were living in presented a climate that ultimately fostered sex trafficking practices. Commenting on these conditions, a Fulbright scholar named Rosga, who was given the task of overseeing researchers on the study of post-war child trafficking in Bosnia and Herzegovina, said: "People often think that all child sex traffickers kidnap their victims, but in many cases the children end up funneled into the system by their own families because of extreme poverty. Very often it's not organized criminals but close relatives or family friends who encourage girls in poverty-stricken families to seek work abroad as an "au pair or waitress."[334] Nicole Lindstrom, who has conducted research in sex trafficking in the Balkans, claims that, "Traffickers capitalize on permeable borders, political and military instability, economic dislocation, and rampant corruption to create efficient supply chains to satisfy the lucrative market for sex workers in Western Europe and the Balkans."[335]

In Kenya, recurrent drought has forced many rural residents to relocate to cities in the hope of eking out a living. Tragically, in some cases, "parents have resorted to sending their young daughters into towns to trade their bodies for money to feed their families…Because food reserves have run out and mothers can no longer afford to feed their children, many decide that the only way out is to 'go to the street'" (IRIN Humanitarian News and Analysis, 2012).[336] This exposes these children to a plethora of deadly communicable diseases.

Reporting on child trafficking practices in Zambia, the United States State Department Trafficking in Persons Report reveals that:

> Zambia is a source, transit, and destination country for women and children trafficked for the purposes of forced labor and sexual exploitation. Child victims, primarily trafficked within the country for labor and sexual exploitation, tend to be female, adolescent, and orphaned. In exchange for money or gifts, relatives or acquaintances often facilitate the trafficking of a child to an urban center for prostitution… Traffickers most often operate through ad hoc, flexible networks of relatives, truck drivers, business people, cross-border traders, and religious leaders.
>
> (United States Department of State Publication 11407 Office of the Under Secretary for Democracy and Global Affairs Bureau of Public Affairs, 2007)[337]

The problem of child trafficking in Zambia is compounded by the porous nature of the country's borders because of her geographical location. Another compounding factor for child trafficking in Zambia is the lax nature of the country's immigration laws. Individuals working with organized human sex traffickers lure Zambian girls and women using the age old bait of false marriage and job offers.

Commenting about the child trafficking activities in Asia, the same United States State Department Trafficking in Persons Report above also states that:

> Japan is one of several destinations and transit countries to which men, women, and children are trafficked for the purposes of forced labor and commercial sexual exploitation. Women and children from East Asia, Southeast Asia, Eastern Europe, Russia, South America, and Latin America are trafficked to Japan for commercial sexual exploitation and male and female migrant workers from China, Indonesia, the Philippines, Vietnam, and other Asian countries are sometimes subject to conditions of forced labor.
>
> (United States Department of State Publication 11407 Office of the Under Secretary for Democracy and Global Affairs Bureau of Public Affairs, 2007)

A significant number of Japanese girls and women have also been identified to be victims of sexual trafficking activities. Sometimes the traffickers use debt to force their victims into prostitution. The girls who enter the sex trade voluntarily soon become disillusioned when they find themselves victims of involuntary indentured servitude. Trafficking in Japan is exacerbated by the reluctance of the Japanese government to comply with standards for eradicating trafficking. Although prosecution of sex trafficking offenders has increased in Japan, the convicted perpetrators are merely given suspended sentences most of the time.

Other factors encouraging sex trafficking around the world include the expansion of the tourism industry, gender discrimination, governments' lax, and ambiguous laws about the rights of the citizenry; expansion of the sexual entertainment industry; and the profit margins attached to this practice. For example, in Sri Lanka, like in most other parts of the world, it is not unusual for foreign pedophiles to woe local young beach boys into sexual practices using money and promises of a lucrative lifestyle.

War caused by political upheavals and other factors is another factor that encourages child sex trafficking. Young girls fleeing regions of conflict inadvertently end up being sex slaves in their destinations. Natural disasters such as the Asian tsunami of 2004 and the Haitian earthquake of 2010 can also leave thousands of young children susceptible to sex abuse and trafficking.

Yet another palpable risk factor for child sex trafficking, particularly against girls, is gender discrimination and subordination in societies that are primarily patriarchal in their set up.[338] Where these gender-based power differentials are endemic, women do not have equal access to education as their male counterparts, rendering them more dependent on their male counterparts for survival. This makes them vulnerable to physical and sexual violence and exploitation. Male control over the sexuality and other areas of women's lives is an allowable and acceptable cultural norm in such societies. Gender-based power differentials often compromise the health, dignity security, and autonomy of their victims. Such practices perpetrate a myriad of violations against women that include sexual abuse of female children, rape, sexual assault, and harassment as well as sex trafficking, particularly of female children.[339]

Economies that are heavily reliant on tourism usually develop a stance that tolerates sex markets. These economies establish, promote, and advertise adults-only holiday resorts, which motivates tourists to make demands to indulge in any type of sexual pleasure they want.³⁴⁰ Such economies that encourage a culture of tolerance for explicit and graphic sexual behavior and images create an environment conducive for commercial sex, culminating into sexual exploitation of vulnerable populations groups. Where society glamorizes explicit sexual practices as part of entertainment, moral barriers to commercial sex are often removed, and sex trafficking increases without regard for the rights or needs of the victims. Legalized prostitution with special offers for tourists seeking special sexual pleasures only serves to increase the demand for commercial sexual services and sexual workers.

The United Nations Children's Fund asserts that each government owes it to itself to ensure that its children enjoy all their human rights. Therefore, governments and local non-governmental agencies must make efforts to urge policy makers to criminalize all forms of child sex trafficking and exploitation and enforce these laws with vigilance. For example, in South Africa, some nongovernmental organizations (NGOs) such as the International Campaign Against Child Trafficking and Molo Songololo have arisen to try and stem child sex trafficking. Legislation such as the Sexual Offenses Act also went into effect in 2007 in South Africa to combat sexual crimes against children such as child sex trafficking and exploitation.³⁴¹ Furthermore, as at the time of writing this book, the Republic of South Africa is in the process of creating a bill called the Prevention and Combating of Trafficking in Persons Bill focused on curtailing and eradicating human and child trafficking in the country.

In an effort to combat child sex trafficking, the United States and Argentina enforced the Trafficking in Persons Protocol in 2007.³⁴² The United States also enacted a federal law in 2000 called the Trafficking Victims Protection Act (TVPA).³⁴³ This law has severe penalties for human traffickers of any type. Victims of trafficking who are not citizens of the United States can receive the same benefits through TVPA as refugees, which allow them to become temporary residents of the United States.

Protection and assistance for victims of human trafficking include granting them provision for housing, education, healthcare services, and job training, and other federally funded services. This is an effort to allow these individuals to start rebuilding their lives afresh. The victims under TVPA are also eligible for the Witness Protection Program. However, in spite of having passed specific and aggressive anti human trafficking laws, the United States is still reported to be:

> A destination country for thousands of men, women, and children trafficked largely from Mexico and East Asia, as well as countries in South Asia, Central America, Africa, and Europe, for the purposes of sexual and labor exploitation. Three-quarters of all foreign adult victims identified during the Fiscal Year (FY) 2008 were victims of trafficking for forced labor. Some trafficking victims, responding to fraudulent offers of employment in the United States, migrate willingly—legally and illegally—and are subsequently subjected to conditions of involuntary servitude or debt bondage at work sites or in commercial sex. An unknown number of American citizens and legal residents are trafficked within the country, primarily for sexual servitude.
>
> (U.S. Department of State, 2009)[344]

Nevertheless, the United States government continues to enforce the laws and to design strategies aimed at eradicating human trafficking of any type. Millions of dollars are being allocated to programs being run by several federal agencies working tirelessly to enhance anti-human trafficking law enforcement efforts and to increase public awareness of the evils of all forms of human trafficking particularly child sex trafficking and its related health problems.

The Perfect Prescription

Child sex trafficking is a serious public health issue that has far-reaching consequences.[345] Victims of child sex trafficking undergo horrendous suffering and brutality, resulting in serious physical and psychological trauma. Apart from the risk of being infected with sexually transmitted diseases, children who are victims of sex trafficking sustain vaginal and anal tearings. They might also suffer other negative outcomes such as sterility, menstrual problems, and hepatitis. Unintended pregnancies are another consequence of sex trafficking. Sometimes pregnant victims of sex traffickers are forced to undergo coerced and dangerous abortions, which expose them to a myriad of complications because the procedures are often conducted in nonclinical settings without proper medical services or resources. The traumatic experiences that sex trafficking victims are subjected to often trigger psychological problems, which include recurrent nightmares, insomnia, and suicidal tendencies as well as drugs and alcohol addictions. People who frequent brothels owned by sex traffickers are in danger of contracting communicable diseases and becoming transmitters themselves.

Individuals who are victims of child sex trafficking are placed in environments that render them at high risk for HIV/STDs infections. Unfortunately, these environments hinder them from accessing any STDs/ HIV/AIDS prevention programs or other restorative programs because, in order to have access to these programs, they would need proof of eligibility, which these individuals might not have. For example, they may be asked to produce proof of their residential address, birth certificate, and a social security card or any other government identification.

Sex trafficking of vulnerable population groups is not a new phenomenon. Tragically, it has been going on for centuries in different parts of the world mainly as a covert or clandestine business. Jonathan Martens, Maciej 'Mac' Pieczkowski and Bernadette van Vuuren-Smyth of the International Organization for Migration (IOM) Regional Office for Southern Africa present the following most heartwrenching account of the senseless criminal sex trafficking of an African young lady that took place early in 19th century South Africa.

> Saartjie Baartman was...a servant on a farm near Cape Town...when a visiting English surgeon, Dr. William Dunlop, promised her fame, fortune, and freedom in a far away land. Baartman readily accepted his offer, and traveled with him to London by ship in 1810. What awaited her in London was neither fame nor fortune nor freedom... Fascinated by the physical features for the people of the Cape, Dunlop chose to exhibit her in the nude in front of large crowds of Londoners, who paid one shilling each to gawk at the "Hottentot Venus" from Africa. When she died...only six years after leaving Cape Town, her body was dissected, her skeleton was removed, and her brain and genitals were pickled and displayed as curiosities in the *Musee de l'Homme* in Paris for the next 160 years.
>
> (Martens, Pieczkowski & van Vuuren-Smyth, 2003)[346]

Later, this story caught the attention of then President of South Africa, Nelson Mandela, who made an official request to have Saartjie Baartman's remains brought back home to South Africa in 1994 for a decent burial among her own people. She had finally found her resting place.

Sex trafficking has continued to thrive over the centuries not only in Africa but all over the world. Recruitment of young people for sexual exploitation by deception continues to plague humanity. Martens and associates further recount the following modern story about child sex trafficking involving African girls:

> Two girls, 16, reported being held up at gunpoint by two white men in Maseru. They were taken to a house somewhere in Qua- Qua. Another two white men were waiting at the house. The men forced the girls to perform oral sex and drink their urine. One girl vomited and was

The Perfect Prescription

terribly beaten. The two girls were kept captive in the house for three days and given only hard bread and milk as food. During the day the two girls were allowed to sleep—during the night they were sexually abused.

(Martens, Piezckowski & van Vuuren, 2003)

The CNN hero for 2010, Anuradha Koirala, started her charity work of rescuing women and girls from sex traffickers in 1993. Millions of female children are sold into sex slavery in India and elsewhere every year as a source of livelihood for the perpetrators. Since then, Koirala has rescued over 12,000 children and women through her organization called Maiti Nepal. She provides shelter for the women and children she rescues. The shelter becomes a place where healing from their traumatic experiences takes place. It is also a place that provides the girls with an opportunity to go to school and develop the skills necessary for accessing gainful employment.

For those who are tested HIV positive when they are rescued, Maiti Nepal provides them with love and dignity and helps them have access to available treatment and resources. Being sold into sex slavery is a girl and woman's worst nightmare, according to Koirala. Because she understands this, she has devoted her life to rescuing as many girls as possible from the nightmare of human and sex trafficking. Sometimes she boldly conducts raids and patrols the India-Nepal border to save the girls from sexual predators. Human and sex traffickers in this area abduct girls who may be as young as 13 and force them to have sex with a minimum of 25 men in a day. If they resist, they are brutally beaten into submission. When Koirala rescues the children, they are often in a terrible shape. Some of them often sustain broken limbs from beatings by their captors.

In her acceptance speech as CNN hero for the year 2010, Koirala said, "We have to end this heinous crime. Please join hands with me to end this crime…Please try to respect the youth. They are the ones who are going to build the next generation"

(Cable News Network, 2012).³⁴⁷ The following is an account of the experience of one of the girls Koirala rescued and adopted. Her name is Geeta. Geeta was only nine years old when she was abducted. She was forced to wear makeup in order to attract male customers. She was also forced to stay awake until 2 a.m., having sex with as many as 60 men in one day:

> I used to be really sad and frustrated with what was happening in my life, she said. The daughter of Nepalese peasant farmers, Geeta—now 26—had been sold to a brothel in India by a member of her extended family. The family member had duped Geeta's visually impaired mother into believing her daughter would get work at a clothing company in Nepal. "The brothel where I was… there [were] many customers coming in every day. The owner used to verbally abuse us, and if we didn't comply, [she] would start beating us with wires, rods and hot spoons."
>
> (Cable News Network, 2012)

It was not until Geeta was 14 that a police officer rescued her and brought her to a safe house compound run by Anuradha Koirala.

God's attitude toward children is that of benevolence. One of the myriad ways he blesses humanity is by giving us children to nurture them, not to destroy them. Children are a heritage from the Lord, which means they are bestowed by him. They are evidence of his favor toward us. Psalm 127: 3-5 tells us that "Lo, sons are a heritage from the LORD, the fruit of the womb a reward. Like arrows in the hand of a warrior are the sons of one's youth. Happy is the man who has his quiver full of them! He shall not be put to shame when he speaks with his enemies in the gate."

Jesus said this about children: "But when Jesus saw it he was indignant, and said to them, "Let the children come to me, do not hinder them; for to such belongs the kingdom of God." (Mark

10:14). Again in Matthew 18:10, He said, "See that you do not despise one of these little ones; for I tell you that in heaven their angels always behold the face of my Father who is in heaven." Jesus also condemned any action aimed at hurting children: "Whoever receives one such child in my name receives me; but whoever causes one of these little ones who believe in me to sin, it would be better for him to have a great millstone fastened round his neck and to be drowned in the depth of the sea" (Matthew 18: 5-6). In Jesus' day, children were not only powerless, they were also vulnerable and without the rights they have in modern day. Jesus' righteous indignation against injustice to children should be our indignation too.

It is true that children do not come without sacrifice on the part of the parents. They are a huge responsibility, but the blessing of having them outweighs the rigors of nurturing them and raising them. When they are young, children can bring laughter and joy in the home, which can outweigh the difficulty of caring for them. A child is priceless in that it is irreplaceable. As children grow in the home, they teach parents numerous lessons in love, trust, maturity, patience, forgiveness, and many others. As they become older, children begin to be responsible for age-specific household responsibilities, and when the parents are old, feeble, and unable to do certain tasks for themselves, older children can be a big help in many ways.

The presence of children in our lives can often constitute the primary reason for continuing to live. As our children build their own families and expand their horizons, our own influence in the world expands too. What a blessing that is if the influence enhances the well-being of mankind. The power to procreate is one of the most sublime privileges given to mankind and should be responsibly undertaken. The Bible likens God to a parent. This certainly elevates the call to parenthood. God's love, actions, and attitude toward his children provide us with a divine template for our own roles as parents. He protects his children, he helps them, and comforts them when they need it (see John 14:26; Isaiah 40:11). He accepts each one of us as individuals and loves us dearly (Jeremiah 1:5; Matthew 7:9-11; Ps. 139:13-16). He guides us in the best direction in life and respects our choices (Deuteronomy 30:19-20).

He will not arm-twist us into obedience because coerced obedience is worthless to him. He, as a responsible parent, not only instructs his children, but disciplines them and empowers them so that they can realize their unique potential (Exodus 17:1-7; Ps. 4:8; Matthew 6:25-34; John 14: 12-13). God cannot and will not sell any of his children for any reason. In fact, he would rather give all he has than see them enslaved or exploited (John 3:16). Therefore, parents and guardians should emulate his benevolence and provide love and security for their children. No child deserves to be sold into child sex or human trafficking.

Parents must protect their children from sex traffickers and other predators. In Leviticus 19:29, Scripture commands parents not to engage their children into prostitution: "Do not profane your daughter by making her a harlot, lest the land fall into harlotry and the land become full of wickedness." All forms of sex trafficking harm and dehumanize the victim.[348] They are also a source of reproach to the communities where they are practiced. The vulnerability of children increases the younger they are and the more dependent they are upon adults for protection and sustenance. The individual who sells them into prostitution makes them victims of every vile sexual act men would like to do to them. A degraded human being has very low self-esteem and this condition can spiral into a host of health problems. When they grow to be adults, children subjected to such violations often have a high propensity toward criminal behavior and violent crime.

The law given by the Lord God against prostituting children was intended to protect the children from these negative outcomes. It was also meant to protect their spiritual wellbeing. Furthermore, the law was a means of protecting the general public because if a prostitute contracted an STD, she would most certainly spread it to her clients who would, in turn, spread it to their next sexual partners and wives, causing an epidemic that could have been prevented by responsible behavior.

According to UNICEF, one way to protect children from traffickers is to ensure that they are given quality care and protection against all forms abuse as:

> Abuse is a contributing factor or even a direct cause of the child being trafficked. Analysis finds that the factors that heighten vulnerability to trafficking are the same as those that increase vulnerability to other forms of violence, abuse and exploitation."[349]

Another method to prevent child trafficking involves distribution of age-appropriate information to children by parents and guardians regarding child trafficking; the tricks and methods child traffickers use to lure children and the suffering the children who are trafficked undergo. Parents and guardians and teachers can arm children with skills that can help them avoid being trafficked. For example, they should avoid talking to strangers and wandering off alone.

Chapter 20

Health and Diet

So, whether you eat or drink, or whatever you do, do all to the glory of God.

(1 Corinthians 10:3)

Our first encounter with Scriptural commandments about food is in the book of Genesis in which we read about God instructing Adam and Eve to eat a vegetarian diet: "And God said, 'Behold, I have given you every plant yielding seed which is upon the face of all the earth, and every tree with seed in its fruit; you shall have them for food'" (Genesis 1:29).

Then after the flood meat was added to the diet of mankind: "Every moving thing that lives shall be food for you; and as I gave you the green plants, I give you everything. Only you shall not eat flesh with its life, that is, its blood" (Genesis 9:3, 4). Later in Leviticus 11 and Deuteronomy 14, more detailed instructions and laws about food types and preparations were added and given to the young nation of Israel just coming out of Egyptian bondage. Meat sources were restricted to only those animals that ruminate or chew the cud for food and have cloven or split hooves. Specific names of the animals whose meat was to be used for food were given. Animals whose flesh was forbidden for food were also specifically mentioned. Their meat, their milk, and eggs were also forbidden as food. Birds that were allowed to be sources of meat excluded scavengers and birds of prey. Fish that was allowed for food had to have scales and fins. The rest were forbidden.

The late Dr. David I. Macht (a pharmacologist, doctor of Hebrew Literature, Johns Hopkins medical researcher, and an experimental biologist who was a pioneer of the methods that are currently being used in measuring pharmacological toxicity) embarked on a landmark research study titled *An Experimental Pharmacological Appreciation of Leviticus XI and Deuteronomy XIV*.[350] The objective of Macht's experiment was to test how much adding and excluding a certain percentage of muscle juices and skeletal extracts from fresh meats of the species of clean and unclean animals, birds and fish (as stipulated in Leviticus 11 and Deuteronomy 14) to plant solutions containing the necessary salts and ions for plant growth would affect the growth of the roots of plants.

Macht used the seedlings of *Lupinus albus* for his research study. *Lupinus albus* is a white-flowered Eurasian herb usually cultivated for forage erosion control. Macht used three sets of seedlings: one set was grown in solutions that were mixed with muscle juices and skeletal extracts from animals that were biblically classified as unclean, the second set was grown in solutions mixed with muscle juices and skeletal extracts from animals biblically classified as clean animals, the third set of seedlings was grown in a saline solution that had no animal muscle juices or skeletal extracts. This third set was the control set of seedlings.

To measure the toxicity of the muscle juices and skeletal extracts used in the experiment, Macht utilized a phyto-toxic index which is a ratio given in percentages. Macht used it to measure the toxicity of the juices and extracts in the solutions and their effects on the growing seedlings. The phyto-toxic index also allowed him to compare the growth rate of the roots of all the three sets of the seedlings.

The results of this experiment demonstrated that the solutions that had muscle juices and skeletal muscle extracts from clean animals, birds and fish, were non-toxic. The growth of the roots of the seedlings in these solutions was not interrupted nor was it adversely affected by adding the juices from clean animals. For example, the seedlings that grew in the muscle juices and skeletal extracts of animals that were biblically classified as clean such as sheep grew 94% as often as the seedling in the control group. The seedlings growing in extracts from oxen grew 91% as often as the control seedlings.

Conversely, the extracts from animals, birds, and fish that were biblically classified as unclean were found to be significantly toxic for root growth when added to the plant solutions. The growth of the roots was found to be significantly inhibited in these solutions. For example, seedlings in pig juice extracts grew only 54% as often as those in the control group and those growing in camel and hamster extracts grew 41% and 46%, respectively. The seedlings growing in horse juice extracts grew 39%. The growth rate of the seedlings in solutions with juices and extracts of clean birds such as pigeons and quails was 93% and 89%, respectively.

Those seedlings that were growing in solutions with juices and extracts from unclean birds such as red tail hawk and crow demonstrated a growth rate of 36% and 46%, respectively. The seedlings growing in juices of fish with scales and fins classified as clean such as herring, pike and shad had a growth rate of 100%, 98% and 100%, respectively. Seedlings growing in extracts of fish listed as unclean such as catfish, puffer and toadfish grew at the rate of 48%, 51%, and 49%, respectively.

The findings of this experiment corroborate the biblical teaching about clean and unclean animals. If the unclean animal juices and skeletal extracts were not conducive for plant growth, it was plausible to conclude that they would also not be conducive for the growth and overall wellbeing of the human body. Therefore, the command not to eat them is appropriate as a health-promoting directive. These findings impressed Macht so much that he exclaimed "all allusions of the Book of Books, to nature, natural phenomena, and natural history, whether in the form of factual statements or in the form of metaphors, similes, parables, allegories, or other tropes are correct either literally or figuratively" (Macht, 1953).

He also added that:

> Such being the extraordinary concordance between the data of the scriptures and many of the modern and even the most recent discoveries in both the biological and physico-chemical sciences, every serious student of the Bible will, I believe, endorse the assertion of Sir Isaac Newton that "the scriptures of God are the most sublime philosophy. I find more sure remarks of authenticity in the Bible than in profane history anywhere."

(Macht, 1953)

Dr. Joe C. Guthrie Jr. conducted a study similar to that of Dr. Macht in which he tested the toxicity of the sources of protein commonly used in Louisiana diets using a research instrument similar to the one used by Macht, a phyto-toxic index.[351] The growth rate of the roots of Mung beans, *Vigra radiata*, was assessed in this experimental research study. Guthrie measured the ratio of growth of non-GMO (non-genetically modified organism) *Vigra radiata* roots growing in broths formed with water and protein from muscle tissues of an array of biblically clean and unclean animals and fish to that of roots growing in a control solution of distilled water that had no animal proteins whatsoever.

Protein sources utilized in the study included beef meats, lamb, deer, pork, chicken, redfish, speckled trout, catfish, fresh blue crab, processed blue crab, white shrimp, fresh red swamp crayfish and processed red swamp crayfish all obtained from local supermarkets and sea food markets. The broth used for testing was prepared by boiling and mixing 90ml of muscle tissue from each of the specimen in 400ml of distilled water. The specimens were tested for pH and for electrical conductivity after being cooled down. The experimental Mung beans seeds were grown in the broth solution, and the control beans were grown in a solution of distilled water without any animal protein juices.

The results of the study demonstrated that protein sources from unclean species had significantly low phyto-toxic indices percentages. The lower the percentage of the toxic index in the findings of this study, the higher the toxic level of the muscle extracts. Lower indices were associated with a poisonous effect on the roots of the seedlings. The lower the indices became, the more poisonous the effect of the solution on growth. The results revealed that protein sources from crab, shrimp and crayfish had remarkably lower phyto-toxic indices compared to those from clean species such as deer, lamb, and beef meats.

The results further revealed that the protein sources listed as clean in the biblical health laws had a significantly nourishing effect on *Vigra radiata* specimens. From the results of this study, it was concluded that a diet consisting of proteins from animals, birds, and fish that are listed as unclean in biblical health laws were harmful to the health of Louisiana residents. These results do not only echo Dr. Macht's findings, they also confirm the biblical dietary guidelines about clean and unclean animals.

Human beings have been endowed with the power of choice by their Creator God. The results of the above studies can either help us rethink our eating habits or they can be relegated to some obscure place or even the trashcan. That is how powerful our power of choice can be. However, this power of choice is not without consequences. Sometimes these consequences can be positive. Other times they can be negative. Our food choices and general dietary habits can determine our health profiles as individuals and as communities.

Our understanding of the relationship between diet and health affects our food choices and ultimately our health, to a large extent. Our nutritional habits and choices can affect the way our bodies function. If not properly handled, these choices can lead to a wide range of chronic diseases such as cardiovascular disease, cancer, osteoporosis, and dental diseases.[352]

The International Federation of Red Cross and Red Crescent Societies claims that there is a global burden of double malnutrition currently threatening humanity.[353] The main focus of nutritionists working in developing nations that have scarce food resources and low income is the scourge of hunger and undernourishment. At the same time and probably not receiving as much attention as low-income nations are those nations that have a significant percentage of diabetes, hypertension and heart problems due to high obesity levels due mostly to dietary excesses.

Sometimes these two can co-exist in the same nation due to income and power differentials. Nevertheless, both forms of malnutrition are harmful to health and well-being. The expanding global food market has resulted in a plethora of food choices, especially in affluent nations. As such, the call to making the right food choices has never been more relevant. Even when there is an abundance of food choices, health can only be enhanced if people know and eat the kind of foods that are health promoting.

Judeo-Christians believe that they did not emerge from some primordial soup but that they were deliberately created by God in his image and for his glory (Genesis 1:27; Isaiah. 43:7). They also believe that God cares deeply about each human being and has a purpose for everyone. He takes the responsibility to guide us through life by his precepts and laws. God separated the nation of ancient Israel from every other nation and designated it as his firstborn. He called Israel his 'first-born son' not his only son: "And you shall say to Pharaoh, 'Thus says the LORD, Israel is my first-born son'" (Exodus. 4:22).

Therefore, God is not Father only to Israel, but he is Father to all nations. Israel was taught moral, spiritual, dietary, and health laws as an exemplar for all other nations. Through Israel other nations would be blessed: "and by you all the families of the earth shall bless themselves" (Genesis 12:3). But Israel had to learn to live as God wanted them to live before they could qualify to be an example to other nations.

Therefore, he gave them laws to live by and to help them abound in health and to become a model worthy of emulating. The Lord God even gave them an incentive for obeying his laws: "If you will diligently hearken to the voice of the LORD your God, and do that which is right in his eyes, and give heed to his commandments and keep all his statutes, I will put none of the diseases upon you which I put upon the Egyptians; for I am the LORD, your healer" (Exodus 15:26).

When this promise was given, Israel had just been miraculously freed from slavery in Egypt, where they had been in captivity for over four centuries. Obviously they had lived in Egypt long enough to be very familiar with the kinds of diseases that plagued the Egyptian people. Modern-day technological advances have been used by scientists to identify and analyze the DNA from mummification samples of Egyptian kings to find out what kind of diseases these individuals died from.

A report by Heather Pringle appeared in the April 2011 copy of Science, the American Association for the Advancement of Science (AAAS), in which cardiologists examined 52 Egyptian mummies for atherosclerosis which can cause stroke and heart attacks.[354] Of the 52 mummies 44 of them still exhibited cardiovascular tissues, which cardiologists could easily examine. The examination of these 44 mummies revealed that 45% of them had "definite or probable hardening of the arteries." These mummies were relatively young, about 40 years old at the time of their death. In his work of the studies of Egyptian mummies, titled Studies in Palaeopathology of Egypt, Sir March Armand

Ruffer, late President of the Quarantine Council of Egypt, reported the following findings:

> At the present time there is perhaps no disease more important to Egypt than that caused by the Bilharzia haematobia. So far no evidence has been produced to show how long it has existed in this country, although medical papyri contain prescriptions against one of its most prominent symptoms—namely, haematuria. The lesions of this disease are best seen in the bladder and rectum, but unfortunately these are just the two mummified organs which 1 have not been able to obtain so far. Nevertheless, in the kidneys of two mummies of the twentieth dynasty, I have demonstrated in microscopic sections a large number of calcified eggs of Bilharzia haematobia, situated, for the most part, among the straight tubules. Although calcified, these eggs are easily recognizable and cannot be mistaken for anything else.
>
> (Ruffer, 1921)[355]

After examining the arteries of the Egyptian mummies, Ruffer reported that "There is no difficulty in recognising completely or partially calcified arteries. Even before they are placed in the softening solution, or at any rate shortly afterwards, their hard, 'osseous' structure is manifest. Arteries...are as rigid as calcified arteries of the present day" (Ruffer, 1921). Ruffer also found that smallpox was prevalent in ancient Egypt. He examined a mummy and reported that "The body was the seat of a peculiar vesicular or bulbous eruption which in form and general distribution bore a striking resemblance to that of small-pox. The portion of skin we were permitted to remove, and which forms the subject of the present note, was taken from the adductor surface of the right thigh." Jeffry Hays, in his article, Health and Health Care in Egypt, reports that:

The Perfect Prescription

In 1910, Marc Armand Ruffer, a French microbiologist, found dried eggs of the schistosomiasis worm in kidneys of two 3000-year-old mummies. Schistosomiasis remains a disease that is prevalent in Egypt today. In other mummies he found gallstones, inflamed intestines, and a spleen that had apparently been enlarged by malaria. Ruffer looked inside ancient blood vessels and found calcified spots—evidence of hardening of the arteries, surprising considering the ancient Egyptians ate a low-fat high-fiber diet with a lot of grains. Ruffer invented a solution of salts for rehydrating ancient tissues.

(Hays, 2008)[356]

Probably most of these diseases were diet related. The Egyptians did not have the dietary guidelines given to ancient Israel. Consequently, they could not have distinguished between clean and unclean animals in their diet. However, even clean animals had to be killed in a prescribed manner in ancient Israel. For example, whoever killed an animal was required to slit its throat to drain the blood out and to prevent the people from eating blood.

In modern day, even clean animals have become a source of diseases because of being mishandled. Bovine or cattle are some of the clean animals mentioned in Leviticus 11. They chew the cud and divide the hooves. However, modern industrial methods of raising these animals have changed their diet, including the way they are slaughtered.

The animals are now being fed with meat and bone meal supplements from their own species as well as other species such as pigs and sheep. Such a diet exposes the animals to diseases found in the tissues and bones of their own kind. These animals are being made into cannibals. The diseases they acquire from such diets are then transmitted to human beings, who consume the flesh of these cattle. The World Health Organization statement on Bovine Spongiform Encephalopathy (BSE) claims that "Strong evidence currently available supports the theory that the agent is composed largely, if not entirely, of a self-replicating protein, referred to as a prion. It is transmitted through the consumption of BSE-contaminated meat and bone meal supplements in cattle feed" (World Health Organization, 2012).[357]

Trichinosis, also called Trichinellosis, is another diet-related disease that is worldwide in prevalence and incidence. In 1966, trichinosis became a notifiable disease in the United States. The Trichinella parasite is often found in game, particularly meat from animals such as bear meat and pork. In the United States, the incidence and prevalence of trichinosis has become less frequent over the years although the threat of an outbreak might not have been completely eradicated.

In 1979, about 61% percent of individuals who had eaten pork sausages became ill with trichinosis in Louisiana.[358] In 1980, outbreaks were reported in Acadia parish, Louisiana, in which nine cases were identified. Another fifteen cases and one fatality occurred in Evangeline and Jefferson Davis parishes in the same year. Efforts have been made by public health professionals to educate the general public about reducing the risk of infection, and observing signs and symptoms of the disease in order to facilitate early diagnosis and timely treatment.

The symptoms of infection with *Trichinella* parasite range from being less obvious to fatal illness, but most of the infections are asymptomatic. The severity of the disease is positively proportional to the amount of larvae the individual has ingested. During the first week after infection, the patient may experience abdominal discomfort accompanied by diarrhea, nausea and vomiting. About one month later, the larvae invade the tissues of the victim, and fever, muscle pain and subungual hemorrhage may begin to occur. When the worms form themselves into cysts in the body tissues, they can remain alive for years.

The Centers for Disease Control and Prevention (CDC) have issued a warning to the general public against consuming raw and undercooked meat in order to avoid being infected with the *Trichinella* parasite.[359] The report claimed that eating even a small portion of undercooked Trichinella-*infected meat* during the cooking process can place a person at high risk for infection. Pigs raised on individual farms are more likely to ingest uncooked garbage as part of their diet compared to their commercial counterparts. As such, they are more susceptible to acquiring the Trichinella parasites. There is no specific treatment for trichinosis once the larvae have attached themselves to the muscles.

Dr. Rex Russell, author of *What the Bible Says About Healthy Living*, informs us that a sudden increase in the population of armadillos occurred a few years ago in the state of Texas and other neighboring states.[360] As a result, some individuals recommended the armadillos as an easily available good source of protein. Food experts designed special recipes that were aimed at making armadillo meat tasty. People's curiosity was aroused and armadillo feasts were held and well attended by those seeking to sample the meat. Armadillos do not chew the cud, neither are their feet split. Therefore, according to Leviticus 11 and Deuteronomy 14, they are classified as unclean and not suitable for food. Before long, several individuals in Texas who had feasted at armadillo feasts became infected with type *Mycobacterium leprae (*M. Leprosy).

Warnings about food in Scripture are not limited to clean and unclean foods. The Scriptures also warn us not to be gluttonous. Even good food should be eaten in moderation, not in excess. In Proverbs 23:19-21, the Bible has this to say about gluttony:

> "Hear, my son, and be wise, and direct your mind in the way. Be not among winebibbers, or among gluttonous eaters of meat; for the drunkard and the glutton will come to poverty, and drowsiness will clothe a man with rags."

The above Scripture gives a stern warning against gluttony in relation to food and drink, although gluttony is generally not restricted to food or drink only but to a lack of self restraint in anything. When surrounded by excess and extravagance, it usually requires godly wisdom and resolve to exercise temperance or self-control. Addictions often manifest themselves as gluttony. Excessive bingeing and drinking is wasteful and can be harmful to our health. The vice of gluttony can also be expensive to support, leading to poverty.

For example, an individual who buys gallons of ice cream costing about $30.00 a week will eventually spend about $120.00 in a month. Excessively eating ice cream can also be harmful to health. The same can be said about a person who buys and ingests multiple packs of alcohol every day. If the individual drives, he can deplete his or her financial resources and be a danger to himself or herself and others. An intoxicated driver is very likely to cause motor vehicle crashes and injure other drivers. Similarly, excessive eating is dangerous as it might lead to obesity, which can lead to other forms of health conditions.

Dr. Russell, quoted above, has spent a lot of time studying the modern benefits of adhering to God's commands and directives for a health-promoting diet. As he scrutinized modern science and nutrition, he discovered an astonishing overlap between the laws of God about clean and unclean animals and general health and wellbeing as did his predecessor, Dr. Macht. Dr. Russell's studies led him to conclude that contrary to popular modern belief, these commands are not obsolete at all. For example, he says, lobsters and all other shellfish were created by God to be cleaning agents of natural water sources. They can ingest and absorb large amounts of pollutants without being sick. But if they are eaten by human beings, they can transmit those same pollutants to those who eat them.

Filter-feeding clams as well as oysters have a concentration of viruses that can cause hepatitis as well as paralytic and neurotoxic shellfish poisoning. Although most of the forbidden animals in the Bible are scavengers that feed on dead decaying flesh, some of them such as horses and rabbits are not necessarily scavengers. But Russell reports that the meat from horses usually contains viruses that are detrimental to optimum human health. Similarly, rabbits are usually agents of tularemia, which is an infectious disease that afflicts human beings.

Concerning pork, Dr. Russell asserts that the pig is inherently filthy, as it will eat almost anything, including feces and decaying flesh. Additionally, the pig's meat is very fatty and the fat harbors most of the toxins. The pig's fat is spread throughout its meat, not isolated as in the case of beef. Dr. Russell further claims that "In the United States, three of the six most common food-borne parasitic diseases of humans are associated with pork consumption. These include toxoplasmosis, taeniasis or cysticercosis (caused by the pork tapeworm Taenia solium) and trichinellosis" (Russell, 1996). He also claims that shellfish can be put in a body of water that is contaminated with cholera-causing bacteria and they will filter all the bacteria and purify the water. Oysters, crabs, shrimp and scallops also filter large amounts of water every day. In chemically contaminated water, catfish usually demonstrate the highest level of contamination. The following is a direct excerpt from Dr. Russell's book:

> Animal fat is also a storage place for toxins and parasites. These toxins are found in the fat of all the animals we eat. Examples include DDT, insecticides, herbicides, antibiotics, hormones and various other chemicals the animals have ingested, breathed or touched. In 1979, a hormone called DES (diethylstilbestrol) was removed from the market because researchers learned that this substance caused cancer in the vagina and cervix in daughters of women who had received the drug to prevent miscarriage. They found that the stockyards throughout the United States injected beef cattle with large amounts of DES because it enabled the animals to gain weight rapidly. And sure enough, the hormone was stored in the animals' fat tissue.
>
> (Russell, 1996)[361]

The epidemic of the Severe Acute Respiratory Syndrome (SARS) that originated in China and quickly spread to other parts of the world was a deadly disease. Researchers in Honk Kong traced the origins of the disease to the consumption of the civet cat, an animal in the unclean list in Scripture. Since then other species have been identified by the World Health Organization as carriers of this disease.[362] These include raccoon dogs, civet cats, Chinese ferret badgers, fruit bats, snakes, and wild pigs. All these are classified as unclean animals, according to the Bible. The individuals who handled these animals were found to be sero-positive for SARS although they were asymptomatic. They were thought to have been contaminated when they handled carcasses of animals that are carriers for SARS.

Sometimes people expose themselves to harmful environments and practices, unknowingly. The common saying that "ignorance is bliss" is founded on the understanding that what we do not know cannot hurt us. However, this is not a true saying because ignorance can also mean that we may not be prepared to recognize and counter that which we do not know if it should threaten us. The Scriptures tell us that "My people are destroyed for lack of knowledge," (Hosea 4:6). Critical knowledge that pertains to health and wellbeing should be sought with diligence.

God did not give reasons for each of the health laws he gave to Israel. The health laws were given for the benefit of the community of Israel. This God who had taken an entire nation of about three million people from the "fiery furnace" of Egyptian slavery using a myriad of unprecedented miracles, and had led them day and night "who led you through the great and terrible wilderness, with its fiery serpents and scorpions and thirsty ground where there was no water, who brought you water out of the flinty rock who fed you in the wilderness with manna" (Deuteronomy 8: 15,16) from heaven for forty years and none among them was undernourished. This was the same God who was giving them laws to preserve their health. During their forty year journey to Canaan, the Israelites' garments did not wear out on them neither did their feet swell on them. God says "For I the LORD do not change," (Malachi 3:6). He is the same always. Israel had put their trust in him, and he had proved himself faithful. We also can trust him.

Scientists have done a lot of commendable work not only to prolong life but to improve the quality of life for humanity through experimentation and other scientific investigations that have yielded unprecedented discoveries of medical remedies for a myriad of diseases. But scientists do not know everything because science is a constantly evolving discipline. Although some new discoveries have been known to confirm earlier scientific discoveries, others have been known to modify and sometimes to completely repudiate earlier discoveries and it is not uncommon for scientists to prove other scientists wrong on a theory. A sustained, dedicated investigation of biblical health laws has revealed truths and principles meant to preserve our health.

As late as 2005 the report from World Health Organization (WHO), Food and Agriculture Organization of the United Nations (FAO) and the World Organization for Animal Health (OIE) indicated that the global prevalence of taeniasis or cysticercosis (caused by the pork tapeworm Taenia solium) obtained from pork consumption was high in Indonesia, India, China, Thailand, Africa, Mexico.[363] Taeniasis or cysticercosis is significantly endemic in some of these nations. This means addressing this issue is not obsolete as taeniasis or cysticercosis is still prevalent in a larger portion of this world, whose inhabitants are in constant contact with each other and with the rest of the world. The report further indicated that in Europe and the United States cases of T. solium taeniosis/cysticercosis were mostly attributed to travel and immigration from places where these health threats are still endemic. The FAO, WHO and OIE also indicate that one of the risk factors for transmission of these pathogens to people is "frequent pork consumption." In 2009, researchers Wenjun Ma, Robert E Kahn, and Juergen A Richt labeled the pig "a mixing vessel for influenza viruses" in their study.[364] These scientists further claimed that:

> Because swine are susceptible to infection with both avian and human influenza viruses, novel reassortant influenza viruses can be generated in this mammalian species by reassortment of influenza viral segments leading to the "mixing vessel" theory... Genetic reassortment among avian, human and/or swine influenza virus gene segments has occurred in pigs and some novel reassortant swine viruses have been transmitted to humans.[365]

The European Food Safety Authority claimed that the H1N1 influenza outbreak initially known as swine flu had it origin in a pig pen.[366] In 2005, the Centers of Disease Control and Prevention (CDC) issued a warning against paralytic shellfish poisoning mainly from mussels, cockles, clams, scallops, oysters, crabs, and lobsters.[367] Another warning was issued against amnesic shellfish poisoning from shellfish and mussels.

There may be some people who may not have been aware of some of the information provided above. This information is provided to underscore what has already been stated in Scripture as far as dietary guidelines are concerned. The idea is not to compel people to stop consuming whatever they want. This information is provided for education purposes from a biblical and public health perspective. It is meant to help people, if they are willing, to exercise caution concerning consumption of foods, which our omniscient God prohibited in his Word for the purpose of optimizing our health.

CHAPTER 21

CHRONIC DISEASES—I

Do you not know that your body is a temple of the Holy Spirit within you, which you have from God?

(1 Corinthians 6:19)

CARDIOVASCULAR DISEASE

Cardiovascular disease is a significantly fatal chronic disease. Although its incidence and prevalence have increased exponentially over the last few decades particularly in developed nations, developing nations have also begun to experience high rates of cardiovascular disease. Risk factors are varied and multiple. However, science tells us that "obesity-associated disorders, such as diabetes mellitus, an atherogenic dyslipidemia, and hypertension, have undoubtedly contributed to create an atherosclerosis-prone environment and thereby the development of cardiovascular disease (CVD)."[368] Other risk factors for cardiovascular disease include improper diet, lack of exercise, smoking, chronic nervous stress, and genetic susceptibility.

A 2000 *Journal of Applied Physiology* research report by Booth and associates claimed that since 1900, the number one killer in the United States has been cardiovascular disease.[369] The exception was probably in 1918 when influenza killed more people than cardiovascular disease. Booth and associates further indicate that in 1996, cardiovascular disease was responsible for approximately 960,000 deaths, accounting for about 60% of all deaths in that year.

The American Heart Association claims that from 1950 to 1996, the number of deaths resulting from heart disease has risen by 37%, which is an increase of 200,000 deaths a year.[370] Although the rates of death from cardiovascular disease decreased by 21.3% between 1986 to 1996, the absolute number of deaths from the same condition only declined by 2% in that same period, which means that cardiovascular disease continues to top the list as a killer.

The battle against cardiovascular disease is an uphill one because the reaction of the medical community has been focused, primarily, on secondary and tertiary prevention and not much on primary prevention. The medical community continues to do a commendable job in applying modern technology to stabilize obvious clinical manifestations of cardiovascular disease. However, the effort to reverse the disease has been unsuccessful because the disease is being treated only after it has become symptomatic and has progressed significantly. Kassirer and Angell, editors of the *New England Journal of Medicine* who advocate measures that are aimed at preventing obesity observe that:

> A progressive fattening of the population is not inevitable. We need to do a better job of educating people about healthful diets, including the calorie content of common foods, without promoting fetishes. Encouraging lifelong, regular exercise in children may well have the greatest effect in terms of preventing obesity, as well as numerous other benefits. If the time children now spend in front of the television eating junk food and watching advertisements for more junk food was instead spent in physical activity, leanness would be virtually ensured.
>
> (Kassirer & Angell 1998)[371]

It is not uncommon for some individuals to entirely blame their genetic endowment for their predisposition to certain diseases. But scientists inform us that although most diseases have a genetic origin, it is also true that only a few people can develop specific diseases such as heart disease as a consequence of a defect in only one single gene. Diseases usually develop as a result of interaction between different genes.

Additionally, although interaction between different genes may place an individual in a category of being susceptible to the etiology of a certain disease, it is also true that disease can develop as a result of interaction between genes and the environment. For example, the high prevalence of diabetes type 2 in the United States has been attributed to the interaction of the environment, behavioral choices and genetic susceptibility. Similarly, cardiovascular disease can also develop due to environmental, behavioral, and genetic factors.

Environmental factors for chronic diseases include protracted exposure to particulate matter saturating the ambient air and behavioral factors such as a sedentary lifestyle and poor dietary habits. Heart disease is another chronic disease that can develop as a result of the interaction among the factors listed above. In a research study to further understand genetic susceptibility to cardiovascular disease among individuals who had diabetes type 2, researcher Lu Qi and associates discovered that "Five single-nucleotide polymorphisms, rs4977574 (*CDKN2A/2B*), rs12526453 (*PHACTR1*), rs646776 (*CELSR2-PSRC1-SORT1*), rs2259816 (*HNF1A*), and rs11206510 (*PCSK9*) showed directionally consistent associations with CHD in the 3 studies" (Lu Qi, 2011).[372] However, although the presence of these genetic markers make an individual susceptible to onset of CVD, adoption of certain lifestyles such as regular exercise and low fat, low sugar dietary habits can mitigate the susceptibility.

Drs. McMillen and Stern in their book *None of These Diseases* indicate that animal fats are the main source of saturated fats leading to an increase in bad cholesterol (LDL or low-density lipoproteins).[373] The saturated fats that we often consume are converted into cholesterol particles by our bodies. A constant consumption of these fats can lead to arteriosclerosis. In societies where meat consumption is low there is a relatively low prevalence of coronary diseases. Cholesterol sticks to the walls of the arteries where it begins to build up into hard plaques with the passage of time. As the hard plaques increase, they begin to narrow the arteries and can, eventually, block off the flow of blood passing through the arteries to carry oxygen to the heart. The result of such an occurrence can be failure by the heart to pump blood to the body tissues. It can also result in the failure of the proper functioning of the heart's electrical system, which can easily lead to sudden death or heart attack.

According to Dr. Rex Russell, the onset of arteriosclerosis can also be exacerbated by an injury to the inner part of the artery.[374] The injury can be caused by a myriad of factors including toxins, viral infection, radiation or any other type of trauma to the inner layer of the artery. The human body is designed in such a way that when an injury occurs to it, it attempts to heal itself. In like manner, when the inner layer of the artery is injured, the artery begins a process of trying to heal itself by laying down plaque or cholesterol at the injured slight.

As the plaque or cholesterol thickens, the opening of the artery begins to narrow, which slows down the blood flow. Then the blood platelets begin to cluster together and begin to form a clot, which, ultimately, blocks the artery, completely. If a coronary artery is blocked, it results to a heart attack. If the artery is a cerebral artery, the result is a stroke.

In societies where meat treatment plants do not follow stringent hygiene and other health regulatory standards, meat consumption should be reduced drastically. In such places, some people have decided to completely avoid consumption of meat altogether in their effort to improve their health. One of the functions of blood in the body is to transport wastes and excretions from the body to excretory ducts of the body in order retain and to regulate the composition of bodily fluids with proper amounts of water, salts and nutrients.

Pulmonary circulation is another bodily system in which the blood plays a vital role as it moves from the heart to the lungs and back to the heart again. The waste-rich blood that is excreted from bodily processes that include cellular respiration is transported to the right atrium of the heart as the blood passes through the superior vena cava. As the red blood cells carry blood to the rest of the body from the heart they pass through tiny vessels known as capillaries where they exchange nutrients and oxygen for cellular waste. These waste products are often eliminated from the body through the body's urinary and respiratory systems. Any type of disruption of this delicate process can lead to significant health problems. For example, deadly infectious diseases can be transmitted from animals to human beings just by ingesting the blood of an animal that has an infectious disease such as tuberculosis or severe acute respiratory syndrome (SARS) or avian flu.

CARDIOVASCULAR DISEASE
CARDIOVASCULAR DISEASE IN EUROPE

A 2008 report of the European Cardiovascular Disease Statistics published by the British Heart Foundation and the European Heart Network paints a very dismal picture of the prevalence and incidence of cardiovascular disease in Europe.[375] Heart disease and disease of the circulatory system also known as cardiovascular disease or CVD are reported to be the main cause of death in all the 48 countries of Europe among women. About 4.3 million people die from this disease each year. Over 50% of deaths among men in Armenia, Georgia, Bulgaria, Azerbaijan, Serbia, Montenegro, Romania, Ukraine and the former Yugoslav Republic (FYR) Macedonia are caused by CVD. Coronary heart disease and stroke are the two main types of CVD.

The World Health Organization (WHO) and the Food and Agriculture Organization (FAO) Report on *Diet, Nutrition and the Prevention of Chronic Diseases* claims that "the high consumption of saturated fats, salt and refined carbohydrates, as well as low consumption of fruits and vegetables" is a dietary practice that constitutes a risk factor for cardiovascular disease.[376] Different research studies such as animal experimental studies, observational research studies, randomized clinical trials and metabolic research studies that have been conducted in different population groups have confirmed a strong association between dietary fat consumption and a significantly high incidence and prevalence of CVD.

The average diet in Europe is nutritionally deficient and poor. Consumption of fruit is below what is recommended by the World Health Organization (WHO) and the Food and Agricultural Organization (FAO), which is supposed to be 400g or more each day per individual. The recommended fat intake a day per individual is 15% and 30% of total energy intake, and the recommended saturated fat intake is about 10% of total energy intake.

The total energy intake is the number of calories taken in daily or total calories supplied by the amount of food eaten in a single day. Unfortunately, most European countries exceed the recommended dose of fat intake daily. This trend has been consistent over the last 30 years. In Eastern Europe, mortality from cardiovascular disease is significantly higher than it is in Western Europe.[377]

Economic Cost of Cardiovascular Disease in Europe

The economic costs of chronic diseases to society can be computed by measuring direct costs associated with healthcare costs and indirect costs related to death and disability.[378] In Europe, in

2006, cardiovascular disease (CVD) was estimated to have cost the European Union healthcare system about €110 billion. About 54% of these costs were incurred by providing inpatient hospital care for people with coronary heart disease. But the economic cost is not limited to direct healthcare alone. There are other aspects of care that require expenditure of public funds such as informal and indirect care for CVD patients. Overall mortality and morbidity costs related to CVD cost the European Union an estimated €41 billion. The economic cost of informal care for individuals with CVD was approximately €42 billion.[379]

One fifth of the overall cost was incurred in costs of care for individuals with CHD and over one fourth of the costs accounted for the care of people who had a stroke. By 2009, the economic cost for CVD had risen to approximately € 192 billion per year. Overall CVD economic cost estimates revealed that 57% of healthcare expenditure was attributed to direct care, 21% to production loss and 22% to informal care. From the above figures, obviously cardiovascular disease remains a major source of morbidity and mortality in Europe.

HEART DISEASE IN DEVELOPING NATIONS

Although chronic diseases have often been perceived as the burden of developed nations, there is, currently, an alarming emergence of personal-lifestyle related chronic diseases in developing nations. This is a direct result of a complex convergence of socioeconomic and behavioral factors.[380] Individual and familial decisions that exacerbate the incidence of heart disease in developing nations include changes in dietary choices, increased alcohol consumption, tobacco use and sedentary lifestyles. Unfortunately, health professionals in developing nations have not been able to recognize the magnitude of the threat of emerging chronic diseases.

One of the reasons for this is that the development of these diseases is not as dramatic and visible as that of infectious diseases these professionals usually deal with. In some developing nations, there is a prevailing viewpoint that being overweight or obese is a sign of opulence and good health.[381]

A woman who gains weight shortly after getting married is usually assumed to have found a good husband. Conversely, if a woman begins to visibly lose weight after marriage, the ability of the husband to properly take care of his wife becomes questionable. Obesity and overweight are rarely seen as health threats by the general public in these areas.

Commenting on the alarmingly high rate of chronic diseases in developing nations, Nugent of the Center for Global Development said "even very poor countries, such as India and Pakistan, and moderately poor countries, such as Russia and China, show higher death rates from chronic disease including heart disease than communicable disease" (Nugent, 2008).[382] Researchers Reddy and Yusuf claim that because the insidious emergence of heart disease in developing nations has not received the deserved attention of local or international public health professionals, there is cause for alarm.[383] There is a genuine fear that the rate of chronic diseases might escalate to overwhelming proportions before any attempt is made to curtail them and their corresponding risk factors.

Other contributing factors to chronic diseases include high rates of urbanization associated with changes in socio-economic and technological profiles of developing nations. These factors have resulted into a significant increase in life expectancy overall. An increase in life expectancy invariably results in an increase in the aged population groups with its age-related diseases which are usually chronic in nature.

In some developing nations, there has been an inverse relationship between eradication of communicable diseases and an increase in the incidence of non-communicable diseases. Other emerging chronic diseases that are beginning to plague developing nations include cancer, diabetes and neuro-psychiatric diseases. Unfortunately, the rise in these diseases has brought a mismatch between the available healthcare services and the rising needs for addressing these diseases. The World Health Organization attributed 28.5% of all deaths in low and middle-income nations to cardiovascular diseases in 1998.[384]

A significant contributor to the increase in heart disease in developing nations has been the widespread adoption of the western diet particularly in urban areas and the abandonment of the indigenous diet, which is mainly based on vegetables and grains. Fast food chains are saturating urban centers in developing nations, tempting office workers to grab quick meals from them.[385]

It is not uncommon for individuals leaving work to opt to buy a takeaway evening meal heavily saturated with fat or refined sugar for their families instead of preparing a traditional, nutritionally balanced meal. These evening meals are consumed in front of TV sets or personal computers after seating in a chair at work the whole day. This is a pathway to a sedentary lifestyle and its related negative health outcomes. Tragically being overweight is considered to be a sign of being less susceptible to disease. The pervasiveness of this viewpoint has become more acute and widespread particularly with the emergence of HIV/AIDS or "slim disease" as it is commonly known in Africa.

It is interesting to note that, in traditional Africa, villagers consumed sugar only once in a while on special occasions. Similarly meat was also consumed on special occasions such as weddings and funerals and other festivals. There were no fast foods restaurants then. Food was made from scratch using fresh, organically grown ingredients. Obesity and diabetes as well as heart disease were not a major concern then. However, even in modern day, women in rural areas of Africa still tend to have a lower body mass index (BMI) compared to their more educated counterparts working and living in urban areas because the former take part in rigorous manual work more often than the latter.

The Bible has something to say about habits that can easily lead to the development of chronic diseases such as heart disease. First of all, the Bible recommends that we live balanced lives, meaning that we should do all things in moderation. It warns us against gluttony and excessive eating in Proverbs 23:20-21 for this can lead to obesity, paving the way for a plethora of health conditions. Fatty foods laden with sugar are especially dangerous for health. We are also admonished to engage in physical exercise during the short period of our existence on this earth (1 Timothy 4:8) because it is profitable for physical well-being.

According to LaRosa of State University of New York Downstate Medical Center, medical science has proved that there is a correlation between heart disease and an elevated level of low-density lipoprotein cholesterol (LDL) also called bad cholesterol in the bloodstream.[386] High cholesterol levels burden the blood causing it to collect in the coronary arteries often leading to coronary heart disease.[387]

This is what God commanded Moses to tell Israel: "Say to the people of Israel, You shall eat no fat, of ox, or sheep, or goat," (Leviticus 7:23). In ancient Israel, animals were free range, eating natural grass. If the warning was appropriate then, how much more relevant is this counsel in modern times when animals are fattened using chemicals in readiness for slaughter? Human bodies are created in such a way that they are able to manufacture all the saturated fat they need for functioning. Therefore, there is no need to consume more saturated fats. Consumption of trans fats is dangerous for cholesterol levels, as they tend to raise LDL while at the same time lowering good HDL.

CHAPTER 22

CHRONIC DISEASES—II

DIABETES

When you sit down to eat ... observe carefully what is before you; and put a knife to your throat if you are a man given to appetite.

(Proverbs 23: 1-2)

Diabetes is a growing global health problem that shows no signs of slowing down in incidence or prevalence. Reports from the World Health Organization about the problem of obesity and overweight worldwide are alarming.

The United States Department of Health and Human Services claims that overweight and obesity are among the 10 leading health indicators of *Healthy People 2010*. In the last couple of decades, there has been an unprecedented increase in obesity in the United States. Over 64% of the adults in the United States are overweight or obese.[388]

The greatest increase was in the group with Body Mass Index (BMI) of more than 30. Along with increase in overweight and obesity rates, there has been a 25% increase in the prevalence of type 2 diabetes in the United States in the past 20 years. Risk factors for diabetes include body mass index, abdominal fat, and weight gain.

Approximately two thirds of adults in the United States have BMI of 27 kg/m² or more. The threat for diabetes among women begins to loom when the BMI starts to exceed 22 kg/m². From 1985 to 2009, thirty-three states experienced obesity prevalence of 25% and above, and nine states had a prevalence exceeding 30%.

Statistics from the World Health Organization indicate that approximately 1 billion adult individuals worldwide are overweight. Among them, about 300 million are clinically obese.[389] Obesity is a major risk factor for the etiology of chronic diseases and their associated disability. The principal reason for the rise in obesity rates involves significant changes in the general lifestyles and behavioral choices of people worldwide. Some of these changes include modernization, urbanization, and nutritional shifts as a consequence of the globalization of the food market.

The relative rise in general income of people worldwide and an increase in diverse population groups living side by side in urban centers around the world has, inevitably, spurred on an unavoidable change in the diet and lifestyle of the general public. As a consequence, traditional diets that have often been high in fiber and complex carbohydrates such as vegetables, whole fruits, potatoes, brown rice, grains, and legumes have given way to quick modern processed foods high in saturated fats and refined sugars.

A dietary trend has emerged that tends to encourage over-consumption of energy-dense, tasty foods that are also nutritionally deficient. These foods are often relatively cheap and served in large portions. Another significant change in the general habits involves a worldwide shift from more physically demanding manual work to less physical office work. Automated transportation systems and passive recreational and physical behaviors such as computer games, watching television programs, and reading encourage a sedentary lifestyle that leads to weight gain and obesity.

Other factors that are likely to contribute to increase in overweight and obesity include metabolic, behavioral, and socio-economic changes. Certain environmental and cultural factors can also be risk factors for obesity. Being overweight and obese can increase susceptibility to various weight-gain related diseases that include high blood pressure, high blood cholesterol, cancer, diabetes, and breathing problems. As the weight increases, so do health risks. However, oftentimes a deliberate loss of weight can reverse these obesity-related health risks.

Type 1 diabetes, which was initially known as juvenile diabetes, is a disease that is commonly diagnosed in young children and youth although adults can, sometimes, also suffer from it. Among adults, it makes up for 5% to 10% of all cases that are diagnosed in the United States.[390] The Centers for Disease Control and Prevention (CDC) claims that type 1 diabetes occurs when there is a significant lack of insulin, as the body does not produce enough of it. Diabetes 1 is also known as insulin dependent diabetes. It can be caused by a virus or an autoimmune disorder.

An autoimmune disorder occurs when the body fails to recognize a particular body organ as its own and attacks it. In the case of type 1 diabetes, the organ is the pancreas. As the body's immune system attacks the pancreas, the Beta cells responsible for manufacturing and secreting insulin begin to die. Therefore, in order for the individual suffering from type 1 diabetes to survive, they need to have a constant supply of insulin by injection. Susceptibility to type 1 diabetes could be exacerbated by autoimmune, environmental, and genetic factors.

The *Action in Diabetes and Vascular Disease (ADVANCE) Type 2 Diabetes* clinical trial research study, sponsored by George Institute of Australia, is reported to be one of the largest clinical trial research studies ever conducted. The participants were 11, 140 adult individuals from 20 different countries at 215 clinical centers located in Australasia, Asia, Europe, and North

America.[391] All the participants of the study had type 2 diabetes. The ADVANCE study claims that there are approximately 246 million individuals worldwide who have diabetes, and most of them have type 2 diabetes.[392]

The highest number of individuals with diabetes is in the Western Pacific geographical areas and Europe. Currently, India has 40 million diabetics, and China has 39.8 million cases of diabetes. Germany has 7.4 million cases, the United Kingdom has over 2 million cases, and Australia has 1.5 million cases. Type 2 diabetes cases have been diagnosed in children, although historically the disease has been more prevalent among individuals over 40 years of age. Usually people with this type of diabetes do not manifest observable symptoms at all. This is the reason most people do not know they have it. But when the symptoms do finally occur, they include extreme thirst, a voracious appetite, inexplicable fatigue, blurred vision, a frequent need to urinate, and wounds that are slow to heal. It is not unusual for male patients who have this disease to manifest erectile dysfunction.

Diabetes can lead to serious complications. An example of a serious complication is the development of cardiovascular disease and stroke, which are a major cause of mortality among diabetics. Heart disease and stroke are the primary causes of death and disability among people with type 2 diabetes. The American Heart Association claims that about 65% of people suffering from diabetes die from some type of heart disease or stroke.[393] Other complications from type 2 diabetes can include nephropathy, which is renal or kidney failure. Nephropathy afflicts about 30% of diabetic individuals.

Often these people end up requiring dialysis or kidney transplant. Neuropathy is a nerve disease or a condition that damages nerves. In diabetics, neuropathy manifests itself with a sensory loss in the feet. This complication can put the patient at risk for amputation. Vision impairment is another diabetic-related complication. Sometimes vision impairment can progress to a complete loss of sight. Peripheral vascular disease and diabetic-related ulceration is yet another complication that can be a result of diabetes. Peripheral vascular disease places diabetics at risk for lower-limb amputation.

The *ADVANCE* clinical trial mentioned above focused on finding out what effect a more intensive blood pressure (BP) lowering effort and tighter glucose control measures would have on the risk of major vascular complications among people suffering from type 2 diabetes. The participants were followed for 5 years after the study. The findings of the *ADVANCE* team demonstrated that the blood pressure lowering treatment regimen based on the fixed combination of the Angiotensin converting enzyme (ACE) inhibitor perindopril and the diuretic indapamide (Preterax®) significantly reduced mortality in patients with diabetes.

The results of the blood glucose lowering part of the study demonstrated that sustained and constantly intense treatment with modified release gliclazide (Diamicron MR®), combined with other necessary drugs, lowered blood glucose progressively and safely. In addition, the strategy applied in this study demonstrated one-fifth reduction in kidney disease and a thirty percent reduced risk of cardiovascular problems. These findings bring hope to people with type 2 diabetes, although there is always the looming problem of accessibility and cost for such treatment regimens.

The National Institutes of Health (NIH) claims that approximately more than 13% of adults in the United States aged 20 and above have diabetes.[394] Tragically, 40% of these individuals remain undiagnosed. Among the elderly, about one third of them are pre-diabetic, which means that they have elevated blood sugar, although it is not yet in the diabetic range.

Catherine Cowie of the National Institute of Diabetes and Digestive and Kidney Diseases (NIDDK), a part of the National Institutes of Health (NIH) had this to say about the prevalence of diabetes in the United States: "We're facing a diabetes epidemic that shows no signs of abating, judging from the number of individuals with pre-diabetes" (Cowie, 2008).[395]

Pre-diabetic individuals have either impaired glucose tolerance or impaired fasting glucose. Impaired fasting glucose means that their fasting glucose level is between 100 and 125 milligrams per deciliter (mg/dL) after an overnight fasting period. Impaired glucose tolerance means that the level of blood glucose after a 2-hour oral glucose tolerance test is between 140 and 199 mg/dL. Although both levels are quite high, they are not high enough to be in the category of diabetes.

The 2005-2006 National Health and Nutrition Examination Survey (NHANES) used the Oral Glucose Tolerance Test to measure the true burden of diabetes and pre-diabetes rates in the United States. The results of the survey demonstrated that the rates of diagnosed diabetes increased in between the surveys they conducted. But undiagnosed diabetes and pre-diabetes rates were about the same. The results also revealed that minority population groups were disproportionately affected by diabetes. In addition, pre-diabetes was more prevalent in men than in women particularly among individuals aged 45 and above.

The U.S.-Mexico Border Diabetes Prevention and Control Project is a collaborative initiative established to determine the prevalence and incidence of diabetes and to identify the associated risk factors in order to develop binational intervention and control programs that respond to the needs of the population groups living along this border.

The prevalence of diabetes is particularly high along the United States-Mexico border where 1.2 million people out of the 7.5 million who live there have diabetes.[396] Seven hundred thousand of the individuals with diabetes live on the U.S. side of the border, and 500,000 live on the Mexican side of the border. About 5.3 million people in this area are either obese or overweight. The prediabetes prevalence is 14% among adults, and the border diabetes-related mortality rates are higher than the national rates. There are also alarming high rates of poverty along this border. Most of the people live below the federal poverty datum line.

Researchers Glayzer and Mitchell present a dismal picture of obesity and diabetes prevalence in the United Kingdom. About one in four adults in England are obese. More than 55% of adults in Wales are either overweight or obese.[397] The Department of Health's online information about the prevalence of obesity in Europe reveals that 58% of type 2 diabetes, 21% of heart disease and between 8% and 42% of some types of endometrial, colon, and breast cancers are attributable to excess body fat.

Endometrial cancer is cancer that starts in the inner lining of the uterus. Although menus in popular restaurants in the United Kingdom are often high in calories, saturated fat, salt, and sugar, almost 30% of household expenses are allocated toward eating out, and about 30% of the people eat out in restaurants and fast foods at least once each week. The alarming rise in the prevalence of obesity and type 2 diabetes in Europe motivated the government in England to announce an ambitious strategy called *Healthy Weight, Healthy Lives* and to be "the first major nation to reverse the rising tide of obesity and overweight in the population by ensuring that everyone is able to achieve and maintain a healthy weight" (Glayzer & Mitchell, 2008).

The strategy includes guiding the customer into making healthier food choices both at home and when eating out. The Food Standards Agency in England has been charged with the responsibility of working with the food industry to help consumers understand nutritional information about the food they choose. All these strategies are for the purpose of encouraging people to make healthier food choices and to adopt better dietary habits.

Astonishingly, Asian countries known for their low BMI are also beginning to grapple with obesity-related diabetes. Prior to 1980, type 2 diabetes rates were between 1% and 5% in Japan.

But recent population-based research studies demonstrate that the prevalence of diabetes type 2 has increased two-fold in Japan in just over two decades.[398] The Japanese lifestyle and diet have changed significantly since the end of World War II. More and more Japanese people have adopted a more sedentary lifestyle than before, and they currently consume more fat than in the past. The consequences of this lifestyle is an inevitable increase in body mass index (BMI) and cholesterol levels, which are often precursors of the development of type 2 diabetes.

In the last two decades, China's economy has soared incredibly, and this has raised the overall standard of living. However, as is the case worldwide, modernization has brought a change in the diet and lifestyle of the general population. Where the people mostly walked or cycled to work, they now drive cars or ride buses and motorcycles. Their diet includes more high-calorie, high fat, and refined sugar products. Inevitably, this lifestyle has brought an increase in obesity and overweight rates. China has also experienced an increase in the incidence and prevalence of type 2 diabetes. Out of an estimated population of over 1.3 billion people, China has 92.4 million adults who have diabetes, making it one of the largest diabetic populations in the world.[399] About 148.2 million (15.5%) adults in China have prediabetes. This condition is a significant risk factor for the development of overt diabetes as well as cardiovascular disease. The Chinese Ministry of Health intends to establish an aggressive diabetes care program in China to curtail the spread of the disease.

ECONOMIC COST OF DIABETES IN INDUSTRIALIZED NATIONS

Diabetes is one of the most costly health conditions to treat.[400] In 2007, direct costs associated with the treatment of diabetes patients were approximately $116 billion in the United States. Another $58 billion was expended on indirect costs that include disability, premature mortality, and loss of productivity. This adds up to a national expenditure of $174 billion. The Los Angeles county expenditure on diabetes-related direct costs alone was approximately $6.4 billion each year. Hospital care is also a major component of the medical costs.

According to Diabetes UK, 10% of the National Health Service (NHS) expenditure goes to diabetes, which is about £1.5 million an hour for England and Wales. This amounts to £25,000 per minute.[401] All together the NHS spends about £14 billion pounds treating diabetes and its associated complications. About 300 people are being diagnosed with diabetes each day in Europe. This means that every five minutes someone is being diagnosed with the disease. One in ten people admitted in hospitals in the United Kingdom have diabetes, and on average their hospital stay costs the NHS an estimated £215.00 each day. Emergency ambulance attendance services cost approximately £220.00 each time they are supplied. Needless to say, diabetes is an expensive disease.

DIABETES IN DEVELOPING NATIONS

DIABETES IN SUB-SAHARAN AFRICA

Type 1 diabetes is a treatable disease in developed nations. But this is not the case in developing nations of sub-Saharan Africa.[402] Type 1 diabetes is a chronic disease that can be fatal if it is not properly treated. Only about 1% of sub-Saharan children with type 1 diabetes live to be six years old after being diagnosed with the disease. The International Insulin Foundation (IIF) based in the United Kingdom is a charity organization committed to prolonging the lives of diabetics in developing nations by supplying them with the insulin they need.

The IIF works with local governments and health departments to provide health services for diabetics. A healthcare system with skilled personnel is critical for treating diseases, such as type 1 diabetes, effectively, and for administering insulin and providing syringes as well as other monitoring equipment for both type 1 and type 2 diabetics.

Data on the epidemiology of diabetes in sub-Saharan Africa are still a little scanty because of lack of cohesive data collecting systems.[403] Nevertheless, available information indicates that there is a significant increase in type 2 diabetes in Africa linked to an increase in obesity, urbanization, development, changes in dietary habits, and changes in lifestyles and behaviors.

The local community is ill prepared to help deal with the problem of chronic diseases in developing nations because, in the past, emphasis was mainly placed on combating infectious diseases. This approach inadvertently neglected the rising incidence and prevalence of chronic diseases. But now chronic diseases should be treated with the same urgency as infectious diseases. In South Africa, estimates of the prevalence of type 2 diabetes are between 3% and 28.7% with the greatest burden of the disease being found among the Indian communities of Durban who have 13% prevalence and the elderly "colored" populations of Cape Town who have a 28.7% prevalence.[404] South Africa is experiencing a remarkable rise in the rates of obesity just like the rest of the global community. About 29.2% of South African men are either overweight or obese and about 56.6% of the women are obese or overweight.

Diabetes in India

Scientists Radha and Mohan of the Madras Research Foundation and Dr. Mohan's Diabetes Center, define type 2 diabetes as "a complex heterogeneous group of conditions characterized by impairment in both insulin secretion and action" (Radha & Mohan, 2006).[405] The recent explosion in the incidence and prevalence of this disease confirms the role environmental factors such as lifestyle play in the development of this disease, although there is also strong evidence that genetic predisposition does contribute significantly to the etiology of the disease. India is experiencing a rise in the fast food industry.

Additionally, there is also an alarming inclination toward a sedentary lifestyle by the general public due to technological advancement, which has brought an inevitable shift in the nature of jobs; from manual labor to less physically demanding work. Physical recreational activities are being replaced by computer video games that require minimal physical activity. As children and youth spend more time playing computer games and sitting in front of television sets instead of engaging in physically demanding outdoor games, their body mass index is likely to increase, placing them at high risk for development of type 2 diabetes.

India reportedly had a significantly low incidence and prevalence of diabetes in the 1970s.[406] However, that scenario has changed drastically with increase in urbanization. Although there is a rise in type 1 diabetes in India, the rise in type 2 diabetes is at epidemic level.[407] In the year 2000, three countries—China, India and United States—were reported to have the highest prevalence of diabetes.[408] India had 32 million people with diabetes in 2000. By the end of the decade, India is reported to have 40 million diabetics. This figure is expected to rise to approximately 69.9 million by the year 2025.

Although obesity rates are relatively low among them, Asian Indians tend to have a larger waist circumference and waist to hip ratios that predispose them to type 2 diabetes. Moreover, "Asian Indians tend to have more total abdominal and visceral fat for any given BMI and for any given body fat they have increased insulin resistance" (Ghosh, et al. 2010).[409] Although genetic predisposition to a health condition increases the risk of developing that condition, there are many ways to mitigate its onset and progression, including controlling environmental factors that are likely to exacerbate the development of the condition. In the case of type 2 diabetes, mitigating approaches include adopting a low-fat, low-calorie diet and exercising regularly for at least

30 minutes a day. These lifestyle modifications can increase the body's sensitivity to insulin in both diabetics and non-diabetics.

The growing fast foods industry in India is one of the main reasons for the alarming increase in type 2 diabetes in the nation. In cities, Indian people have started depending more on readily available fast foods that are rich in calories and saturated fat and refined sugar than the traditional diet. Historically, in India, type 2 diabetes used to be associated with the affluent, but it has now permeated the ranks of the poor.

ECONOMIC COST OF DIABETES IN DEVELOPING NATIONS

In developing nations, a proper quantification of the economic cost of diabetes is hampered by limitations in related data.[410] However, available data indicate that, in Tanzania, the combined projected growth loss between 2005 and 2015 as a result of diabetes-related mortality rates as well as heart disease was estimated to be US $2.5 billion.

In India, providing treatment for everyone who has diabetes might cost approximately US $13.8 billion. That constitutes about one fourth of the country's entire health expenditure. Production loss for untreated diabetics amounts to about US $20.4 billion in India. In Latin America and the Caribbean, the number of people who died from diabetes in 2000 was estimated to be 339,035 which represented a total loss of 757,096 discounted years of productive life in individuals aged 65 and younger.[411]

In monetary value, the cost was about $3 billion. Permanent disability associated with diabetes causes a loss of approximately 12,699,087 years, which in monetary terms is approximately US $50 billion. Temporary disability causes an estimated 136,701 loss of years among the working class, amounting to approximately US $763 million. Treatment associated with insulin and oral medication costs US $4,720 million and hospitalizations cost approximately US $1,012 million. Diabetics' medical consultation and care for complications related cost about US $2,508 million and US $2,480 million, respectively. Diabetes, therefore, places a heavy economic burden on both developed and developing nations, worldwide.

WEIGHT LOSS PROGRAMS

There is currently a plethora of weight loss programs, particularly in industrialized nations in an effort to stem the unprecedented rise in obesity rates. Diet fads have a long history. Some early dietary plans included taking laxatives and purgatives to reduce obesity.[412] The stubborn steady increase in obesity and its side effects has introduced as sense of desperation, which makes people susceptible to all forms of obesity cures.

Dinitrophenol, currently being used as a strong pesticide and herbicide, was a recommended weight loss remedy in the mid 1930s. Later it was discovered that this "cure" was responsible for speeding the body's metabolism rate to a dangerous point where the body literally burned itself up. Severe side effects associated with ingesting the drug were reported. Twelve women were reported to have become temporarily blind after taking the drug. Most of the people who took a large dose of the drug experienced severe adverse health effects. By 1938, dinitrophenol was banned because of its severe side effects.

The human chorionic gonadotropin (HCG) was an obesity cure of the mid 1950s. A daily injection of this hormone was reported to reduce hunger which, ultimately, led to eating less and resulting in weight loss. Adverse side effects began to be reported regularly about the drug until the reports caught the attention of the Food and Drug Administration (FDA), which responded by requiring producers of HCG to put a label on the drug; warning the public against using it as a remedy for weight loss or fat redistribution therapy in 1974.

Although the diet and weight loss industry is a billion-dollar business, overweight and obesity rates continue to rise. People often try one weight loss program, lose some weight, only to gain it all back again. Then they go and try another program, and the cycle continues. The problem is that there is no magic pill for sustained weight loss. It takes a great effort, determination and commitment to change a behavioral pattern in order to lose weight. Often this change requires a lifetime of self-discipline. A well-balanced diet and a viable exercise program can set one on the way to weight loss. Most people do not have a comprehensive understanding of the extent to which food can impact our health. As a result, they fall prey to eating disorders of one kind or another, including eating either too little or too much.[413]

Developing nations are often beleaguered by malnutrition problems in the form of lack of foods with proper nutrients such as calcium, iron, folic acid, and vitamins. This situation is particularly intense in rural areas where the effects of frequent famine as a result of drought are acutely felt. Developed nations are also plagued by problems of either under nourishment or over nourishment due to numerous food products flooding the food markets. Often this leads to nutrition-related problems such as obesity or anorexia.

Anorexia is a disorder that occurs often in pre- or post-puberty phases of life. The emphasis on being thin in a culture that is contending with an unparalleled obesity epidemic has caused some overweight and obese individuals to become victims of eating disorders in their effort to lose weight. Sometimes these people feel obligated to adopt strenuous exercise and weight loss programs while eating virtually nothing in order to lose their excess weight. It is not unusual for people who are obsessed with losing weight to end up being anorexic. The National Alliance on Mental Illness defines anorexia as "a serious, occasionally chronic, and potentially life-threatening eating disorder defined by a refusal to maintain minimal body weight within 15 percent of an individual's normal weight" (NAMI, 2012).[414]

The Perfect Prescription

A lot of health challenges are related to obesity, including high blood pressure and hypoglycemia. Hypoglycemia occurs in people who are physically inactive but who eat large amounts of fats, sugars, and meats. This type of diet can enhance the development of type 2 diabetes in most cases. Avoiding and controlling diabetes includes observing a low-fat diet and exercising. Exercise is a good way of maintaining a good body shape and preventing health challenges. But exercise should be properly planned and executed, because intense workouts and misuse of exercise equipment can tax the body and cause avoidable injury.

The general public in the United States and around the world is curiously interested in issues related to food and diet. Digital Video Discs (DVDs) and books explaining the obesity issue and how to reverse or avoid it are flooding publishing houses and bookstores. They are also selling very well. There is also an unprecedented surge in weight loss and diet programs. Unfortunately, some of the programs lure their clients by promising drastic weight loss in unrealistically short periods of time. Sometimes these weight loss programs are so rigorous and demanding on the body that although people adopt them and lose weight for a while, they regain the weight right back because they cannot keep up with the demands of the program for a long time. It becomes too taxing on their bodies.

Other times the programs themselves are viable, but people do not know exactly how to follow them. As a result, they end up being ill or fatigued, and they are unable to continue the program. Often they experience a promising initial loss of weight, but that could only be due to excessive loss of water, and the weight quickly comes back. Some weight programs focus on behavioral and dietary changes. For people who are genuinely committed to changing their eating lifestyle, these programs can be beneficial. Programs that involve exercise and proper eating plans that give people a well-rounded, reasonable routine that is easy to adhere to and is sustainable can lead to a realizable weight goal.

The media exerts a lot of influence on the general public and how they perceive dieting, exercise, weight loss, nutritional choices, and body images. A certain body image, usually represented by a thin model or celebrity, is often glamorized in the media as the ideal body structure. This pressurizes people into trying all types of programs to lose weight to gain at least a semblance of the advertised body image they crave.

Unfortunately, people are also bombarded by relentless advertising for snacks, fast foods, candy and soda, which continues to woo them to eat and drink more of these products. Food industries spend billions of dollars advertising their products so that commercials often become the primary nutrition advice the public is exposed to. Either way, people can go too far. They can end up under eating or over eating to the point of hurting their health. The federal government, working through the United States Department of Agriculture and the Department of Health and Human Services, publishes a Food Pyramid with Dietary Guidelines every five years. However, as authors Jain and Schneider pointed out, "The recommendations may not be transferable to different cultures and ethnicities, and may not address special nutritional needs of pregnant mothers, vegetarians, lactose intolerant individuals, young children or other special populations"[415] (Jain & Schneider, 2007). It is also not clear from the pyramid how many servings of a recommended food product should be consumed at each meal. The New Food Pyramid not only emphasizes eating healthy, it also has a recommendation for daily physical activity.

Biblical dietary guidelines do not stipulate how many servings an individual should have per meal either. But, being sensitive to the fact that people might tend to overeat even with healthy foods, Scriptures advise us to do all things in moderation, including eating. Some religious groups who have adopted biblical diets and other health lifestyles have witnessed remarkably positive health outcomes.

Reporting on the health profile of the Amish people, Jeannine Stein observes that a pocket of Old Order Amish people who live in Ontario has remarkably low rates of obesity although their diet is high in calories and sugar.[416] They are at 4% obesity rate. This group of people keeps its weight low because of its lifestyle, which consists of manual and vigorous work activities. Men and women spend most of their work time doing physically demanding chores such as lifting, shoveling, digging, and shoeing horses. They also do a lot of gardening, feeding farm animals, and other similar manual activities. However, Amish communities that have moved away from less strenuous occupations have experienced a notable rise in obesity.

Long-term studies of Seventh-day Adventists in California have demonstrated that Adventists live several years longer than other Californians. It has been found out from prospective studies of Adventists that maintaining a lean body shape throughout one's lifetime is critical for optimum health and longevity.[417] When researchers into the lifestyle and eating habits of this population group broke down the health habits of these individuals in statistical analyses, they found out that among many other health promoting habits observed by this population group was a regular participation in a great deal of physical activity. They also discovered that their diet was mainly grain and plant-based. They were also committed to maintaining a medium body weight. They also consumed grains such as brown rice, which contain anti-oxidants and lignens necessary for the health of the cells.

Most Christians believe that regular physical exercise is an essential component of good health and that some type of physical labor is fundamental for optimum health. People can reap benefits from regular health-promoting physical activity, whether rigorous or moderate. Even among individuals who are advanced in age and are quite frail, physical mobility and functioning can be enhanced through moderate physical activity. The benefits of physical activity, therefore, cannot be over-emphasized.

In 2002, the United States Department of Health and Human Services released the following dismal statistics reflecting some of the negative health outcomes of sedentary lifestyles:[418] approximately 12.6 million people in the United States have coronary heart disease, and another 1.1 million people suffer a heart attack in each given year. An estimated 17 million people are diabetics and 90-95% of them have diabetes type 2. Over sixteen million people are pre-diabetics, and 107,000 individuals are diagnosed with colon cancer each year. Over 300,000 people suffer from hip fractures every year, and 50 million people have high blood pressure.

Overall, more than two-thirds of the entire population of the United States is either overweight or obese. Regular exercise significantly reduces the risk of developing or dying from the above conditions. Most of the deaths from chronic diseases are linked to a sedentary lifestyle.

The Bible tells us that "for while bodily training is of some value, godliness is of value in every way, as it holds promise for the present life and also for the life to come" (1 Timothy 4:8). Note that this Scripture does not negate the importance of physical exercise. Rather, it indicates that physical exercise is relevant for this temporary life. If physical exercise is of benefit to our physical bodies, which are temples of the Holy Spirit then as good stewards, we need it.

Dr. Mary Ruth Swope, an expert in health nutrition, posits that "Modern day research scientists are proving God's word regarding dietary matters to be without error" (Swope, n.d.).[419] While the Bible does not directly address the problem of overweight and obesity or weight loss, it encourages us to take care of our health and our bodies. It also counsels us against gluttony, which can lead to being overweight or obese.

For example, in Proverbs 23:1-3 the Bible says, "When you sit down to eat...observe carefully what is before you; and put a knife to your throat if you are a man given to appetite. Do not desire his delicacies, for they are deceptive food." Putting a knife to the throat if given to gluttony is caution against unrestrained appetite. Being gluttonous is not a good way to take care of one's body: "Do you not know that your body is a temple of the Holy Spirit within you, which you have from God? You are not your own; you were bought with a price. So glorify God in your body" (I Corinthians 6:19-20). Science also admonishes us against eating too much sugar-based foods. Scripture tells us that "If you have found honey, eat only enough for you, lest you be sated with it and vomit it" (Proverbs 25:16) and in Proverbs 25: 27 it says that "It is not good to eat much honey." The Bible does not mention sugar by name since this is a new product that was only discovered in the 1800s. Honey was the sweetest substance in ancient Israel. Therefore, whether, it is honey or real sugar, it should all be consumed in moderation to protect health and well-being.

We live in an age when suggestions to adopt biblical counsel on health are not often heeded or taken seriously. Biblically oriented lifestyles are usually perceived as being archaic and obsolete. One professor refused to enroll her toddler into a Christian preschool facility for fear that religion would truncate his creativity by putting him in a so-called mold that would "standardize" his thinking capacity.

She said that she wanted her son to have an unbridled imagination and creativity free from so-called restrictions imposed by religion-based training. An assistant professor at a separate private university claimed that religion was not for intellectuals. This viewpoint seems to echo Karl Marx's statement about religion being "the opium of the masses."[420]

It is also not uncommon to watch movies or read stories that depict religious people as an ignorant and gullible group of individuals. Their leaders are portrayed as being exploitative individuals, expertly manipulating their followers for personal gain. These are not the only reasons for the rejection of religion. Some reasons are related to pain and suffering.

For example, people often ask: "How can a loving God allow so much pain and suffering in the world?" Other times, rejection of Christianity is related to disillusionment in cases where a loved one did not get healed in spite of ardent intercessory prayers being offered on their behalf. Sometimes those who are viewed as intellectuals develop an objection to anything that has its source in religion because they have been trained to be "critical thinkers." Some of them become serial cynics who question the existence of all things that cannot be empirically verified or quantified in order to avoid believing error.

Professor R. Reno claimed in his article, *An Error Worse than Error*, that sometimes truth outruns our powers of reason.[421] Unfortunately, often critical reason is critical and not creative. Reno further contents that critical thinking thrives in parsing arguments and examining premises and filtering beliefs, but critical reason will only pull down and not build up. Critical reason may succeed in clearing and weeding out the undergrowth of error, but it has no capacity to plant seeds of truth. The danger is that the mind trained in critical reasoning might fear error so much that although it may have the capacity to doubt, it may lack the capacity to believe. Critical reasoning fosters a mind-set that hastens toward finding reason, any reason at all, to avoid nurturing convictions particularly about things that cannot be empirically proven; things that need faith to believe them. Reno tells of his own personal experience as a critical thinker:

> In my experience, although the modern university is full of trite, politically correct pieties, for the most part its educational culture is cautious to a fault. Students are trained-I was trained-to believe as little as possible so that the mind can be spared the ignominy of error. The consequences: an impoverished intellectual life. The contemporary mind very often lives on a starvation diet of small, inconsequential truths, because those are the only points on which we can be sure we're avoiding error.

The Perfect Prescription

(Reno, 2010)

Some of the great intellectuals and thinkers of our times have acknowledged the existence of a Creator God. For instance, Blaise Pascal, the French mathematician, once remarked that: "There is a God shaped vacuum in the heart of every man which cannot be filled by any created thing, but only by God, the Creator, made known through Jesus" (Lamont, 1997).[422]

An additional reason for hesitancy to accept biblical-based instructions is related to perceptions about the church. As Philip Yancey aptly observes, "the church has led the way in issues of justice, literacy, medicine, education, and civil rights. But to our everlasting shame, the watching world judges God by a church whose history also includes the Crusades, the Inquisition, anti-Semitism, suppression of women, and support of the slave trade" (Yancey, 2002).[423]

Could it be that the rejection of biblical health laws is, partly, a consequence of the church's historical mistakes articulated above? However, it must be noted that one does not have to convert to Christianity to benefit from biblical health laws. Nonbelievers can readily apply these laws to their own lives and improve their health and well-being. For example, an individual does not have to be a believer to benefit from eating in moderation. If they are properly understood and applied, biblical health laws can be an astonishing blessing to all mankind.

Living by biblical directives can be a challenge, particularly if popular opinion insists that doing so is a sign of intellectual deficiency. Ancient Israel experienced this peer pressure as well and often balked under its weight. When they finally arrived in the Promised Land after the original generation had died off on the way, Israel discovered that they were surrounded by idol worshippers—nations that had visible monarchs ruling over them. Israel was the only theocracy. They perceived themselves as the odd ones out, the only ones who bowed down and worshipped an invisible God. Sometimes they found it frustrating to worship this invisible God.

As they observed the worship practices of the surrounding nations, the Israelites began to long for the same worship practice and political governance. Their uniqueness became an albatross to them. Finally they began to demand to the Prophet Samuel that they wanted a king like other nations around them. They wanted a king they could touch and see—someone visibly present and less mysterious, even after the Prophet warned them about the ensuing problems of being ruled by another human being. They insisted on choosing mortal man to govern them and with that Israel started on a journey of steady spiritual and political decline until finally they were displaced and carried off into exile and slavery.

Among the kings who ruled Israel were some who feared God and attempted to do what was right in spite of their human frailties and weaknesses such as King David. Because King David took God at his word and loved him, God strengthened the nation of Israel under him. David ruled Israel gloriously and ushered it into its Golden Age under his son, King Solomon. God rewarded him by establishing an everlasting dynasty for him. The Messiah, the Lord Jesus Christ, came from the lineage of King David. This God who honored the faith of fellow mortal men like King David is still the same today. He still honors those who take Him at His word including His word about health promoting principles. If ministers of religion can emulate their counterparts the priests of ancient Israel by leading their congregations in promoting healthy lifestyles as depicted in the Bible, the world's health status will be changed for the better. There is more to ministry than preaching the word much as that is very important. People need to learn more about taking care of their health.

CHAPTER 23

SMOKING

And whatever you do, in word or deed, do everything in the name of the Lord Jesus, giving thanks to God the Father through him.

(Colossians 3:17)

Smoking is becoming a global concern. Parents around the world are frantically trying to find ways to prevent their children from adopting the habit. But there is very little they can do to protect them from being exposed to secondhand smoke, particularly in societies that allow smoking in public places. What used to be a habit mainly for adults has now been adopted by teens and young adults in alarming proportions. Both developed and developing nations are contending with the issue of smoking among both young people and adults. Health professionals all over the world have been disseminating information to educate the general public about the harmful effects of cigarette smoking.

In the United States, a large prospective study was conducted by Rogot and Murray over a period of 16 years—between January 1954 and December 1969 among United States veterans aged 31-84 years to assess the association between tobacco use and mortality rates.[424] Earlier studies such as the one conducted by Dorn in 1959 confirmed the fact that people who smoked cigarettes had a higher risk of dying from smoking-related ailments that include lung cancer, respiratory diseases, ulcers, liver cirrhosis, and cardiovascular health problems.[425] The results of the Rogot and Murray prospective study demonstrated a significantly positive association between tobacco smoking and lung cancer as well as heart disease, stroke, and other chronic lung diseases.

According to the Centers for Disease Control and Prevention, the association between cigarette smoking and lung cancer started as a mere suspicion among British healthcare employees in the 1920s. The employees noticed that almost all of the patients who developed lung cancer were also cigarette smokers. Epidemiologists' interest was aroused by this suspicion, which prompted them to start investigating a potential association between cigarette smoking and lung cancer between the 1930s and 1960s. Two epidemiologists involved in this work were Sir Richard Doll and Dr. A. B. Hill.[426] Sir Richard used a prospective case-control study method in which he measured the history of smoking among a group of lung cancer patients and compared it with a group of patients who did not have lung cancer over a period of four years. Richard and Hill later utilized a cohort of British physicians as participants in a research study to explore mortality rates of these doctors in relation to their smoking habits.[427]

Over the ensuing years, they collected information about the cause of their deaths. The findings of both research studies revealed a significantly positive association between cigarette smoking and lung cancer. As a result of these findings, Sir Richard stopped smoking himself. Because of the findings in his research in this area Sir Richard was awarded the United Nations Award for Cancer Research in 1962 and the gold medal of the European Cancer Society in 2000.

The Perfect Prescription

The World Health Organization (WHO) report reveals alarming statistics about the effects of smoking, worldwide. For example, the WHO report indicates that smoking-related diseases kill 1 in 10 adults worldwide.[428] In the United States alone smoking is responsible for the death of one in five people, annually. Tragically, approximately 47.5% of all men smoke, which is over a third of the global male population. Projected statistics for 2030 reveal that if the current smoking trend continues, smoking will kill one in six people, worldwide. The WHO reports that every eight seconds, a human being dies from tobacco use. About 15 billion cigarettes are being sold every day, which means that approximately 10 million cigarettes are sold every minute. In Britain, about 12 times more people have died from smoking than from the ravages of World War II.

Quoting the 1982 United States Surgeon General's report about smoking, the American Cancer Society stated that "smoking is the major single cause of cancer mortality [death] in the United States" (American Cancer Society, 2012).[429] This is the case even though there are many other risk factors for cancer such as air pollution, radon, food additives, and pesticides. Echoing the report from the Office of the Surgeon General, the U.S. Department of Health and Human Services cautioned that:

> Smoking causes coronary heart disease, the leading cause of death in the United States. Cigarette smoking causes reduced circulation by narrowing the blood vessels (arteries) and puts smokers at risk of developing peripheral vascular disease (i.e., obstruction of the large arteries in the arms and legs that can cause a range of problems from pain to tissue loss or gangrene). Smoking causes abdominal aortic aneurysm (i.e., a swelling or weakening of the main artery of the body—the aorta—where it runs through the abdomen).
>
> (U.S. Department of Health and Human Services, 2004)[430]

The U.S. Department of Health and Human Services also reported that smoking is a causative factor for lung cancer and that there are more deaths caused by tobacco use each year than by human immunodeficiency virus (HIV), illegal drug use, alcohol use, motor vehicle injuries, suicides, and murders combined. Furthermore, an estimated 90% of deaths from chronic obstructive lung disease are a result of smoking.

Individuals who smoke one half packet of cigarettes everyday are at high risk for heart attacks and cancers. Drs McMillen and Stern, in their book *None of These Diseases,* claim that chain smokers suffer "up to 34 times more laryngeal cancer and 72 times more lung cancer."[431] Cigarette smoke contains over 40 carcinogens (cancer causing agents). When a person smokes a cigarette, the smoke goes into the lungs where all these chemicals are absorbed into the bloodstream, to be dissolved into the blood. The blood circulates these chemicals to all the organs of the body. This is the reason why cigarette smoke can also cause other cancers such as cancer of the cervix, the stomach, the kidneys, the breast and pancreas, and many more.

Cigarette smoke contains toxins that undermine health and well-being, such as carbon monoxide, benzene, phenol, ammonia, cyanide, nitro benzene, arsenic, methanol, and many more. About 200, 000 Americans die each year from cigarette-smoke induced heart attacks. Drs. McMillen and Stern have dubbed cigarettes in a packet "a fistful of coffin nails" because people who smoke heavily shorten their lives by a total of approximately 8 years.

Every single cigarette that is smoked reduces the life expectancy of the smoker by five minutes. Therefore, if an individual smokes 12 cigarettes in a day, their life is shortened by 60 minutes (12 cigarettes x 5 minutes). If they smoke 24 cigarettes in one day, they deduct 2 hours from their life expectancy each day. Smoke from cigarettes makes the arteries grow narrower and the blood cells stickier than they should be. This makes it easy for the cells to cluster in the narrow passage of a coronary artery and to block it, which could easily cause a heart attack. If the blocked vessel is a cerebral artery, the individual could suffer a stroke. These types of heart attacks tend to be quite serious because the victim's blood already has low quantities of oxygen due to the presence of smoke toxins. Therefore, when the heart demands more oxygen, the supply is too inadequate to revive it. Such heart attacks are often fatal.

Cigarette smoking is one of the most significant public health challenges in the United States. Cigarette smoke contains nicotine, which is an addictive drug. When people smoke, the nicotine is absorbed in the linings of the mouth and the lungs via blood circulation. It is also distributed to the heart and the brain using the same method. The nicotine then stimulates feelings of calmness, relaxation, and alertness all at once. People who want to stop smoking experience a host of unpleasant withdrawal problems that adversely affect their physical and psychological functions. The tars that are contained in cigarette smoke add to its carcinogenicity. Decades of research finally convinced cigarette manufacturers of the deadliness of the tars in the cigarettes, and motivated them to add filters to reduce tar intake. But, apparently, this addition changed the taste of the product, making it less appealing to smokers. Therefore, in order to restore product acceptability, the manufacturers had to add a certain amount of "safe" tar and nicotine in the cigarettes. Smoking does not only affect the smoker. It also affects individuals in close proximity to the one who is smoking by being exposed to secondhand smoke.

Long-term exposure to secondhand smoke is as bad for health as actually smoking cigarettes and causes similar health problems. Nonsmoking spouses of individuals who smoke have a high risk of lung cancer as well as heart problems. The children of smokers are also at high risk for cigarette smoke-related diseases because of constant exposure to cigarette smoke. Research studies have revealed that in Hawaii, 11% of the population is at risk of being exposed to secondhand smoke in their homes, and about 14% of children are at risk of being exposed to secondhand smoke.[432]

Secondhand smoke, which is also known as environmental tobacco smoke (ETS), is generally applied to any smoke from tobacco that non smokers are exposed to.[433] In their research report, Behan, Eriksen and Lin define environmental tobacco smoke as "the exposure of a nonsmoker to the combustion products of cigarettes and other tobacco products" (Behan, Eriksen & Lin, 2005). There are two types of ETS. The first one is the mainstream smoke, which is the smoke that smokers produce when they inhale and then exhale on a cigarette. The second one is what is known as the side stream smoke, which is the smoke that drifts into the environment from a lit cigarette or pipe. In a typical smoky room, about 85% of the smoke may be stream smoke. Environmental tobacco smoke (ETS) is a source of significant morbidity and mortality among those who have never smoked but have often found themselves in close proximity with individuals who smoke.

The 2006 report from United States Surgeon General had the following to say about secondhand smoking:

> The health effects of secondhand smoke exposure are more pervasive than we previously thought. The scientific evidence is now indisputable: secondhand smoke is not a mere annoyance. It is a serious health hazard that can lead to disease and premature death in children and nonsmoking adults...it can also cause heart disease and lung cancer in non-smoking adults and is a known cause of sudden infant death syndrome (SIDS), respiratory problems, ear infections and asthma attacks in infants and children.
>
> (Report of the Surgeon General, 2006)[434]

The Office of the Surgeon General working in tandem with the U.S Department of Health and Human Services and

The Perfect Prescription

other public health organizations in the nation has continued to disseminate information to enlighten the general public on the health risks of smoking. In an effort to underscore the harmfulness of environmental tobacco smoke, the office of the United States Surgeon General released a report, which cautioned that:

> There is no risk-free level of exposure to secondhand smoke. Nonsmokers exposed to secondhand smoke at home or work increase their risk of developing heart disease by 25 to 30 percent and lung cancer by 20 to 30 percent. The finding is of major public health concern due to the fact that nearly half of all nonsmoking Americans are still regularly exposed to secondhand smoke.
>
> (Report of the Surgeon General, 2006)[435]

Environmental tobacco smoke continues to threaten the health of everybody who comes in contact with it. Unfortunately, its health risks are worse for infants and young children exposed to it in indoor settings. The only way to completely protect them is not to expose them to smoke at all and to make homes, automobiles, work environments, and other public buildings frequented by non smokers smoke-free zones.

In the United States, monetary costs of health care expenses related to environmental tobacco smoking and those costs associated with morbidity and mortality are estimated to be over $10 billion. Between 2000 and 2004, cigarette smoking as well as exposure to cigarette smoke cost the United States $96.8 billion in the form of productivity loss.[436] An economic loss represented by a dollar amount is only part of the loss caused by cigarette smoke to society. People who smoke ultimately experience personal and family hardships associated with this habit, such as imminent onset of chronic diseases, emotional drain associated with those illnesses and death. These are unquantifiable and sometimes irrevocable losses not only to the family but to the community. They cannot be measured in economic terms.

Cigarette smoking continues to increase ominously, particularly among teenagers and young adults. What is more alarming is that the teenage and young adult population groups are not in any way concerned about the repercussions of these behavioral choices. Teenagers perceive smoking as a habit that enhances their standing and status among their peers. About 90% of current adult smokers picked up the habit in their teens.[437] Advertisements by tobacco companies in the form of T-shirts and ball caps that bear cigarette brand names continue to lure teenagers and young adults to adopt cigarette smoking. The infiltration of cigarette smoking is currently global in magnitude.

SMOKING IN DEVELOPING NATIONS

Tobacco use is beginning to increase in an unprecedented and disconcerting manner in developing nations. Developing nations are the new targets of cigarette smoking advertisements. These advertisements seem to be succeeding quite well.

In Ethiopia, most of what scientists and public health professionals know about the incidence and prevalence of smoking has been derived from studies conducted in the urban areas of the country. In the last two decades, Ethiopia has witnessed a disturbing rise in cigarette smoking rates. The effects of this rise are beginning to be keenly felt through an increase in tobacco-related diseases and deaths in the country. Often, in developing nations, the socio-economic status is a great predictor of tobacco use. In these nations, at the beginning of a tobacco-smoking epidemic, the rates tend to be high among individuals in high-income brackets. But as smoking begins to increase and saturate the country, it starts to seep down into low-income bracket communities as well, steadily making inroads into all socioeconomic groups of the country.

In Cambodia, about 67% of the male population living in urban areas smokes.[438] In rural areas, the percentage is higher at 86%. Street advertising of tobacco smoking rose by 400% in Cambodia between 1994 and 1997, and in 1997 one third of imported goods to this country was composed of cigarettes. The government is facing an uphill battle trying to control smoking, particularly among young adults who view the habit as an appealing adventure.

The Western Pacific Region, which is composed of East Asia and the Pacific, is reported by the World Health Organization (WHO) to have the highest smoking rates.[439] Approximately two thirds of the male population smoke tobacco in this region. About one in three cigarettes produced is consumed in the Western Pacific Region. Among the global teenage population aged between 13 and 15, one in five smoke in this region. Approximately between 80,000 and 100,000 children and young adults start smoking each day worldwide, and fifty percent of these live in Asia.

Children who start smoking in their adolescence are likely to continue smoking in their adult years. The WHO claims that children are influenced to start smoking by advertisements that glamorize tobacco smoking: " Through both its direct and indirect advertising, the tobacco industry associates cigarette smoking with athletic prowess, sexual attractiveness, professional success, adult sophistication, independence, adventure and self-fulfilment" (Ross Hammond, 2000).[440] This obviously catches the eyes of the young impressionable minds and lures them toward adopting this dreadful habit.

In Malaysia, about 30% of the children and young adults aged between 12 and 18 smoke. Smoking is rising not only among male teens but among females as well in this nation. Reports from the WHO Fact Sheet for 2002 further reveal that in the case of tobacco smoking advertising, Malaysia has been dubbed the "indirect advertising capital" of the world. Some of the tobacco industry's most blatant efforts to target young people can be seen in Malaysia. Spending on tobacco advertising is extremely high in Malaysia.

In 1997, the tobacco industry spent about $90 million in advertising. In 2000, two tobacco firms alone reportedly spent more than US $40 million. The situation in Malaysia is similar to that found in the Philippines, where 40% of adolescent boys smoke. There is no national policy or law in the Philippines prohibiting minors from procuring cigarettes. Approximately 20,000 smoking-related deaths occur each year in the Philippines.

Although smoking rates are still relatively low in Africa, tobacco use is beginning to increase at a faster rate on this continent than elsewhere in the world. In Kenya, the habit starts quite early in life.[441] Peer pressure, colorful and incessant advertising, and age are among the greatest influencers of starting the habit of smoking among older teenagers and young adults in Kenya. Parents and teachers' smoking habits influence the younger children. In a study conducted by Schoenmaker and associates in Ethiopia among individuals aged 15 years and above, it was revealed that 11.8% of the men were smokers.[442] Among women, the rates were significantly low (0.2%). The average daily cigarette consumption per person was 6.6 cigarettes a day.

SMOKING DURING PREGNANCY

The concentration of cotinine, an alkaloid and metabolite found in tobacco can be vertically transmitted to the fetus in utero through maternal tobacco smoking during pregnancy. "It has been estimated that the total nicotine dose received by children whose parents smoke is equivalent to their actively smoking between 60 and 150 cigarettes per year" (Hawamdeh, Kasasbeh & Ahmad).[443]

An assessment of schoolchildren for levels of salivary cotinine concentrations in a Jordanian population revealed that the levels of cotinine correlated significantly with the smoking habits of the children's parents particularly the mothers. Cigarette smoking during pregnancy can also increase prenatal mortality and premature labor as well as placental abruption. Smoking during pregnancy can also be a risk factor for congenital damage to the respiratory system of the fetus. The rapidly developing delicate respiratory system of the fetus is considerably sensitive and susceptible to being damaged by substances such as nicotine and cotinine. Other health conditions that can be caused by maternal smoking during pregnancy include suppression of the fetus' immune system as well as impairment of leukocyte function. Mild neurological developmental problems have also been found to be associated with smoking during pregnancy.

A 1974 study by Harlap and Davies conducted among more than 10,000 infants demonstrated that infants whose mothers were smokers during pregnancy had been admitted into one hospital or another for treatment of bronchitis or pneumonia, particularly in winter, at a rate that was 28% higher than their counterparts whose mothers were not smokers.[444] The rate of bronchitis and pneumonia among infants exposed to smoke increased as the number of cigarettes smoked by the mother increased during pregnancy.

In 2004, scientists conducted a population-based cohort study in which they followed 58,841 singleton births in Finland using data from nationwide registries.[445] The births were followed over a period of 7 years to assess associations between maternal smoking habits during pregnancy and risk for childhood asthma. The results revealed that maternal tobacco smoking during pregnancy significantly increases the risk of asthma for children during the first 7 years their lives.

Smoking has also been repeatedly implicated as a risk factor for stillbirths. The risk of stillbirths increases as the rate of maternal smoking increases. In a Swedish research study, over 526,000 pregnant women were observed during their first and second pregnancies to assess the role of smoking habits on the risk of subsequent stillbirths.[446] The women's information about their smoking habits was gathered by the researchers from standardized antenatal records. The participants were categorized as nonsmokers, moderate smokers, and heavy smokers- three categories. Birth registers that kept unique registration numbers of the mothers allowed the researchers to access information about births. The results of the study indicated that women who smoked in their first and second pregnancies had a significantly increased risk of stillbirth in the second pregnancy.

The women who stopped smoking from their first pregnancy to the second pregnancy had a lower risk of stillbirth. From these results the researchers also believe that there are numerous adverse effects of maternal smoking during pregnancy including neonatal deaths, pre-term births and intrauterine growth retardation. Smoking has also been implicated in stunted fetal growth and placental disruption, which are some of the main causes of stillbirths.

The report from the Scientific Committee on Emerging and Newly Identified Health Risks (SCENIHR) in Europe examined the adverse health effects of smokeless tobacco, which includes moist snuff, chewing tobacco, dry snuff, and nasal snuff.[447] Apart from containing addictive substances, smokeless tobacco products (STP) also contain carcinogens such as nitrosamines. These carcinogens primarily target the pancreas in their destructive work. They also are high risk factors for oral cancer. These diseases can shorten one's life expectancy and undermine productivity.

THE BIBLE AND TOBACCO SMOKING

Because of what it does to the health of not only those who smoke it but also those who find themselves, inevitably around smokers such as children and spouses, tobacco smoking does not honor God. It hurts the body, which the Scriptures expressly call the temple of the Holy Spirit. One does not have to be a believer in God to acknowledge that tobacco smoking has brought untold suffering to those who have found themselves inextricably held in its grip.

The practice of tobacco smoking was non-existent in Bible times. Therefore, the Bible does not directly address or mention tobacco smoking by name. However, since the Lord God wants us to enjoy good health, it is logical to conclude that he does not sanction any type of habit that is injurious to our health including smoking. In 1 Corinthians 10:31 the Bible tells us that "So, whether you eat or drink, or whatever you do, do all to the glory of God." No one can honestly say that they smoke in order to glorify God. Because of the myriad health problems associated with tobacco smoking, it cannot be classified as one of the habits that bring glory to God.

Tobacco is not a natural food that can be readily given to children. It is a harmful substance. Sometimes it is tempting to defend smoking by pointing to the fact that most Christians who speak against smoking have other vices such as unhealthy eating habits that include food addictions. Some people argue that because some great preachers like Charles H. Spurgeon enjoyed smoking cigars, they also can. That may be true, but it does not make it right either. Those were mortal men who were susceptible to making wrong decisions and sinning. The fact is that tobacco smoke hurts the health and well-being of any person who inhales it and those around them.

Public health interventions against cigarette smoking in the United States have focused on discouraging the general public from smoking altogether. Other interventions by public health professionals have included putting pressure on government to enact policies and enforce laws that forbid the sale of tobacco products to minors. Because of this pressure from public health professionals, laws have been enacted that place restrictions on indoor smoking. Another public health intervention method has included proposals to increase cigarette prices and to impose significant taxes on cigarettes as a deterrent strategy. All these strategies are focused on promoting the health of the general public by reducing their exposure to an injurious substance. This is an approach that has its foundation in biblical health laws. It is another echo of biblical health-promoting principles.

CHAPTER 24

HIV INFECTION AND CIRCUMCISION

He that is eight days old among you shall be circumcised; every male throughout your generations, whether born in your house, or bought with your money from any foreigner who is not of your offspring,

(Genesis 17:12)

Some societies observe the practice of infant male circumcision. A few days after the male child is born it is circumcised for various reasons. In the 1900s, in the United States, the practice of infant circumcision began to flourish because it was generally viewed as a necessary procedure by both physicians and parents.[448] However, over the years, some physicians began to question the benefits of the practice. Debates arose between parents and physicians about the health benefits of infant circumcision. Some parents wondered why "genital mutilation" should be practiced on infants. In response to the emerging debate of the 1930s about circumcision, a myriad of research studies have been conducted by different researchers and scientists to prove or disprove the claim that the practice of infant circumcision has any health benefits at all.

In 1932, Dr. A. L. Wolbarst reviewed 1,103 fatal penile cancer cases. In his findings, there was not a single Jewish man found to have had a case of penile cancer.[449] Subsequent studies and reviews of cases of penile cancer were conducted including the one conducted by Dagher in which the findings of the review indicated that there was not a single circumcised man who had been found with the disease out of the 521 cases reviewed.[450]

In 1900, Dr. Hiram Wineberg conducted a research study at New York's Mount Sinai Hospital to assess the incidence and prevalence of cervical cancer among Jewish women.[451] The findings of the study revealed that these women were relatively free from cervical cancer. Dr. Ira I. Kaplan and R. Rosh replicated the study in 1947 at New York's Bellevue Hospital. The study was reported in the 1947 June issue of the *American Journal of Roentgenology*. Their findings were consistent with those of Dr. Wineberg: cervical cancer was virtually nonexistent among Jewish women.[452]

In 1954, another milestone study that was conducted to assess rates of cervical cancer among women in Boston found that cancer rates among non-Jewish women were eight and a half times more than among Jewish women.[453] Scientists attributed the low incidence of cancer among Jewish women to the practice of routine circumcision among their males.

However, other scientists repudiated these claims about the health benefits of male circumcision. For example, in his 1967 response to advocates of circumcision, Dr. Morgan, in the *Medical Journal of Australia*, called the procedure "the cult of circumcision" and that "those in favor of the operation are almost without exception intense, humourless and terrifyingly evangelical" (Morgan, 1967).[454]

He further contended that "soap and water" was the only reason why some population groups have a low incidence of penile cancer. According to Dr. Morgan, population groups with a high incidence of penile cancer had questionable hygiene standards. It was about hygiene not uncircumcision. Other researchers including Zoossmann-Diskin of Australia echoed Dr. Morgan's views and vehemently refuted the practice of circumcision as a preventive procedure against cancer of the cervix. In 1994, Warren and Bigelow wrote an article in the *British Journal of Sexual Medicine*, contending that:

> We do not know why this operation (circumcision) was carried out, but many writers have suggested that it was a sacrificial rite. No doubt human sacrifice was widespread, and it seems likely that substitutes for this practice included the sacrifice of domestic animals and mutilations of the human body, of which circumcision is just one example. Circumcision would usually have been carried out as an initiation ordeal at about the time of puberty, but there was a tendency for the age at which it was performed to shift earlier, so that Jewish ritual circumcision has been carried out on the eighth day of life since biblical times.
>
> (Warren & Bigelow, 1994)[455]

In 1966, the United Nations took a stand regarding the routine circumcision of male babies by questioning whether the infant child had freedom of speech as indicated by the United Nations Convention on the Rights of the Child. The United Nations Convention on the Rights of the Child, Article 13, Part 1 stated that: "The child shall have the right to freedom of expression... [*infant circumcision circumvents the child's freedom to decide for himself what parts of his body to keep, and his freedom of sexual expression by permanently and unnecessarily diminishing his sexual sensations*]."[456] Emboldened by the stand taken by the United Nations Convention on the Rights of the Child, the American Academy of Pediatrics issued the following statement concerning routine neonatal male circumcision in 1971: "there are no valid medical indications for circumcision in the neonatal period. The present committee has undertaken a review of data to support arguments 'pro' and 'con' circumcision of the newborn, and finds no basis for changing this statement" (American Academy of Pediatrics, 1971).[457]

Shortly afterwards the Report of the Ad Hoc Task Force on Circumcision which evaluated the practice of neonatal male circumcision claimed that "There are no medical indications for routine circumcisions, and the procedure cannot be considered an essential component of health care....The skin is a protective organ, and any break in its integrity affords an opportunity for initiation of infection" (Thompson, et al. 1975). [458]

In 1989 the Academy examined new research on the association of circumcision with the incidence of urinary tract infection (UTI) and issued another statement in which it stated that "Newborn circumcision has potential medical benefits and advantages as well as disadvantages and risks" (American Academy of Pediatrics, 1989).[459] The latter statement seemed to be softening the Academy's earlier stance about circumcision. Over three decades, the American Academy of Pediatrics published five policy statements on neonatal circumcision. The latest one was published in 1999 and states that:

> Existing scientific evidence demonstrates potential medical benefits of newborn male circumcision; however, these data are not sufficient to recommend routine neonatal circumcision. In circumstances in which there are potential benefits and risks, yet the procedure is not essential to the child's current well-being, parents should determine what is in the best interest of the child. To make an informed choice, parents of all male infants should be given accurate and unbiased information and be provided the opportunity to discuss this decision. If a decision for circumcision is made, procedural analgesia should be provided.
>
> (American Academy of Pediatrics, 1999)[460]

Concerning risk of urinary tract infection (UTI) in uncircumcised infants that American Academy of Pediatrics stated that "All studies that have examined the association between UTI [urinary tract infection] and circumcision status show an increased risk of UTI in uncircumcised males, with the greatest risk in infants younger than 1 year of age. Evidence regarding the relationship of circumcision to STD [sexually transmitted diseases] in general is complex and conflicting" (American Academy of Pediatrics, 1999).[461]

In an article that appeared in the *Archives of Pediatrics & Adolescence Medicine* of June 2010, Dr. Aaron A.R. Tobian and his associates challenged the American Academy of Pediatrics (AAP) vacillating policies on male circumcision. They contended that more research has been conducted in the previous four years to re-evaluate the AAP policy regarding routine neonatal circumcision including three randomized clinical trials focused on the assessment of the benefits of circumcision to health. Dr. Tobian and his team's report revealed that:

> Circumcision decreases human immunodeficiency virus acquisition by 53% to 60%, herpes simplex virus type 2 acquisitions by 28% to 34%, and human papillomavirus prevalence by 32% to 35% in men. Among female partners of circumcised men, bacterial vaginosis was reduced by 40%, and *Trichomonas vaginalis* infection was reduced by 48%. Genital ulcer disease was also reduced among males and their female partners. These findings are also supported by observational studies conducted in the United States.
>
> (Tobian, 2010)[462]

Dr. Tobian and his team acknowledge that there have been concerns that the results of the three randomized trials conducted in Africa may not be applicable to the United States because the modes of transmission differ to a certain extent. For example, the primary route of transmission of HIV from one individual to another in Africa is via heterosexual intercourse while, in the United States, significant infection with HIV infection is acquired through intravenous drug use and men having sex with men. However, even in the United States there is a significant percentage of HIV infection occurring through heterosexual intercourse that could be prevented by circumcision.

Statistics by Dr. Tobian and his team indicate that African Americans represent 13% of the entire population of the United States. But they account for approximately 48% of all HIV infections, and in some inner cities, the rates of infection are almost on the same level as those observed in Africa. Infection with HIV through heterosexual exposure is becoming the leading route of HIV transmission among African Americans. The incidence of HIV among teens and young adults in Washington, D.C., is 38%. This means that the benefits of circumcision demonstrated in the African randomized clinical trials can be applicable to other HIV high-risk heterosexual groups in the United States and other areas where HIV infection is endemic.

Nevertheless, critics contend that the African findings of adult circumcision trials may not justify neonatal circumcision, but Dr. Tobian's team reports that a significant number of observational studies conducted in Africa included participants who were circumcised in their infancy. The team also asserts that the remarkable consistency of the results of both observational and randomized controlled clinical studies demonstrate that the concern about circumcision as a preventive procedure against STDs including HIV is unfounded.

This consistency establishes the long-term prophylactic effect of male circumcision. Commenting on the benefits of circumcision, Dr. McMillen observes that "If the tight, unretractable foreskin is not removed, proper cleansing cannot be readily performed. As a result many virulent bacteria, including the cancer-producing Smegma bacillus, can grow profusely" (McMillen, n.d.).[463]

The Perfect Prescription

A publication called *Horizons*, founded by the Population Council in collaboration with other organizations and institutions such as the International Center for Research on Women, the International HIV/AIDS Alliance, the Program for Appropriate Technology in Health, the University of Alabama, and Tulane University, and supported by the U. S. Agency for International Development and the Office of Health and Nutrition, Global Bureau, states that a growing body of scientific findings has demonstrated that male circumcision is considered to be associated with reduced risk of HIV infection in sub-Sahara Africa.[464] The report confirms that although most of the studies on male circumcision and its health benefits were conducted in Africa, the findings are relevant and may can be applicable to other parts of the world where HIV infection is expanding.

The effort by public health officials to advocate male circumcision as a preventive intervention against HIV infection is growing. The World Health Organization (WHO) claims that its decision to advocate mass circumcision was a result of having reviewed various research studies that proved that medical male circumcision reduced HIV infection significantly. Basing their position on research about the health benefits of male circumcision, both the WHO and USAIDS concluded that male circumcision should be considered an efficacious intervention method to curb HIV infection in the most susceptible regions of the world.

The WHO further asserted that "There is compelling evidence that male circumcision reduces the risk of heterosexually acquired HIV infection in men by approximately 60%" (WHO, 2012).[465] Consequently, WHO and USAID have adopted male circumcision as one of the intervention methods against the spread of HIV in countries where it is endemic, particularly in those countries where circumcision has not been a routine procedure. However, individuals who are already infected with HIV are exempted from medical male circumcision unless it is recommended by a physician for particular medical reasons.

If circumcision has no health benefits, as some critics claim, it would be morally and scientifically inappropriate for the World Health Organization and the United States Agency for International Development (USAID) to advocate and implement mass circumcision programs in Africa and elsewhere as an intervention strategy against the spread of sexually transmitted diseases (STDs), including HIV. Encouraging people to undergo an unprofitable invasive surgical procedure would be unethical. It would also be a breach of the very human rights, which the World Health Organization has been upholding all along. In addition, it would be an unnecessary waste of resources.

The United Nations Programmme on AIDS (UNAIDS) and the World Health Organization (WHO) have developed a toolkit that provides guidelines on conducting mass circumcision. The toolkit includes types of procedures to be utilized, key policies and cultural issues to be taken into account during the program. The key policy options established include indentifying priority populations for this undertaking such as all male adults, young male adults, adolescent males, newborn males, and males at high risk for HIV infection.

All services must be delivered in hospitals, clinics, mobile vans, and in private, nongovernmental medical locations with surgeons, family physicians, and clinical officers presiding over the operations. This intervention strategy has received strong political commitment and leadership from governments of target nations as well as financial help from private organizations including the Melinda and Bill Gates Foundation, which injected $50 million into the program.[466]

Having suffered unprecedented loss of human capital due to AIDS, many sub-Saharan African countries are in an economically desperate condition and are ready to cooperate with the international community to reduce the incidence of HIV. It brings them some hope that there could be an end to the HIV/AIDS nightmare. It is, therefore, not surprising that they have responded positively to the mass circumcision intervention strategy.

The following news report form Zambia National Broadcasting Company of June 18, 2009 indicated that:

> The Zambia Police Service says plans are underway to introduce a mandatory circumcision policy for all male recruits. Kamfinsa Police training school commanding Officer, Malcom Mulenga, says male circumcision will help prevent HIV and AIDS cases in the Police service. Mr. Mulenga says the Zambia Police Service has continued to lose qualified manpower as a result HIV/AIDS. He was speaking when the American government handed over a Voluntary Counselling and Testing centre to the Zambia Police Service. At the same function, Home Affairs deputy Minister, Misheck Bonshe, welcomed plans by the Zambia Police Service to circumcise male recruits. And the United States Charge d' Affairs for Zambia, Michael Koplovsky, said his government has set aside K1.5 billion for the construction of health centres for police officers.
>
> (Zambia National Broadcasting Company, 2009)[467]

According to a report from Integrated Regional Information Networks (IRIN) Humanitarian News Analysis, which is a service of the United Nations (UN) Office for the Coordination of Humanitarian Affairs, thirteen sub-Saharan African countries have adopted the mass circumcision program and have included in it their national HIV prevention policies.[468] These countries are depicted below:

Kenya has focused its male medical circumcision effort on the Nyanza province, which has the highest prevalence of HIV/AIDS and where only 40% of the men have been circumcised. By the end of 2009, over 90,000 men had been circumcised in Kenya. By 2013, it is hoped that about 1.1 million of Kenyan men will have undergone the procedure.

Zambia:

Zambia happens to be one of the hotspots of HIV infection in sub-Saharan Africa. Food production at household level in Zambia has been adversely affected by inadequate labor due to the impact of HIV/AIDS, which is affecting the most productive age group. This scenario is common in other sub-Saharan African countries as well. Only about 13% of the male population is circumcised. However, plans are underway to circumcise approximately 250,000 men every year. In 2009, 16,000 men were circumcised at eleven sites. The goal is to have 300 sites offering these services by 2014.

Swaziland:

The prevalence of circumcision is 8%. Government aims to step up circumcision among 80% of men aged 15 to 24 by the year 2014. Swaziland has the highest HIV prevalence in the world. By the end of 2009, only about 5,000 men had undergone the procedure.

Botswana:

By April 2009, more than 4,300 men had been circumcised in Botswana. The Ministry of Health in Botswana continues to scale-up circumcision practices and services and aims to reach approximately 460,000 HIV negative men and boys below the age of 49 by 2012.

Zimbabwe:

In April of 2009, Zimbabwe launched the pilot phase of the circumcision intervention strategy, in which 1,818 men were circumcised. The country established an official national male circumcision policy in November 2009.

Rwanda:

The government of Rwanda embarked on a mass male circumcision exercise in its army where HIV/AIDS prevalence is 4.5% compared to the national prevalence of 3%. The nation is being urged to scale-up circumcision across the rest of the population groups especially among the youth.

South Africa:

The government of South Africa had the draft of the national circumcision policy completed by December 2009. The male circumcision HIV intervention strategy is moving much more slowly in this country in spite of the fact that South Africa has the world's largest HIV positive population. Approximately 35% of South African men are circumcised. Only one site is providing the services, Orange Farm, near Johannesburg, where more than 14,253 men were circumcised in 2009.

Namibia:

A draft of the national circumcision policy was presented to parliament in 2009. Five circumcision sites have been identified and two of them are in operation. Surgical health professionals are being trained to undertake the process. The unit cost per circumcision procedure is quite prohibitive in Namibia at US $88 for an adult male and US $72 for a newborn. These costs could hamper progress. Government is being urged to lower the cost.

Lesotho:

This small mountain country has already approved a national policy for circumcision although it has not yet been launched.

Nevertheless, the circumcision program has already started and approximately 4,000 men are being circumcised yearly at both government and private clinics in Lesotho. A countrywide Non-Governmental Organization (NGO) called Puisano Outreach Organization is promoting male circumcision as a tool for prevention against HIV throughout the country.

TANZANIA:

Overall, male circumcision is well accepted in this nation. Any procedure that has the potential to reduce or eradicate HIV/AIDS on the African continent is likely to be well received because that is where the burden of the disease is greatest. All that is required is to make sure that the program is well explained and understood by the target population groups to increase compliance. About 70% of men are already circumcised in this nation. A national policy is being developed and three sites have been set up to provide circumcision services.

MOZAMBIQUE:

Currently, no formal government circumcision policy exists. However, an existing HIV prevention approach already includes male circumcision. Five sites have been designated to provide services in order to scale-up the program.

MALAWI:

Data analyses are being conducted in this nation to form a foundation for a proper circumcision strategy. Meanwhile an NGO named Banja la Mtsogolo is already providing male circumcision services in its clinics with the help of its 19 trained clinicians.

UGANDA:

This is one of the nations that has hosted a number of research studies that confirmed the association between circumcision and reduction in HIV infection rates although only about 25% of its male population is circumcised. At the time of the report from IRIN, Uganda still had no national male circumcision policy nor had it started service delivery.

The Bible tells us that God instituted the practice of male circumcision. He made the following covenant with Abraham:

> As for you, you shall keep my covenant, you and your descendants after you throughout their generations. This is my covenant, which you shall keep, between me and you and your descendants after you: Every male among you shall be circumcised. You shall be circumcised in the flesh of your foreskins, and it shall be a sign of the covenant between me and you. He that is eight days old among you shall be circumcised; every male throughout your generations, whether born in your house, or bought with your money from any foreigner who is not of your offspring.
>
> (Genesis 17:9-12)

In response, Abraham obeyed the commandment of the Lord:

> Then Abraham took Ish'mael his son and all the slaves born in his house or bought with his money, every male among the men of Abraham's house, and he circumcised the flesh of their foreskins that very day, as God had said to him. Abraham was ninety-nine years old when he was circumcised in the flesh of his foreskin. And Ish'mael his son was thirteen years old when he was circumcised in the flesh of his foreskin. That very day Abraham and his son Ish'mael were circumcised; and all the men of his house,

those born in the house and those bought with money from a foreigner, were circumcised with him.

(Genesis 17:23-27)

And the people of Israel have honored and observed that commandment ever since the day it was given. The succeeding generations after Abraham were to circumcise every male infant who was eight days old. Every time God gives instructions to His people, He does so because He wants them to enjoy good health and have a close fellowship with Him. Jesus said He had come to give abundant life. God's man-ward movement is for the benefit of all mankind all the time. Although, in the New Covenant, it is true that circumcision is not required for salvation or for making the believer righteous, it has medical and health benefits, which have been verified by many research studies cited earlier in the book.

Why was the rite of circumcision to be conducted on the eighth day? Scientists Zeigler and Oakes present the following reasons as propounded by the scientific community:[469]

1. Blood Clotting Proteins (Prothrombin) are continually produced in the liver;
2. The Liver needs Vitamin K to make clotting proteins;
3. Vitamin K is produced in our intestinal tract;
4. When a baby is born the Vitamin K levels are similar to that of the mother;
5. Infants are born without the required bacteria in their intestines to produce Vitamin K;
6. It takes about five days for the bacteria to build up in order for the baby to start producing its own Vitamin K and;
7. Between zero and six days the level of Prothrombin drops to 30 percent of normal.

(Zeigler & Oakes, 2008)

According to scientists, the greatest risk of profuse bleeding occurs between the second and sixth days of the infant's life. God told Abraham and Moses to conduct neonatal circumcision for male infants on the eighth day when the risk of profuse bleeding would be low. That was over 4,000 years ago, and it is still relevant for health promotion. Health professionals are now beginning to use it to combat sexually transmitted diseases. God's truth does not need to be defended. It defends itself.

When the practice of neonatal circumcision was adopted by western doctors, they often did the surgery almost immediately after the baby was born, even before the eighth day while the baby and its mother were still in hospital. The doctors were puzzled to notice that it was not uncommon for the babies to bleed profusely after the surgery. It was in the 1900s that scientists discovered that vitamin K was necessary for blood clotting and that the bodies of babies did not start making vitamin K until after they were five days old.

Dr. Rex Russell recounts an experience he had in his first surgical cases involving circumcising a neonate.[470] After he had finished conducting surgery he bandaged the wound and left the baby to rest. After a while, he came back to check on his patient only to find that the bandage was drenched with blood from the wound. Vitamin K had to be administered to the patient to help the blood start to clot. The bleeding was significantly reduced, though it continued for another couple of days.

Specialists conducted some tests to find out whether the baby was a hemophiliac. He was not a hemophiliac. The established procedure at the medical institution required that male babies should be circumcised during the first three days after birth. During this time, vitamin K, the blood clotting agent, is absent in the blood of the neonate, hence the profuse bleeding from the surgery.

We know that God does not coerce anyone into doing anything. He prefers that we exercise our power of choice. Therefore, in spite of the benefits of routine circumcision, if the parents of the neonate have misgivings about having the baby circumcised, they should have the right to decide against it. But it is important for them to learn from the pediatrician how to thoroughly clean the foreskin of the baby's penis and to teach him how to do it properly for himself when he is of age. If they decide to have the baby circumcised, they need to have it done in a clinical setting where a trained physician will perform and monitor its healing process. Additionally, if there is no consensus between the parents about circumcising the baby, it may be prudent not to do it.

Chapter 25

Elder Abuse

You shall rise up before the hoary head, and honor the face of an old man, and you shall fear your God: I am the Lord.

(Leviticus 19:32)

When a society views the elderly population as a source of wisdom and as custodians of societal values on which the cultural stability of a community is dependent, it learns to honor and respect them. But if old age is viewed as a "loss, a decline from the best in life, a major demographic problem, a drain on the economy, something which could overwhelm the health system" (Conference of European Churches, 2007)[471] then a way is opened for elder resentment, abuse, and ill-treatment.

This perception can also instigate discrimination known as ageism against the elderly, which can be exacerbated by the functional disability of the elderly as well as other forms of impairment, which compel them to be more dependent on others for activities of daily living. The more dependent they become, the more they are perceived as a source of annoyance.

The World Health Organization describes elder abuse as "a single or repeated act, or lack of appropriate action occurring within any relationship where there is an expectation of trust, which causes harm or distress to an older person."[472] Another definition of elder abuse from the Encyclopedia of Aging is "the careless, indifferent, or malicious lack of attention by a designated or implied caregiver that results in harm from an elder's basic human needs not being met"[473] and because negligence usually involves inaction or lack of action on the part of the perpetrator, it is difficult to quantify. It can only be detected when its cumulative effects are seen on the victim. Elder abuse is multidimensional, which means that it takes many forms including physical abuse, psychological abuse, financial exploitation, emotional abuse, medication abuse, abandonment, and exploitation or marginalization of the interests of elderly people reflected in social and economic policies that exclude or ignore their well-being.[474]

Elder physical abuse takes place when an elderly person sustains injury through hitting, slapping, kicking, burning, or being coerced into doing something they would rather not do. Sometimes physical abuse may go unnoticed even in the presence of telltale marks on the body of the elderly individual since, most of the time, it is assumed that the elderly have unstable balance and can easily trip and fall or bump themselves against some fixture and sustain a bruise or injury. Those entrusted with the responsibility of protecting the elderly from abuse should watch for the following signs of abuse:[475]

1. If the elderly person is not being properly taken care of they usually have open wounds, particularly if they are mostly bedridden. The wounds might also be an indication that they have been stabbed or burned by a cigarette or hurt by any other injurious weapon.
2. If an elderly person has welt marks on the body, it could be a sign that they are being beaten with a belt or a stick or any object that is likely to produce welts on a human being.

The Perfect Prescription

3. Sometimes elderly people who are not properly cared for might have unexplained sprains, broken limbs, gashes or fractures. These could be caused by being pushed by the abuser or being shoved. Other forms of physical strain exerted on them can injure them in similar manner.
4. When the abuser punches the elderly person, they might sustain a black eye. Other times they have scratch marks. Some of these injuries can be quite severe such as a broken nose or limb.
5. Sudden hair loss manifesting itself as patches on the head should be able to arouse suspicion of elder abuse as well. Abusers might grab the elderly person by the hair and remove some of it leaving visible patches.

Another common form of elder abuse is sexual abuse, which involves coercing an elderly person to take part in any type of sexual act.[476] A sexually abused elderly person may have bruises around the genital and breast area, indicating that force was used to get the person into submission. An abused elderly person can also suddenly develop unexplained venereal disease or any other related infection in the genital area as a result of being infected by the abuser. In some cases they could manifest anal and genital bleeding from constant sexual abuse.[477] Blood on their clothes can also be a sign of being abused, and so can torn undergarments.

Elder abusers can sometimes subject their victims to emotional abuse. Emotional abuse is a kind of behavior that can cause harm to the elderly person's self-worth and psychological well-being. This type of abuse can include name-calling. It can also be in the form of deliberately embarrassing the elderly person by making snide remarks about them. Abusers can even destroy their victim's property on purpose and stop them from socializing with their friends or other members of their family.

When the elderly person is constantly subjected to that kind of treatment, they might respond by developing a demeanor marked by emotional agitation or they may become significantly withdrawn and refuse to communicate. Other times they might manifest such strange behavior as biting whoever comes close to them, or they may start rocking themselves in an effort to comfort themselves. It is also not unusual for them to develop aggressive behavior marked by insulting and threatening, or they may choose to totally ignore their family members and other acquaintances. Often they might insist that they be left alone or they might even isolate themselves by sitting away from everybody else.

There are times when those who are entrusted with caring for the elderly neglect and ignore them. Elder neglect includes the caregiver's failure to satisfy the basic needs of the elderly person, such as giving them the food they need at the right time or failure to provide them with shelter or housing or clothing. Those who are charged with the responsibility of monitoring the well-being of an elderly person should make sure that the elderly person has no injuries that are not being properly cared for.[478]

Neglected elderly people usually have unexplained wounds or injuries to their bodies. They can also have unexplained sunken eyes as well as cheeks mostly due to weight loss as a result of not being properly fed. A neglected elderly person often wears dirty clothes and has unkempt hair. If they do not have their aids such as a walking cane or walker even when their medical history indicates that they should use them all the time, it is a sign that their wellbeing is not seriously taken into consideration. They are being neglected. There are also cases in which elderly people are left alone in the home with no one to monitor them or provide the care they need. This is called abandonment.

Elderly abandonment can include leaving the elderly at bus stops, airports, or any other public place alone. When the elderly are thus abandoned, they may suffer incredible agitation, fear, and psychological anguish, which can worsen their health condition. In countries where there are few social services to address the needs of the elderly, their children are expected to take care of them.

The Perfect Prescription

If they have no children of their own, their closest next of kin is expected take care of them. In countries where there are government programs, the well-being of the elderly is often left in the hands of public programs entrusted with such responsibilities. In either case, it is possible for elderly people to suffer at the hands of those who are supposed to care for them.

Financial exploitation is another type of abuse the elderly can be subjected to. Often this occurs when an elderly person's money, property, and assets are misused by the caregiver.[479] Financial exploitation constitutes the unauthorized expenditure of the elderly person's funds by the caregiver. Financial exploitation of the elderly often includes misusing their credit cards and personal checks by buying items they did not authorize. It can also take the form of outright stealing of cash and other valuable household items from the elderly by the caregiver or whoever the perpetrator may be. Sometimes financial exploitation takes the form of forging the elderly individual's signature in order to make unauthorized purchases. Oftentimes financial exploiters coerce the elderly into changing their wills to favor the abuser or to hand over rights to their assets to the caregiver.

The list of elder abuse is almost endless. Medication abuse is another significant type of elder abuse. This can include overmedicating the elderly person, or it can take the form of dispensing medication that is not necessary or appropriate. Other times medication abuse is under-medication of an elderly individual so that they are deprived of necessary medication. Sometimes the abuser can use under-medication as a form of punishment for so-called deviant behavior or as a type of blackmail or death threat. Such a threat might be a threat against the elderly that that they will die unless they surrender their medication to the abuser. Over-medication can be used to keep vocal elderly people sedated and unable to voice their opinions or needs.

Exploitation and marginalization of elder interests can also occur through social and economic policies. This is often "a process and a state that prevents individuals or groups from full participation in social, economic and political life and from asserting their rights. It derives from exclusionary relationships based on power" (Economic and Social Commission for Western Asia, 2007).[480] In such cases, public health professionals should advocate for policies that encourage elder participation in policy making undertakings to make their voices heard and to ensure that their right to live with dignity is upheld.

Elderly people should also be allowed to actively participate in planning, designing, and implementing programs related to ageing. This allows them to speak about ageing from experience and from an informed vantage point. Policies that promote or tolerate socioeconomic and healthcare disparities and other practices that fuel elder discrimination and marginalization should be identified, challenged, modified or completely eliminated.

In traditional Africa, the elderly were taken care of by their children. Elders were always treated with great respect in African communities. They were the people who were summoned for advice whenever conflict arose, whether it was familial or inter-tribal in magnitude. However, in the changing socioeconomic landscape of Africa, younger generations have migrated to urban centers to find education and employment leaving the elderly to fend for themselves.[481]

The coming of the AIDS pandemic has placed unprecedented responsibilities on the elderly population group of Africa. It has also significantly changed their role. The decimation of a significant proportion of Africa's younger productive generation means that their orphaned children have to be put in the care of their grandparents since there are not enough public programs to cater for the needs of all the orphans. The elderly are now contending with a multifaceted tragedy of losing the economic support of their deceased children, taking care of their HIV infected children as well as taking care of the orphans whose parents have already succumbed to AIDS. These elderly people also have to deal with their own personal age-related health problems. HelpAge, an international organization standing up for the rights of older people, recounts the following story from an elderly lady in Kenya:

> My daughter died and left behind four orphans. She was unmarried and her brothers have refused to take responsibility over the orphans. As their grandmother, I could not stand aside and watch them suffer. I decided to take care of them. Unfortunately, I do not have enough strength to till land and generate food and money for our up-keep. I rely on assistance from the Misyani HelpAge, which provides some food and medical assistance to me. I am forced to share the little food I get with my grandchildren since I cannot eat alone as they watch.
>
> (Help-Age 2001)[482]

In the above story, elder abuse is manifesting itself in the refusal of surviving grown children to assume the roles of guardians for their deceased siblings' children. Local and international organizations are making coalitions in an effort to address the plight and abuse of these elders of Africa by formulating appropriate intervention strategies and proposing enactment of policies to protect the rights of the elderly population groups where they do not exist.

Elder abuse in the healthcare sector in Kenya has been identified as a source of concern. Often the elderly patients are unable to satisfy the payments for health care introduced in government hospitals because they have no source of income. This means that they cannot always have access to healthcare services when they need them. As a consequence, they turn to traditional healers and midwives whom they perceive to be more amiable and less expensive than government hospitals.

Cases of abandonment that involve the elderly are, reportedly, increasing in Kenya. Some of the elderly people who manage to pay for hospital care are often left abandoned there by their children or relatives. Approximately three in twenty of these elderly individuals are left abandoned. Medical care for them is also often delayed by the intricacies of a bureaucratic system trying to establish whether they qualify for a fee waiver or not.

According to the National Center on Elder Abuse, there are also thousands of elderly people being abused all over the United States, but there are no official national statistics.[483] Therefore, the actual figure of abused elders is unknown. One reason for the absence of state statistics is due to lack of a uniform or standardized reporting system. The other reason no national comprehensive statistics related to elder abuse are collected is because of a lack of a large-scale nationwide tracking system.

Statistical estimates about the problem of elder abuse depicted below have been garnered from private investigators over the years. Between 1 and 3 million elderly people over 65 have been injured, ill treated, or exploited in one way or another. The rate of elder abuse is between 2% and 10%, and about 1 in 14 incidents of elder abuse take place at home. Other estimates indicate that about 5 million cases of elder financial extortion and exploitation take place every year.[484,485] As indicated above, the actual prevalence rate is unknown since about 20% of elder abuse cases go unreported. But estimates indicate that approximately 472, 000 elders were abused in 2000. Some elderly people experience significant forms of abuse or potential neglect in long-term facilities as well.[486]

Elder abuse rates are higher in certain areas than in others. According to a report by Hamilton and that of the Maine Department of Health and Human Services, "Maine, the nation's oldest state in median age and second most rural state, has a rate of elder abuse estimated to be above the national average" and that "Maine's elderly suicide rate is among the highest in the United States."[487,488] But tragically, only one in fourteen occurrences are reported, which means that most elder abuse events go unreported and undetected.

The Perfect Prescription

Elder abuse is a hidden problem within most societies because the perpetrator might be a member of the family of the victim who also might even be functioning as a primary caregiver and on whom the victim is totally dependent for various needs. In cases where the abuser is a child or spouse of the abused person, the victim usually chooses to withstand abuse rather than risk losing the ties they may believe to have with the abuser. Usually the victim might opt to handle the problem within the family than to involve the legal system. Other times the victim might tend to underestimate the impact of the abuse on their general health. It is also possible that the victims fear that if they report the abuse, their living arrangements may change and that they might have to be institutionalized.

Consequently, the prevailing abuse may seem, to them, more bearable than the thought of being taken to an unfamiliar institution. There are also times when the victims have a tendency to blame themselves for having "instigated" the abuse or the abuser might convince them that if they did not do some "stupid" things there would be no need to hit them or to take away the cane or walker from them or to withhold their medication. The victims might also be afraid that no one will believe their story of abuse. It is their word against the word of the abuser and so they prefer to keep quiet.

Healthcare abuse of the elderly has been reported to be perpetrated by "unethical doctors, nurses, hospital personnel, and other professional care providers."[489] When looking for signs of healthcare abuse by health care providers, one must analyze things such as charges for health care services that were not provided. Other healthcare abuse evidence may take the form overcharging or double billing for healthcare services or getting kickbacks for elderly patient referral to a certain type of provider or for prescribing certain types of medications.

Healthcare abuse is also the tendency to deliberately over medicate the elderly patient or under medicate them. It is giving fraudulent types of treatment regimens aside from what the elderly patient needs or is already receiving. It can take the form of insurance fraud, which is a means of obtaining payment from the elderly person's insurance carrier in a fraudulent manner.

The Nursing Home Abuse News once reported that abuse is "an unconscionable act that is perpetrated upon older individuals who are unable to protect themselves against physical, emotional, sexual, or financial abuse."[490] What is most reprehensible about this practice in nursing homes is that the victim pays the institution where the abuser might be employed to provide services meant to improve the well-being of the elderly person.

Signs of institutional abuse and neglect include the presence of a constant pungent smell of urine or feces on the elderly individual or in their room or wherever their living area may be within the healthcare institution or the presence of hazardous material in the elderly individual's living area. Other forms of institutional abuse of the elderly manifest themselves in obvious dehydration and malnutrition in the elderly individual. In this type of abuse, the elderly individual is not properly or adequately dressed most of the time, and they have a disheveled appearance and are dirty and unkempt.

In Japan, elderly people have traditionally received care from family members. The wife to the elderly person's son often assumed the role of caregiver for her elderly in-laws. But the increase in urbanization and job opportunities has raised the percentage of women in the workforce. This has resulted in a major shift in these traditional values.[491] Daughters-in-law who are in regular employment are finding the roles of being caregivers stressful and burdensome. This tension, which is exacerbated by high expectations, has prompted the transfer of domestic caregiving of the elderly to a formal, community-based system.

Although the levels of elder abuse are still lower in Japan than in other industrialized nations, it is beginning to increase at a significant rate with 32% of abusers being the sons of the abused and 21% are their daughters-in-law. Reporting on the alarmingly rising rate of elder abuse in Japan, Elaine Lies (2004) writing for Global Action on Aging, wrote about a case of a 78-year old Japanese woman who lived with the family of her son in Gunma, Tokyo. During the months she was in their care, her bedding was never changed regularly and her food was left on the side of her bed. Inevitably, her situation deteriorated to a point where she had to be hospitalized. She died shortly afterwards.

The World Health Organization (WHO) claims that elder abuse is a global problem that requires global intervention methods. One public health intervention strategy recommended by the WHO is aggressive community education to raise awareness of the magnitude of the problem. Another proposed intervention strategy involves screening for signs of elder abuse in geriatric service institutions and social services. Public health officials are working toward multi-agency partnerships aimed at preventing the abuse of elderly people.

Christian values have a different view about ageing. Among true believers, ageing is not contemplated upon with apprehension or trepidation. It is not a negative phenomenon. All generations, including the elderly, are a vital part of the fabric of society, a resource necessary for its effective functioning and wellbeing. Each period in an individual's life has something unique to offer humanity. According to the Bible, old age is a blessing. The Bible speaks of old age as a splendor or beauty or honor: "The glory of young men is their strength, but the beauty of old men is their gray hair" (Proverbs 20:29). Again it says, "You shall rise up before the hoary head, and honor the face of an old man, and you shall fear your God: I am the LORD" (Leviticus 19:32).

One of the fundamental principles of Christian ethics on which hangs the foundation of the dignity of every human being is the directive or commandment "You shall love your neighbor as yourself" (Matthew 22:39). This inherent dignity of every human being is not based on what the individual has achieved or their capabilities. It is based on what human beings are according to Scripture. The Bible speaks with final authority on how we ought to treat other human beings as it does on most other subjects. Loving my neighbor as I love myself entails the understanding that the other human being, regardless of age difference or any other difference, for that matter, has the same intrinsic value that I have. This is exemplified in Genesis 1:26-27 where the Bible says:

> "Then God said, 'Let us make man in our image, after our likeness; and let them have dominion over the fish of the sea, and over the birds of the air, and over the cattle, and over all the earth, and over every creeping thing that creeps upon the earth.' So God created man in his own image, in the image of God he created him; male and female he created them."

Man in this case refers to mankind. Implied in this Scripture is the fact that we are all made equal since we all came from the same source. We are made in the image of God regardless of our physiological, biological, and other differences. Each one of us reflects the image of God no matter how distorted that may seem to outward observers. In the Book of Ruth, the Bible gives us an account of how Ruth, the Moabites young woman and Naomi's widowed daughter-in-law, committed herself to taking care of her ageing, widowed mother-in-law during the time of her vulnerability and loss. Ruth's selfless love was abundantly rewarded. She became an ancestor of the Messiah, the Lord Jesus.

The commandment in Exodus 20:12 exhorts us to, "Honor your father and your mother, that your days may be long in the land which the LORD your God gives you." This commandment must be obeyed whether the parents grow old and are no longer able to participate in gainful employment or productive labor. We have an obligation as children and families to support and care for the elderly who need it, and to encourage them to utilize their specific capabilities to strengthen family and neighborhood relationships. This can foster a sense of belonging and of being needed, which is very important for psychological and physical health. The elderly people's wisdom and experience is "a treasure which is often underestimated or even unrecognized, but which is of great benefit to society as a whole."[492]

Scripture tells us how our Lord Jesus Christ, in the throes of the most ignominious and excruciatingly painful death on the cross, remembered to assign the care of his mother to his close disciple, John. We will never be called to endure what he endured, but this is one of the many examples he left that is worthy emulating.

When elderly people are valued, it becomes easy for them to get to a point where they can be reconciled with their own memoirs and life stories even as they prepare themselves, psychologically, as the shadow of death lengthens on them. When elderly people become so incapacitated that they require to be institutionalized in a skilled care facility outside their homes, those who place them in such institutions should not feel guilty if they have done the best they could for their elderly parent.

Chapter 26

Asthma

Incline your ear, and come to me; hear, that your soul may live.
(Isaiah 55:3)

Asthma is a chronic lung disease. It is an airway health disorder, which, if not properly managed or treated, can severely impair daily living. It can even be fatal. Asthma can impair or reduce the level of participation in family life activities. It can also contribute to a significant loss of productivity. Asthma affects approximately three hundred million people worldwide.[493] The incidence and prevalence of asthma has been steadily rising in the last three decades in both developed and developing nations. Researchers are baffled by this alarming rise. Recently, Africa, Asia, and Latin America have experienced a considerable surge in the incidence and prevalence of asthma. The Global Initiative for Asthma defines asthma as:

> Asthma is a chronic inflammatory disorder of the airways in which many cells and cellular elements play a role. The chronic inflammation is associated with airway hyperresponsiveness that leads to recurrent episodes of wheezing, breathlessness, chest tightness, and coughing,

particularly at night or in the early morning. These episodes are usually associated with widespread, but variable, airflow obstruction within the lungs that is often reversible either spontaneously or with treatment.

(Global Initiative for Asthma, 2011)[494]

The onset of asthma is often facilitated by genetic susceptibility or predisposition usually working in concert with environmental factors. Genes interacting with other genes or genes interacting with environmental factors can increase the risk of onset of asthma. Obesity is another factor that increases the risk of development or expression of asthma.

A study conducted in 2008 by Emily Rosenbaum of Fordham University, New York, aimed at determining whether differential exposure to potentially harmful conditions in the neighborhood and the home can have observed differences in the incidence and prevalence of asthma.[495] This study was conducted in New York among ten different racial and ethnic groups. Its results demonstrated that Puerto Rican households had the highest levels of asthma followed by other Hispanic population groups and then African Americans. The researchers attributed these findings, largely, to dilapidated and deteriorating housing conditions. Low social order and lack of cohesion in the neighborhood were also found to be other risk factors for the high prevalence of asthma.

In a different research study that explored racial differences in asthma among young children, investigators Hill and associates made the following comment about the results of their research study: "The burden of asthma disproportionately affects children living in economically disadvantaged urban communities. The relationships between ethnicity, genetic differences, lower socioeconomic status, poor medication adherence, greater exposure to environmental triggers, and absence of regular asthma care all contribute to this disparity" (Hill, Graham & Divqi, 2011).[496]

This explains why the prevalence of asthma is higher among poor communities in developed nations. In developing countries, the prevalence of asthma is higher among the affluent than among the poor. The association between obesity and the development of asthma in developing nations is statistically significant even when other risk factors and confounders are controlled.[497]

Other studies have claimed that, in infants, the prevalence of asthma tends to be higher in male babies than in female babies. But in adulthood, there is a switch in prevalence. Then women have a higher prevalence than men.[498] This switch has been attributed to the fact that male infants' lung size is smaller than that of female infants, but in adulthood, male lungs are often larger than female lungs.

1. Air Pollution and Asthma

At birth, babies' lungs are considerably underdeveloped and not fully functional. A baby is born with only one-tenth of the sum total of an adult's alveoli. Drs. Thomas Bateson and Joel Schwartz of the National Center for Environmental Assessment, Office of Research and Development, and Departments of Environmental Health Epidemiology, Harvard School of Public Health, respectively, claim that from birth, the infant experiences an exponential alveoli growth or multiplication: "During this period, the lung undergoes significant morphogenesis; respiratory bronchioles develop, as do the epithelium and the immune cell populations. Alveoli multiply from 24 million at birth, to 257 million by the time the child is four. The development of alveolar does not take place until the 32-36th week of gestation" (Bateson & Schwartz, 2008).[499]

It is during this period that the baby's developing lungs are particularly vulnerable to injury by air pollutants. Any injury to the lungs can have long-lasting negative outcomes. Because the breathing of young children is remarkably different from that of adults, exposure to pollutants has different health effects and outcomes on them. Usually adults breathe through the nose, which has the capacity to filter inhaled particles and gases because it is lined with hair. But little children breathe primarily through the mouth, which makes them inhale larger amounts of pollutants than adults even when both are breathing the same air in the same environment.

Because young children tend to have a larger lung surface per unit of body weight than grownups, they also have the capacity to inhale more air per unit of body weight.[500] Additionally, children spend more time outside their homes and are more active than adults particularly during favorable weather conditions. They spent their time in vigorous physical activities that include constant running. Therefore, their exposure to outdoor air pollutants can be quite high. The deep breathing that accompanies high levels of physical activity pulls air pollutants further into the lungs more quickly and in large quantities. In their research study, Ginsberg and associates found that "in the pulmonary region of the lung, particle dose can be two- to fourfold higher among young children as compared with adults" (Ginsberg, Foos and Firestone, 2006).

Exposure to certain air pollution and certain allergens can also increase the likelihood of the development of asthma. For example, traffic-related air pollution is significantly associated with the development of asthma and atopy as the research study conducted by Studnicka and associates in Vienna, Austria, among eight rural communities demonstrated.[501]

Atopy is a genetic predisposition that makes some people easily develop immediate hypersensitive reactions when they come in contact with common environmental antigens. It is often commonly manifested as allergic rhinitis. In three German communities NO_2 (nitrite), levels outside the homes of the study participants significantly predicted the development of hay fever, wheezing and allergic rhinitis.[502]

In a research study conducted among Dutch school children, van Vliet and associates found that asthma was more prevalent among children who lived about 100 meters (about 109.4 yards) from the highway than among those who lived farther away.[503] Traffic intensity was also found to be significantly associated with chronic respiratory problems. Children brought up in high air pollution locations have often been found to have limited lung function. There is often a close association between air pollution and the development of asthma.

Children whose parents are asthmatic are also more vulnerable to the development of asthma, particularly when they are also regularly exposed to home air pollutants. According to United States Environmental Protection Agency, people in the United States spend more time indoors than outdoors compared to their counterparts in developing nations. This gives them a longer exposure to indoor air pollutants, making them more susceptible to developing respiratory problems including asthma.

People living in developed nations spend about 90% of their time indoors, at school, at work, and at home.[504] Poor indoor air quality can not only trigger asthmatic attacks in an individual who already has asthma, but it can also hasten the development of asthma in susceptible individuals especially children. Some of the indoor air pollutants that are likely to accelerate the development of asthma include dog and cat dander, dust mites, mold, environmental tobacco smoke, irritant chemicals, and fumes resulting from household activities such as cooking.

Chemical odors emitted from these activities can easily trigger asthmatic attacks. Scented soaps, detergents, and perfume can aggravate asthmatic attacks as well. Cockroach allergens from cockroach droppings can also increase the risk for the development of asthma. Children living in inner cities in the United States have a range of cockroach allergy rates of between 17% to 41%.[505, 506]

2. Bacterial and Viral Infection and Asthma

In early life, infection with respiratory syncytial virus (RSV) and para-influenza virus can lead to symptoms that resemble childhood asthma.[507] Respiratory syncytial virus causes infection of the lungs and the respiratory tract. Para-influenza virus and other related viruses can cause an array of respiratory problems whose symptoms can vary from those of a common cold to influenza-like pneumonia. Wheezing illnesses and asthma in all age groups are closely linked to viral infection such as respiratory syncytial virus and parainfluenza virus.

Matthew M. Huckabee and R. Stokes Peebles Jr. conducted a meta-analysis of some of the most recent studies that explored the contribution of viruses to the development of asthma.[508] One of the studies they reviewed was conducted by Wu and associates among a cohort of 95,310 children enrolled in the Medicaid program and born between 1995 and 2000. These children were followed over the next viral seasons from infancy or zero years until age 5 ½. The objective of this study was to find out whether the birth of the infant in relationship to the winter virus peak season could alter its risk of developing early childhood asthma. The findings of this study demonstrated that: "Timing of birth in relationship to winter virus season confers a differential and definable risk of developing early childhood asthma, establishing winter virus seasonality as a causal factor in asthma development. Delay of exposure or prevention of winter viral infection during early infancy could prevent asthma" (Wu, et al., 2008).[509]

The study also found that the development of asthma was further exacerbated by genetic susceptibility. Another finding in the same study was that a virus that is likely to cause bronchitis is also able to cause asthma. Another study conducted by Janssen and associates endeavored to explore the complexity of respiratory syncytial virus (RSV) susceptibility and to identify the genes and other biological pathways that play a role in its development among 470 children who were hospitalized for RSV bronchiolitis.[510] It was discovered that single-nucleotide polymorphisms (SNPs) in innate immune genes played a significant role in determining susceptibility to RSV bronchiolitis among the children. Additionally, the RSV was found to lead to the development of asthma. These studies confirm that environmental exposure, including viral infection, can lead to the development of asthma.

3. Occupational Substances and Asthma

The current global workforce is comprised of approximately 2,600 million individuals. This number is growing continuously. An estimated 75% of this workforce is in developing nations.[511] The working population is composed of approximately 60-70% of the world's adult males and about 30-60% of the world's adult females. Forty million individuals join the workforce, annually. Any workplace hazards, therefore, become a threat to one of the most productive and significantly large proportions of the population of the world.

Occupational asthma is more prevalent in developed nations than in developing nations because of the presence of and sustained exposure to a myriad of occupational substances that can trigger onset of asthma.[512] Unlike in developing nations, workers in developed nations usually perform their duties in confined places. Therefore, any exposure to occupational hazardous materials tends to be higher than in the general environment.

Individuals with occupational asthma have higher levels of hospitalization and mortality than their healthy counterparts. Evidence indicating that the workplace contributes significantly to the burden of asthma is increasing. Exposure to certain occupational substances that include isocyanates and irritants can adversely affect airway responsiveness and trigger development of asthma. Immunogenic substances that include platinum salts can also stimulate onset of asthma. Currently, there are more than 300 substances that are associated with the development of occupational asthma in previously healthy individuals.[513]

Occupational asthma is difficult to differentiate from other forms of asthma except that it usually occurs in adults. Asthma is known as the most common occupational disorder in developed nations. According to research findings by Rémen and associates, occupational asthma takes two forms:

1. The Reactive Airways Dysfunction Syndrome (RADS). This type of asthma is usually induced by acute inhalation of irritant substances. It is a persistent asthma syndrome that occurs after being exposed to high levels of irritants particularly in poorly ventilated work places.

2. The immunological type whose latent period after exposure to irritant substances varies. This is the most frequent type of occupational asthma. It occurs after a latency period during which sensitization takes place.

(Remen, et al. 2010)[514]

Occupations that are closely associated with the development of asthma include agriculture, painting, cleaning jobs, and plastic manufacturing occupation. When employees in these occupations are removed from exposure to the substance that triggers asthma as soon as the symptoms manifest themselves, they often recover completely. However, if they continue being exposed to the trigger substance over a protracted period of time, the disease can become severe and even persist after exposure to the substance has been halted. Therefore, early recognition of the development of the disease is a critical step toward prevention of severe and persistent asthma. Usually individuals who develop occupational asthma first develop rhinitis before they develop bronchial symptoms.

The study by Rémen (2010) and associates further claims that occupational exposures to asthma triggers are reported to be responsible for between 10% and 15% of new developments of asthma cases in adults, with notable differences across occupational sectors. For example, hairdressers have a high risk of developing occupational asthma and other respiratory diseases because of being constantly exposed to several agents that are likely to irritate their airways. In France, hairdressing represents the fourth most common cause of occupational asthma in women.[515] The agents considered to be responsible for causing occupational asthma among hairdressers are bleaching agents and persulfate salts.

Dr. Jane Hoppin claims that very little is known about the respiratory health risk of applying pesticides to agricultural products on commercial farms.[516] A study was conducted by Dr. Hoppin and associates aimed at assessing pesticide application as a risk factor for asthma among farm female workers in North Carolina and Iowa.[517] The results of the study demonstrated a significant increase in the prevalence of occupational asthma in women who applied or mixed pesticides. This underscored the likelihood of constant exposure to pesticides as a risk factor for the development of occupational asthma.

4. Exposure to Tobacco Smoke and Asthma

Smoke produced by cigarettes, cigars, and pipes has a deleterious effect on the respiratory system. When an individual inhales smoke, irritating and harmful substances from it penetrate and settle into the linings of their airways. These substances cause significant damage to tiny hair-like structures in the airways called cilia. Once the cilia are damaged, they are unable to perform their function of ridding airways of dust and mucus causing mucus and dust to accumulate in the airways.

This can trigger an asthmatic attack, especially in individuals who already have asthma. Exposure to secondhand smoke and active smoking also play a significant role in the actual development of asthma.[518] Tobacco smoke negatively affects the natural immunity by depressing it, and predisposing it to respiratory diseases. Tobacco smoke also increases the risk for immunoglobulin E-mediated sensitization. Immunoglobulin E (IgE) is one of the immunoglobulins found in the skin and mucous membranes.

Active tobacco smoking has also been implicated as a risk factor for developing new asthma especially in individuals with rhinitis. Drs. McMillen and Stern have the following to say about the effects of smoking: "In the lungs, a spring-like protein, elastin, forms a suspension system that keeps the tiny air tubules expanded. Smoking causes enzymes to break down elastin and smoking blocks the body's ability to repair this breakdown. The lung's elastic suspension disintegrates, and the tubules collapse. Over several years, the smoker slowly suffocates" (McMillen & Stern, 2000).[519]

In an article that appeared in the 2004 copy of the *European Respiratory Journal*, scientists reported that in most industrialized nations, approximately 25% of adult individuals who have asthma are current cigarette smokers.[520] Prenatal and early childhood chronic exposure to tobacco smoke increases the risk of developing asthma-like symptoms among young children. Infants whose mothers smoke are four times likely to develop wheezing early in their lives. A study by Willers and associates reveals that: "The chance of developing asthma and allergy might be determined during fetal life because there are potential mechanisms by which environmental factors, such as maternal diet and lifestyle, can influence the development of the airways and immune system of the child *in utero*" (Willers, et al. 2008).[521]

Therefore, both maternal smoking during pregnancy and exposure of children to environmental tobacco smoke are risk factors for development of asthma in early life. Environmental smoke or second hand smoke contains numerous toxic chemicals that have adverse effects on general health as well as respiratory health.

5. Diet and Asthma

Researchers in the Global Allergy and Asthma European Network (GA²LEN) explored three key dietary areas to determine whether they are likely to trigger allergic respiratory problems in a child. These areas were breastfeeding, ingestion of certain nutrients and probiotics.[522]

The findings of this research study revealed that an infant who is exclusively breastfed, whose diet constitutes breast milk only with no other liquids for the first four months of its life, is protected from cow's milk protein allergies until it is 18 months old. The study also found out that exclusive breastfeeding for a period longer than four months reduces the risk of asthma development until the baby is six years old. Another finding indicated that in cases where the mother is unable to breastfeed due to health problems, hypoallergenic formula combined with avoidance of solid foods for four to six months is a source of protection from development of asthma.

Hypoallergenic formula prevents the development of allergies triggered by cow's milk protein before the age of five years and further protects the infant from eczema until the baby is four years old. Other studies assessing the potential relationship between diet and development of asthma have found that infants who were fed cow's milk or soy protein have a significantly higher incidence of wheezing compared to their counterparts who were exclusively breastfed.[523]

Further research has demonstrated that diets high in processed food, fats found in margarine and vegetable oil, and diets low in fruit and vegetables and n-3 polyunsaturated fats such as those found in fish have considerably contributed to the increase in the prevalence of asthma.[524] A second area that is linked to the development of allergic reactions and triggering development of asthma is associated with the actual individual components of diet.

Antioxidants such as vitamin C, vitamin E, and selenium obtained from consumption of fruit and vegetables have a protective effect against respiratory diseases including asthma. An increase in the consumption of fruit such as apples as well as green vegetables, and avoidance of consumption of margarine and other related fats has been found to improve the health of asthmatics. Probiotics and prebiotics have a promising effect in protection against development of allergies by positively affecting the bacteria in the stomach that stimulate and boost the immune system. Probiotics have been found to reduce the risk of atopic disease. Atopic disease is a genetic predisposition to developing immediate allergic reactions such as asthma and rhinitis due to the presence of an antibody in the skin or in the blood.

6. Asthma in Developing Nations

There is, currently, little awareness in developing nations about asthma and its associated debilitating effects. Nevertheless, reports from the World Health Organization indicate that most of the world's population especially in developing nations gets its energy from solid fuels such as wood, cow dung, coal, and crop waste.[525] Cooking activities carried out in enclosures using such solid fuels on open fires and stoves without the help of chimneys leads to significant indoor air pollution. The byproducts of the combustion of these solid fuels have adverse health outcomes because they are capable of penetrating deep into the lungs when inhaled.

A study by Padmavati and Joshi found a substantial deposition of carbon in the lungs of patients exposed to biomass smoke.[526] Necropsies or autopsies of non-smoking women exposed to biomass smoke who had cor pulmonale, which is an enlargement of the right ventricle of the heart resulting from long-term lung disease, revealed that all had respiratory health problems including emphysema, chronic bronchitis and tuberculosis. A study conducted in rural China in which 93% of the sample used wood or hay for cooking found a significantly positive association between exposure to biomass smoke from wood and hay and prevalence of wheezing and asthma. The World Health Organization (WHO) further claims that indoor pollution from solid fuels is:

> Responsible for 2.7% of the global burden of disease. Globally, indoor air pollution from solid fuel use is responsible for 1.6 million deaths due to pneumonia, chronic respiratory disease and lung cancer, with the overall disease burden (in Disability-Adjusted Life Years or DALYs, a measure combining years of life lost due to disability and death) exceeding the burden from outdoor air pollution fivefold. In high-mortality developing countries, indoor smoke is responsible for an estimated 3.7% of the overall disease burden, making it the most lethal killer after malnutrition, unsafe sex and lack of safe water and sanitation.
>
> (Desai, Mehta & Smith, 2004)[527]

A growing number of studies are also finding an association between exposure to solid fuel combustion products and respiratory diseases such as lung cancer, chronic obstructive pulmonary disease (COPD) and asthma as well as airflow obstruction.[528]

7. Economic Cost of Asthma

Due to its chronic nature, which demands continuous direct and indirect treatment and management, asthma often results in loss of productivity. The economic cost of asthma can be quite substantial. In addition to the actual experience of poor health by individuals who have asthma, this disease, like any other chronic disease, imposes a significant financial burden on the afflicted individuals, their families, and healthcare institutions.[529]

Approximately 15 million Americans have asthma, including 9 million children younger than 18. Between 1980 and 1995, the prevalence of asthma and asthma-related emergency room visits for adults and children younger than 18 increased 74% and 36%, respectively.[530] Corso and Pertig observed in their study that asthma is: "One of the most common causes of school absenteeism, a major cause of disability and/or restricted activity among children, and is one of the leading causes of hospitalizations among children. In addition, children with asthma continue to suffer as adults, affecting not only their quality of life but their lifetime productivity as well" (Corso & Pertig, 2004).[531]

However, when asthma is properly managed by applying the recommendations made by related disease management programs, hospitalizations and emergency visits are significantly reduced. In the United States, it is estimated that both the direct and indirect annual cost of asthma among children aged 5 to17 is about $2.8 billion or $1,098 per individual child.[532] Of the $2.8 billion, $919 million or $364 per child constitutes indirect costs associated with parents' loss of productivity at work and $1.5 billion or $600 per child constitutes direct healthcare expenses. All costs inflation adjusted to 2006. The total lifetime cost of asthma expenses for individuals born after 2000 was estimated to be $7.2 billion. This includes direct medical costs at $3.2 billion and $4 billion in work/productivity loss.

In some developing nations, hospitalization of patients with asthma is the only means of assessing the severity of the burden of asthma.[533] This means that the severity of the burden of asthma can only be measured using hospitalization data because no other type of data are available since individuals with less severe cases of asthma do not go to hospitals. But comprehensive information about the general incidence and prevalence of asthma is not available due to lack of cohesive data collection programs.

The Asia-Pacific region has few data describing the economic burden associated with the prevalence of asthma. A study reported in the 2006 issue of the *European Respiratory Review* conducted by Lai and associates attempted to provide more information on the economic cost of asthma by investigating and reporting the per-patient direct, indirect and societal cost of asthma in the Asian region.[534]

The findings of the study revealed that asthma indeed takes a tremendous economic toll on this region. Although there are substantial variations between different countries in the region and although the overall economic cost is lower than that reported by Western countries such as the United States and Europe, "the economic burden on countries in the Asia-Pacific region is higher in relation to *per capita* healthcare expenditure or *per capita* GDP, (Lai, 2006)." The costs associated with urgent care, according to the study by Lai and associates, accounted for approximately 60% of all direct costs.

Even for a nation such as Singapore, which had the lowest economic burden compared to other Asian countries, the percentage of medical expenses were still threefold higher than those of the United States at 32%. Developing nations in the same category as those of the Asia-Pacific region experience considerable costs associated with asthma due to poor programs and methods employed to control the disease leading to urgent healthcare utilization. The insufficient use of effective asthma control therapy was the cause of increased need for hospitalization of patients, which, in turn, increased healthcare expenditure.

The Global Initiative for Asthma observes that the prevalence of asthma in South America especially in Peru, Brazil, Uruguay and Paraguay is higher than the average of all countries, worldwide.[535] The high prevalence of asthma in these nations is not proportional to industrialization but rather to poverty.

Asthma levels are higher in poor cities where most of the people belong to low socioeconomic statuses.

This makes economic impoverishment a risk factor for development of asthma in this region. Lack of integrated asthma control programs and methods intensify this problem. Lack of government funded pharmaceuticals has placed three fourths of the pharmaceutical market in the hands of the private sector, making the cost of medical care prohibitive and often unobtainable, adding to the economic burden of the disease. Mortality from asthma is quite high in South America although variations exist across countries.

In Brazil, where there is an increased availability of inhaled corticosteroid therapy, mortality rates have been considerably reduced. The implementation of asthmatic educational programs and management guidelines is helping improve the health of asthmatic children from low socioeconomic communities in this area. In some South American cities, air pollution is quite high. This contributes to general morbidity and mortality rates associated with respiratory problems that include asthma. Government and public health professionals acknowledge that air pollution is a source of health concern and are designing strategies to reduce air pollution levels in the affected areas.

The Report from the Global Initiative further reveals that the prevalence of asthma is generally low in West Africa. However urban communities are beginning to experience a substantial increase in the prevalence of asthma compared to their rural counterparts. The increase has steadily risen over recent decades.

In 1975 researchers could not detect a single case of asthma among a group of 1,000 Gambian children and adults. But by 1997, 3% of the rural community of the Gambia reported asthmatic symptoms. Increased urbanization is likely to significantly increase the prevalence of asthma in the near future in this country. A major problem associated with managing asthma in these places is the scarcity of disease control programs and therapeutic remedies.

It is also true that often asthmatic symptoms have been confused for other infectious diseases in Africa. This could result in misdiagnosis and mistreatment of asthma, which could contribute significantly to morbidity and mortality from asthma. For example, the overlapping symptoms of asthma with those of tuberculosis can make it practically difficult to diagnose asthma. Social and economic problems that beleaguer the relatively young African countries are another problem in treatment of asthma. These problems include lack of comprehensive healthcare infrastructures equipped well enough to deal with the burden of existing infectious diseases, let alone emerging chronic diseases such as asthma. Additionally, poor nutrition and housing intensify the burden of disease.

In South Africa, asthma is the third most common cause of hospitalization in children after pneumonia and gastroenteritis. The burden of asthma has increased in recent decades just like in most other African nations. However, due to the proliferation of the mining industry, South Africa also experiences mining-related diseases that include pneumoconiosis, but occupational asthma is on the increase as well. Occupational asthma has become a frequently reported occupational respiratory disease in South Africa. Changes in healthcare services that include improved access to quality asthma management and education have been recommended and are being pursued. Most asthma-related deaths in South Africa occur outside the hospitals because of lack of transportation and poor home management techniques for individuals with acute asthma. Asthma is a global problem that has considerable global social and economic implications.

The Bible speaks to us with authoritative finality when addressing great and dynamic issues. For example, it informs us that "So God created man in his own image, in the image of God he created him; male and female he created them," (Genesis 1:27).

This is not a suggestion. It is a statement of fact. God did not only create us, he endowed us with physical bodies that have amazing reparative capabilities. If we obey his counsel, we have a greater chance of living healthy lives. The Bible does not specifically give counsel on prevention of asthma, but it gives guidelines for promoting overall health, which have the potential to reduce the incidence and prevalence of asthma as well. The basic components of good health include clean fresh air, good hygiene, exercise, a healthy and nutritious diet, clean water, regular rest, enough sleep, reducing levels of stress, positive thinking and living in an environment that is free from toxins and pollutants.[536] If properly observed, all these factors can work in concert to reduce levels of toxins in our bodies and optimize our health.

Although genetic factors are important determinants of the development of asthma (and other diseases) in susceptible individuals, these genetic factors are usually reinforced by environmental factors such as lifestyle. For general health to thrive, our environment should be free from harmful substances such as tobacco smoke, pet dander, dust, cockroaches, mold, and mildew. The effects of multiple chemicals and toxins interacting within our bodies include an increased susceptibility to a myriad of diseases. The elimination of health-threatening environmental factors mitigates the onset of diseases including asthma and other health conditions. The following is an insightful excerpt from a publication:

> Exposure to air pollution, water contamination, toxic substances, heavy metals, endocrine disrupters, and carcinogens turn God's cycle-of-life design into a truncated lifeline… Our own bodies, as temples of God, need to be purged of pollution and toxic matter… Our waste should not accumulate in a landfill so that it poisons the land and people living nearby. Our daily living should not use or release toxic pollution or chemicals that cause environmental degradation and human illness.[537]

The Perfect Prescription

The biblical injunction about ridding our homes of mold and mildew and burying deadly waste indicates that God wants our homes and other surroundings to be hygienic and sanitary so that our health can thrive. After the Fall, our bodies became subject to death. But for the time allocated to each one of us on this earth, between birth and death, God has provided principles necessary for healthy living. This is not to insinuate that everyone who has asthma contracted it by slighting biblical counsel. Biblical counsel is never condemnatory. It is cautionary. When road traffic officials warn against texting while driving, they are not necessarily accusing all of us of texting while driving. Rather, they are helping us avoid what could easily endanger our lives. They are merely providing advice for optimizing our health and well-being, and so is biblical counsel. In this case, biblical counsel serves to emphasize the fact that if we have a person who has asthma in our home, one way to help them is to ensure that their surroundings are free from items that can easily trigger an asthmatic attack. This is true of any other disease. If we know what can exacerbate the condition of the sick among us it is only reasonable to ensure that we avoid it and maintain an environment that optimizes their health.

Chapter 27

Cost Saving in Healthcare: A Biblical Perspective

He sent forth his word, and healed them, and delivered them from destruction.

(Psalm 107:20)

We have seen that the preventive health approach as taught in Scripture has always yielded positive outcomes. It has helped reduce healthcare costs wherever it has been applied effectively. Simple and basic health practices include adopting a healthy diet and observing stringent hygiene standards such as washing hands before handling food and after using the bathroom.

Other basic health-promoting practices include drinking clean and safe water as well as observing appropriate garbage removal and treatment standards. All these help eradicate disease-carrying agents and vermin. In addition, safety rules at home, on the road, and at work promote health and well-being and reduce the burden of injury and disease as well as related health care expenses.[538] Diseases that are difficult to cure or manage such as chronic diseases are often a result of lifestyle choices or voluntary behavioral choices. This means that it is possible to prevent them or to delay their onset by adopting appropriate health-promoting habits.

There is an obvious link between health and behavioral choices. As such, the impact of disease can also be mitigated by good lifestyles and health-enhancing behavioral choices. Alan G. Kraut, Executive Director of the Association for Psychological Science, claims that there is no longer any doubt about the effect of behavior on health and that: "Many leading health conditions—such as heart disease; stroke; lung disease and many cancers; obesity; AIDS; suicide; teen pregnancy; drug abuse and addiction; depression and other mental illnesses; neurological disorders; alcoholism; violence; injuries and accidents originate in behavior and can be prevented or controlled through behavior" (Kraut, 2009).[539]

In the light of the above observation, it is critical to understand behaviors that improve health and those that impair it in order to succeed in disease-prevention strategies. More positive results can be achieved through aggressive and detailed public education campaigns aimed at cautioning the public against adoption of health-impairing behavioral choices. Kraut further asserts that through public education about health-related behaviors, the general public can come to understand and tackle questions about their health such as:

> What are the best ways to manage diabetes and arthritis? How do genes and the environment influence behavioral traits such as aggression and anxiety? What goes into the decision to avoid risky sex? What is the best combination of cognitive behavioral therapy and pharmacological treatment for depression? How can we use virtual reality environments to lessen the effects of post-traumatic stress disorder?
>
> (Kraut, 2009)

The Centers for Disease Control and Prevention (CDC) are alarmed by the escalating health costs attributed to treatment and management of an array of health disorders. This has prompted them to propose a national collaboration, which includes employers as a means for reaching and improving the health of millions of individuals working for them. This is an effort to develop a community of people that is engaged in cutting health risks and promoting general health.

One approach is associated with tobacco cessation. But there are many other approaches that can be adopted. The CDC have articulated that there is a dire need to assist all types of employers to design and implement viable strategies to help improve the health of their employees which will, ultimately, reduce risky behavioral choices and the burden of disease at the workplace and in the communities where their employees live. According to the CDC, "The United States cannot effectively address escalating health care costs without addressing the problem of chronic diseases" (Centers for Disease Control and Prevention, Updated 2012).[540] The total annual economic impact of the burden of preventable chronic diseases in the United States is more than $1 trillion.[541]

About 75% of United States healthcare expenditure goes to chronic diseases, most of which are preventable. Although most employers have been significantly concerned about the unbridled healthcare expenses, they have lacked the skills and tools to address the issue. In 2005, the CDC funded the Health and Productivity Management (HPM) Project conducted by Thomson Medstat in association with the Cornell University Institute of Policy Rresearch, which was designed to identify organizations that had "improved employee health and reduced costs through HPM initiatives, learn how these organizations have achieved these outcomes, and formulate indicators of promising practices in HPM to the business community," (Thomson Medstat, 2006).[542]

A later evaluation of the project revealed that although organizations did not often publish HPM efforts, some organizations reported having experienced a significant reduction in health risks. The organizations have also experienced remarkable cost savings due to the implementation of HPM campaigns and programs.

The Milken Institute and Partnership to Fight Chronic Disease, an independent economic organization whose mission involves designing and implementing strategies to improve the lives and economic conditions of different population groups in the United States and around the world, claims that "the most common chronic diseases are costing the economy more than $1 trillion, annually" and that "that figure threatens to reach $6 trillion by the middle of the century."[543] The Institute analyzed the financial drain caused by treatment of seven common chronic diseases, namely: cancer, diabetes, hypertension, stroke, heart disease, pulmonary conditions, and mental illness. They also analyzed the financial expenses associated with treatment and management of various forms of cancer. Their results indicated that in 2003, health care expenses for treating these seven diseases amounted to $227 billion for Americans who were non-institutionalized, and more than 50% of Americans are afflicted by one or more chronic diseases. The Institute asserts that although the scenario appears overwhelmingly formidable, aggressive lifestyle changes across the board such as regular exercise, weight control, improved nutrition, and reduction in tobacco smoking could remarkably reduce the health care expenses for chronic diseases cited above.

People have a general awareness that tobacco use, unhealthy food choices and bad dietary habits, alcohol consumption, and a sedentary lifestyle are detrimental to health. They also are aware that regular exercise is good for health, but, tragically, they continue to engage in these self-destructive behaviors. This puzzling scenario has piqued the interest of researchers, particularly those in the discipline of decision science who are now engaged in exploring and analyzing what role cognitive factors can play in influencing individual judgment and choices.[544]

The Perfect Prescription

The researchers are further studying how emotional and social factors can work in concert with cognitive factors to further affect people's judgment and decision-making, particularly in health matters. This means that there is a possibility that the process of decision-making could be predicted or even improved.

Currently there is a need for infrastructure support of behavioral research in order to further promote behavioral interventions and treatments of chronic diseases using behavioral changes. A strategy should be designed and implemented to facilitate communicating what are termed as "gain-framed" messages to the general public so that they can be empowered to take control and protect their own health.

An example of "gain-framed" health messages is: "If you exercise regularly, you will be able to lose weight." This is a more positively framed message that challenges the listener to choose gainfully than if one was to say: "if do not exercise you will not prevent obesity." This approach would have to start with population groups who are most at risk for certain chronic diseases to reduce the rate of onset of these diseases.

Commenting on the benefits of preventive health strategies in the February issue of the 2008 *New England Journal of Medicine*, scientists admitted that:

> Indeed, some evidence does suggest that there are opportunities to save money and improve health through prevention. Preventable causes of death such as tobacco smoking, poor diet, physical inactivity, and misuse of alcohol have been estimated to be responsible for 900,000 deaths annually—nearly 40% of total yearly mortality in the United States. Moreover, some of the measures identified by the U.S. Preventive Services Task Force, such as counseling adults to quit smoking, screening for colorectal cancer, and providing influenza vaccination, reduce mortality either at low cost or at a cost savings.
>
> (Cohen, Neumann & Weinstein, 2008)[545]

A report of the Synthesis Project from the Robert Wood Johnson Foundation by Sarah Goodell and associates on the cost savings and cost-effectiveness of clinical preventive care observed that:

> Preventive services can reduce the prevalence of a targeted disease or condition and help people live longer, healthier lives. There is wide agreement that preventive care provides important health benefits. Many preventive services offer good value for increasingly scarce health care dollars. Benefits for many preventive services come at a relatively low cost and much preventive care is cost-effective.
>
> (Goodell, Cohen & Neumann, 2009)[546]

This scenario indicates that preventive health is worth pursuing, otherwise healthcare costs will keep escalating to unacceptable levels. Like any other program or system, when implemented effectively, preventive health offers advantages to the entire community. It has been observed by public health professionals that implementation of preventive health programs is one of the greatest challenges in preventive health.

Designing an effective preventive health program requires a systematic, unbiased approach to the entire process. Since public health professionals have been endowed with the academic skills that qualify them to effectively address burdens of disease in communities, they are in a strategically appropriate position to aggressively promote preventive health. In their article on threats to global health and opportunities written for change, authors Ulrich Laaser and Leon Epstein inform us that:

> An important development in modern public health conceptualization has been the recognition of the principle that it includes not only the classical elements of prevention in terms of environmental threats and spread of communicable disease, but also the planned action of health care systems in their responsibility for the health of

all individuals that make up a community. Consequently, public health practice has extended to areas such as the primary prevention of chronic disease, its early diagnosis, and treatment in order to avoid disability in all its forms.

(Laaser & Epstein, 2009)[547]

1. Preventive Health in Developing Nations

In developing nations, millions of people suffer from preventable diseases and other health problems. Often these are associated with malnutrition and poor hygiene practices. Women in the child-bearing age group experience complications associated with childbirth because of lack of access to comprehensive health resources.[548] Intra-country health disparities are attributed to lack of a proper health care system exacerbated by lack of funds. Inter-country health disparities are a consequence of differences in healthcare expenditure, lack of access to technology necessary for medical research, as well as a lack of skilled manpower.

In some developing countries, the annual healthcare expenditure per individual is about US $10.00. Tragically, in these countries, palpable healthcare disparities also exist between the poor and the rich, with the rich having more access to available subsidized government healthcare services than the poor. Strategies to bridge this gap should include empowering the poor through education to adopt personal and familial preventive healthcare methods at home that include avoiding risky behavioral choices. Another strategy is to introduce innovative and collaborative community approaches such as those adopted by Ghana and India in which intensive training of local community leaders and health workers has been utilized to meet the health needs of the poor. In China and Indonesia, the poor often pool their resources together to help each other when they fall ill.

Dr. Robert Sharpe, Scientific Director for International Associations against Painful Experiments on Animals, applauds the public health work of Lemuel Shattuck and Edwin Chadwick who, by observing different communities, discovered that people who lived in squalid and crowded conditions with little food were much more susceptible to contracting infectious diseases and to die from them.[549]

It is to individuals such as Shattuck and Chadwick and their studies that we deeply owe the relative improvement in our life expectancy. It was their findings that led to the enactment of laws aimed at improving nutrition, hygiene, and sanitation in residential and work places of vulnerable communities. This ultimately led to a rapid fall in mortality rates from infectious diseases. These two are among some of the famous scientists who successfully championed the cause of community public health as a preventive measure.

Developing nations carry a disproportionately heavy burden of preventable, infectious, and chronic diseases. Although modern medicine can treat and manage these diseases, it is powerless to eradicate them if the environment and habits that cause them remain the same. Better individual and community health can be achieved by adopting the same methods that were proposed by both Shattuck in the United States and Chadwick in England.

Author Brian Inglis in his book *Diseases of Civilization* aptly observes that: "The chief credit for the conquest of the destructive epidemics...ought to have been given to the social reformers who had campaigned for purer water, better sewage disposal and improved living standards. It had been their efforts, rather than the achievement of the medical scientists, which had been chiefly responsible for the reduction in mortality from infectious diseases" (Inglis, 1983).[550]

The pattern of disease has changed in developing nations. While they have traditionally contended with infectious diseases, they are now witnessing a remarkable rise in preventable chronic diseases such as heart disease, cancer, diabetes, and strokes. Muir and Parkin reported in the January 5, 1985, issue of the *British Medical Journal* that 80% to 90% of cancers are regarded as preventable. The same applies to most other chronic diseases such as heart disease, stroke, and diabetes.[551]

Anand and Associates in their 2008 article, which appeared in the *Pharmaceutical Research Journal*, claimed that "Instead of our genes, our lifestyle and environment account for 90–95% of our most chronic illnesses."[552] The above claims indicate that the bulk of premature and preventable diseases in the United States and elsewhere around the world can be avoided. Failure to tackle the underlying or root causes of these main health problems will only increase their incidence and prevalence, and will keep draining national resources, leaving not enough funds for other developmental programs.

A noteworthy example of the benefits and efficacy of preventive health was demonstrated between 1996 and 2001 when a federally funded landmark clinical trial was conducted by researchers at the George Washington University (Maryland, US) and the University of Pittsburg Medical Center (Pennsylvania, US) to determine if lifestyle changes could be utilized as a form of intervention to prevent the onset of Type 2 diabetes in individuals at risk for the disease.[553]

The study was called Diabetes Prevention Program (DPP). The participants were overweight individuals with impaired glucose tolerance and at risk for developing full-blown diabetes. During the course of the study, the participants were required to change their behaviors and lifestyles by adopting a prescribed healthy diet, exercising moderately and routinely, and losing some weight. Some of the foodstuffs the participants were required to eat during this period included fruit such as apples, oranges, and purple grapes. The vegetables included spinach, beans, zucchini, cabbage, and romaine lettuce. The participants were also asked to abandon consumption of unhealthy foods with high sugar content such as glazed doughnuts, ice cream, and high fat content foods during the study.

Case managers of the above study who delivered the intervention had frequent contact with the participants to help them achieve their goals. A sixteen-week core curriculum was distributed to individual participants. The curriculum covered the topics that included physical activity, nutrition, and behavioral self-management techniques. Individual toolboxes were developed for each participant to help them identify and overcome specific barriers to achieving their goals during the study. The case managers were chosen from the same ethnic groups as the participants. The DPP staff was provided training, feedback, and support through an extensive, centralized network that included standardized training. The staff also had access to local experts in nutrition and exercise.

Further, the DPP staff was required to participate in monthly individual and regional conference calls with lifestyle staff to provide them with the guidance and consultation necessary in the study. This clinical trial required extensive local and national network to provide the needed training, feedback and clinical support for the interventionists of the study. The results of this clinical trial, which were published in 2002, demonstrated a 58% reduction in the incidence of diabetes among all participating ethnic groups of both genders. The participants who were aged 60 and above benefited the most from the lifestyle changes by having their risk of onset of diabetes reduced by 71%. The following is part of the report of the findings of the clinical trial:

> Many of the fifty-seven million Americans at high risk for type 2 diabetes could be spared some, perhaps all, of the suffering from the disease. Rather than being consigned to a future of chronic illness, they could slow or conceivably halt the progression from prediabetes to diabetes. By contrast, if those prediabetic populations did nothing to change their behavior, they would in all likelihood develop type 2 diabetes within ten years; possibly go on to have

heart attacks or strokes; potentially lose their limbs, eyesight, and kidney functioning; and probably die years before their time... The DPP study showed that if every one of those fifty-seven million people with prediabetes were able to make the lifestyle changes that the study participants made, ten million would sharply lower their risk of developing type 2 diabetes. And the study results were surprising in other ways as well. The DPP showed that lifestyle interventions could be more effective prevention tools than taking medication.

(Brink, 2009)

Although prevention may be labor intensive and costly initially, it reduces the likelihood of disease, which, in turn, reduces healthcare expenses, significantly. Properly planned prevention strategies can be an investment that can yield real cost effective returns over a long period of time for the money spent upfront to forestall disease. The Protecting the Next Pregnancy project was another preventive intervention strategy in which investigators worked with women who were identified as heavy alcohol consumers during their previous pregnancy.[554]

The goal of the study was to prevent drinking alcohol during pregnancy with the anticipation that this would improve the birth weight, length of gestation, and developmental outcomes of the next or subsequent pregnancy. The participants' previous pregnancy was labeled as the index pregnancy in this study. The participants in the project were women who had consumed from four drinks a week constituting 0.3 ounces of absolute alcohol a day to 16 drinks a week during their index pregnancy.

The average rate of alcohol consumption in the study was 1.2 ounces of absolute alcohol per day. The participants were randomly assigned to either a control group or an experimental group and were followed for up to five years. The women in the experimental group were exposed to five sessions of brief but intensive intervention sessions, which were based on cognitive behavioral approaches, while those in the control group were only given standard clinical care without intervention sessions.

The counselors who presided over the experimental group started their intervention sessions by reviewing the definition of a standard drink. Then they assisted the participants in setting goals of abstaining from or reducing alcohol consumption and taught them ways to achieve the goals. Besides the five experimental sessions, other booster sessions were conducted over the follow-up period of five years.

The women in the control group were only advised that "You can have a healthier baby if you cut back or stop drinking during pregnancy" (Hankin, 2008). The findings of this study demonstrated that the women in the experimental group drank significantly less than their counterparts in the control group during their subsequent pregnancies. While 25% of women in the control group drank at least 0.3 ounces of absolute alcohol each day, only 11.8% of the participants in the experimental group drank at that level. Among the participants who continued to drink alcohol during their subsequent pregnancies, the women from the experimental group had reduced their overall alcohol consumption to half that of their counterparts in the control group.

This reduced consumption of alcohol led to improved birth outcomes, fewer low-birth weight babies, and still fewer premature births among the participants in the experimental group. In addition, the babies born to women from the experimental group exhibited better neurobehavioral performance by the age of 13 months compared with babies born to women from the control group.

This brief intervention, therefore, not only protected subsequent pregnancies but reduced the healthcare costs that would have been associated with more low-birth weight and premature babies' needs. Preventive health care truly pays dividends. More effort should be channeled toward preventive health care, particularly as stipulated in the Scriptures.

ENDNOTES

CHAPTER 1

1 Douglas S. Winnail, "Defeating disease: How the Bible can help." Tomorrow's World. Accessed August 16, 2010, http://www.tomorrowsworld.org/cgi-bin/tw/tw-mag.cgi?category=Magazine 19&item=1104107931

2 Foley, John, P. Ed., "Jefferson Cyclopedia: A Comparative Collection of Views of Thomas Jefferson." Vol. 1, pp. 402 in *Jonas's Heath Care Delivery in the United States*. 5th Ed. Springer Publishing Company. 1995

3 Redwanur M.Rahman, "Human rights, Health and the State in Bangladesh." *BMC International Health and Human Rights*, 6:4 (2006). doi:10.1186/1472-698X-6-4

4 World Health Organization, 2010. *Definition of Health*. Geneva, Switzerland. 2010, http://www.who.int/occupational_health/publications/healthy_workplaces_model_action.pdf

CHAPTER 2

5 Association of Schools for Public Health, 2010. *What is Public Health?* Michigan, United States. 2010,http://www.whatispublichealth.org/ and http://allegancountycoa.org/docs/HD/ED/HDED20100712_FAQs.pdf

6   James M. McGinnis & Christopher DeGraw "Healthy Schools 2000: Creating Partnerships for the Decade." *Journal of School of Health*, *61* (7), 292-207 (1991).
7   Tony Truong. "Advanced preventive medicine in the Bible." Accessed October 30, 2010. http://www.ucalgary.ca/uofc/Others/HOM/Dayspapers2000.pdf
8   World Health Organization. *Poor Sanitation Threatens Public Health* 2008. Geneva, Switzerland. Accessed August 1, 2011. http://www.who.int/mediacentre/news/releases/2008/pr08/en/index.html

CHAPTER 3

9   Mary-Jane Schneider *Introduction to Public Health*. (Jones and Bartlett, Publishers, Inc. Sudbury, MA, 2004)146, 339. Print.
10 Public Health Functions Steering Committee, 1995. *Public Health in America*. United States. Last Modified 2008. Accessed August 1, 2011. http://www.health.gov/phfunctions/public.htm
11 Douglas S. Winnail, "Defeating disease: How the Bible can help."Tomorrow's World. Accessed 16 August 2010,http://www.tomorrowsworld.org/cgi-bin/tw/tw-mag.cgi?category=Magazine 19&item=1104107931
12 J.C. Geiger, "The Lure of Medical History." *California and Western Medicine*,39 (6), (1933): 406-409. Accessed 4 August 2011. http://www.ncbi.nlm.nih.gov/pmc/articles/PMC1658878/pdf/calwestmed00430-0047.pdf
13 P.K. Mills, W.L. Beeson, R.L. Phillips, & G.E. Fraser, "Cancer Incidence among California Seventh-day Adventists, 1976-1982." *The American Journal of Clinical Nutrition*, 59 . suppl. (1994): 1136S-1142S
14 R.L. Philips, L. Garfinkel, J. Kuzma, W.L. Beeson, & T. Lotz, "Mortality among California Seventh-day Adventists for Selected Cancer Sites." *Journal of National Cancer Institute*, 65.5: (1980):1097-1107

15 J.E. Ernstrom, "Health Practices and Cancer Mortality among Active California Mormons." *Journal of the National Cancer Institute*, 81.23: (1989): 1807-1814
16 Congregational Health Ministries. *Health and Welfare Ministries, General Board of Global Ministries*, The United Methodist Church, New York, New York. In Andrea C. Lomboy, 2009. Medical Rural Hospital Flexibility Program (FLEX) Agreement through the Virginia Rural Health Resource Center. Essex County, Tappahannock. United States. Accessed 17 December 2012, http://www.vdh.state.va.us/healthpolicy/primarycare/ruralhealth/documents/cha-summary-essex.pdf
17 Angelique C. Harris, "Sex, Stigma, and the Holy Ghost: The Black Church and the Construction of AIDS in New York." *Journal of African American Studies*, 14. (2009): 21-23. doi 10.1007/s12111-009-9105-6
18 UNICEF, World Conference of Religions for Peace & UNAIDS, *What Religious People can do about HIV/AIDS. Action for Children and Young People.* United Nations Children's Fund (UNICEF), 2003. New York, United States. Accessed 4 November 2010, http://www.unicef.org/adolescence/files/Religious_leaders_Aids.pdf
19 6th Annual Health & Wellness Fair, *Congregational Health Assessment Findings Pilot Program- Bath County* 2009. New York, New York. Accessed 21 November 2012 from http://www.virginiaheartattackcoalition.org/pdf/Bath_AndreaLomboy.pdf
20 Harold G. Koenig, *The healing power of faith: Science Explores Medicine's Last Great Frontier.* (1999) Simon & Schuster, New York, NY. Print.
21 R. Saxey, "A physician's reflections on Old Testament medicine. Notes and comments." *Journal of Mormon Thought.* (n.d.). 124, 128. Accessed 31 October 2010. https://dialoguejournal.com/wpcontent/uploads/sbi/articles/Dialogue_V17N03_124.pdf
22 Jordan S. Rubin, *The Great Physician's R_x for Health and Wellness: Seven Keys to Unlock Your Health Potential (2004).* Thomas Nelson. Nashville, TN. 1979. Print.

Chapter 4

23 National Vital Statistics Report, 2009. *Cause of Death*. United States. Accessed 22 November 2012, http://www.cdc.gov/nchs/ and http://www.asap-care.org/epidemiology_of_dying.htm

24 World Health Organization Factsheets. *Cancer*. United States. Accessed 7 September 2010. http://www.who.int/mediacentre/factsheets/fs297/en/index.html

25 Douglas S. Winnail, "Defeating disease: How the Bible can help."Tomorrow's World Accessed 16 August, 2010. http://www.tomorrowsworld.org/cgi-bin/tw/tw-mag.cgi?category=Magazine 19&item=1104107931

26 World Health Organization. *Malaria is alive and well and killing more than 3,000 African children every day*. United States. Accessed 22 September 2010. http://www.who.int/mediacentre/news/releases/2003/pr33/en/

Chapter 5

27 Mary-Jane Schneider *Introduction to Public Health*. (Jones and Bartlett, Publishers, Inc. Sudbury, MA, 2004). Print

28 Lana Skrtic "Hydrogen Sulfide, Oil and Gas, and People's Health." (MA Thesis. University of California, Berkeley. 2002).

29 Sanford Lewis. *Beyond the Chemical Century: Restoring Human Rights and Preserving the Fabric of Life*. (1999). (Jamaica Plain, MA)Web. Print.

30 B. Ostro "Outdoor Air Pollution. Assessing the Environmental Burden of Disease at National and Local Levels. Series 5" World Health Organization. Geneva. 2004. Accessed 9 August, 2011. http://www.who.int/quantifying_ehimpacts/publications/ebd5/en/index.html

31 B. Ostro. "Outdoor Air Pollution: Environmental Burden of Disease at National and Local Levels, Series, No. 5." 2004. World Health Organization. Accessed 22 November, 2012. http://www.who.int/quantifying_ehimpacts/publications/ebd5.pdf

32 World Health Organization. *Metrics: Disability-Adjusted Life Years (DALY)*. Accessed 8 September, 2010. http://www.who.int/healthinfo/global_burden_disease/metrics_daly/en/index.html

33 Frank Raes. "Climate Change Policy Making." Conference of the Parties to the UN Framework Convention on Climate Change (COP 17). Joint Research Centre, European Commission. Durban, South Africa. November 28th-December 9th 2011. 4th Updated Version. Accessed December 18 2012 http://ies.jrc.ec.europa.eu/uploads/fileadmin/Documentation/JRC-CC-COP17.pdf.pdf

34 Jeffery Chanton. "Global Warming and Rising Oceans." 2002. American Institute of Biological Sciences. Accessed 16 September 2010. http://www.actionbioscience.org/environment/chanton.html

35 Naomi Oreskes. "Beyond the Ivory Tower: the Scientific Consensus on Climate Change." *Science*, 306 (5702) (2004): 1686. DOI: 10.1126/science.1103618. Web. 9 August 9, 2011. http://www.sciencemag.org/content/306/5702/1686.full

36 Word Health Organization. *Indoor air pollution: national burden of disease estimates*. United States. Accessed September 2010. http://www.who.int/indoorair/publications/nationalburden/en/index.html

37 Gregory A. Wellenius, et al. "Particulate Air Pollution and Hospital Admissions for Congestive Heart Failure in Seven United States Cities." *The American Journal of Cardiology*, 97, (2006): 404-408.

38 A. Bhatnagar. "Environmental cardiology: studying mechanistic links between pollution and heart disease." *Circulation Research*, 99 (7) (2006): 692-705.

39 R.D. Brook. "Cardiovascular effects of air pollution." *Clinical Science (Lond)*, 115(6) (2008):175-187.

CHAPTER 6

40 United States Geographical Survey. *The water in you. Water Science for Schools*. Modified 2012. Accessed 3 January 2011. http://ga.water.usgs.gov/edu/propertyyou.html

41 Lenntech. *Water facts and trivia*. Water Treatment Solutions. Accessed 2 November 2010. http://www.lenntech.com/

water-trivia-facts.htm and http://www.dads.state.tx.us/texercise/programs/fitforhealthofit/factsheets/HydrationFacts.pdf

42 Katherine E. Bliss. "Enhancing U.S. Leadership on Drinking Water and Sanitation: Opportunities within Global Health Programs. A Report of the CSIS Global Health Policy Center." Center for Strategic and International Studies. 2009. Accessed 13 September 2010. http://csis.org/files/publication/090924_Bliss_WaterHealth_Web.pdf

43 World Health Organization. *Health Through Safe Drinking Water and Basic Sanitation*. Accessed 7 September 2010. http://www.who.int/water_sanitation_health/mdg1/en/index.html

44 Matsuura, K. "United Nations Educational, Scientific and Cultural Organization (UNESCO) in Action. International Year of Freshwater Launched." 2003. Accessed November 2010 http://unesdoc.unesco.org/images/0013/001335/133510e.pdf

45 United Nation Millennium Declaration. *Resolution adopted by the General Assembly*. 2000. Accessed 23 November 2012. http://www.un.org/millennium/declaration/ares552e.htm

46 A. Pruss-Ustum, R. Bos, F. Gore & J. Bartram. "Safe Water, Better Health: Costs, Benefits and Sustainability of Interventions to Protect and Promote Health." World Health Organization. 2008. Accessed 13 September 2010. http://whqlibdoc.who.int/publications/2008/9789241596435_eng.pdf

47 Mukesh Yadav. "Hospital Waste—A Major Problem." *JK-Practitioner 8* (4). (2001): 276-202

48 Thomas L. Constable. "Notes on Leviticus". 2010 Edition. 2010. Web. 3 January 2011. http://www.soniclight.com/constable/notes/pdf/leviticus.pdf

Chapter 7

49 World Health Organization-Geneva. 1985. *Public Health Implications of Alcohol Production and Trade*. Geneva, Switzerland. 1985. Accessed 14 December 2010. http://whqlibdoc.who.int/offset/WHO_OFFSET_88.pdf

50   Thomas M. Brown, Marcos Cueto, & Elizabeth Fee. "The World Health Organization and the Transition from International to 'Global' Public Health." *American Journal of Public Health* 96.1 (2006): 62-72.
51   R. Room, T. Babor, & J. Rehm. "Alcohol and Public Health." *Lancet*, 365. 9458 (2005): 519-530. PMID: 15705462 [PubMed - indexed for MEDLINE
52   Glucksman, E. (1994). "Alcohol and Accidents." *British Medical Bulletin, 50* (1) (1994): 76-84.
53   Jones, W. Keith. "A Murine Model of Alcoholic Cardiomyopathy. A role for zinc and metallothionein fibrosis." *American Journal of Pathology*, 167.2 (2005): 301-304.
54   Mayo Clinic. 2008.Cardiomyopathy. *U.S. News*. December 12. 2008. Print.
55   Health Encyclopedia. "Alchoholic Hepatitis." University of Rochester Medical Center. Last Modefied December 20, 2012. http://www.urmc.rochester.edu/encyclopedia/content.aspx?ContentTypeID=85&ContentID=P00655
56   S.I. McMillen, S.I. & David Stern. *None of These Diseases (3rd ed)*. Grand Rapids, MI: Flemming H. Revell, 2000.
57   National Institute on Alcohol Abuse and Alcoholism, *Cognitive Impairment and Recovery from Alcoholism*, Alcohol Alert, No. 53. 2001. Accessed 13 June 2013. http://pubs.niaaa.nih.gov/publications/aa53.htm
58   Clive Harper. "The Neuropathology of Alcohol-Related Brain Damage." *Alcohol and Alcoholism*, (2009):1-5, doi: 10.1093/alcalc/agn102
59   Azheimer's Australia. "Alcohol Related Dementia." Help Sheet.2010. Last Modified 2010. Accessed 25 November, 2012. http://www.fightdementia.org.au/understanding-dementia/alcohol-related-dementia.aspx
60   Primal Chowdry, & Priya Gupta. "Pathophysiology of Alcoholic Pancreatitis: An Overview." *World Journal of Gastroenterology*, 12.46 (2006): 7421-7427. ISSN 1007-9327

61 National Institute of Health National Institute of Alcohol Abuse and Alcoholism (NIAAA) (1998). "Economic Costs and Drug Abuse Estimated at $ 246 Billion in the United States." *NIH News*, May 13, 1998 Accessed December 20, 2012.(Last Modified, n.d. http://www.niaaa.nih.gov/news-events/news-releases/economic-costs-alcohol-and-drug-abuse-estimated-246-billion-united-states

62 National Association for Children of Alcoholics (n.d.). "Information on Drugs and Alcohol." Last Modified 1998. Accessed 25 November, 2012. http://www.nacoa.net/impfacts.htm

63 Antonia Abbey, et al. (2001). "Alcohol and Sexual Assault." National Institute on Alcohol Abuse and Alcoholism (NIAAA) Alcohol Health and Research World 2001. Last Modified, n.d. Accessedd 10 October 2010. http://www.athealth.com/Practitioner/ceduc/alc_assault.html

64 Bijil Arackal & Vivel Benegal. "Prevalence of sexual dysfunction in male subjects with alcohol dependence," 2007. *Indian Journal of Psychiatry, 49* (2), 109-112. doi: 10.4103/0019-5545.33257

65 Mendelson, J. H., & Mello, N. K. "Medical progress, Biologic concomitants of Alcoholism," 1979. *New England Journal of Medicine, 301*, 912-921

66 The Magazine of FEANTSA-The European Fedeation of National Organizations Working with the Homeless AISBL (2011). "Homeless in Europe. Homeless, Health, Health and Homeless: Overcoming the Complexities." 2011. Accessed November 25, 2012 from http://www.feantsa.org/files/freshstart/Communications/Homeless%20in%20Europe%20EN/PDF_2011/Homeless_in_Europe_Spring_2011.pdf

67 F.G.Moeller, & D.M. Dougherty. "Antisocial Personality Disorder, Alcohol and Aggression." *Alcohol Research and Health, 25*.1 (2001): 5-11.

68 B. Subra, et al. "Automatic Effects of Alcohol and Aggressive Cues on Aggressive Thoughts and Behaviours." *Personality and Social Psychology Bulletin*, 36.8 (2010): 1052-1057.

69 M.S. McCloskey, & M.E. Berman. "Alcohol Intoxication and Self-aggressive Behavior." *Journal of Abnormal Psychology*, 112.2 (2003): 306-311. Print.
70 S.L. Mercer, et al. "Translating Evidence into Policy: Lessons Learned from the Case of Lowering the Legal Blood Limit for Drivers." *Association of Educational Psychologists*, 20.6 (2010): 412-420. doi:10.1016/j.annepidem.2010.03.005. Print.
71 Centers for Disease Control and Prevention (2012). "Impaired Driving: Get the Facts." Last Modified October 2012. Accessed 25 November, 2012. http://www.cdc.gov/motorvehiclesafety/impaired_driving/impaired-drv_factsheet.html
72 L. Blincoe, et al. (2002). "The Economic Impact of Motor Vehicle Crashes, 2000. Washington (DC): Dept of Transportation (US), National Highway Traffic Safety Administration (NHTSA)." Accessed December 20, 2012. http://www.cita-vehicleinspection.org/Portals/cita/autofore_study/LinkedDocuments/literature/NHTSA%20the%20economic%20impact%20of%20motor%20vehicle%20crashes%202000%20USA%202002.pdf
73 Jack Dearden, & Jason Payne. "Alcohol and Homicide in Australia. Trends and Issues in Crime and Criminal Justice, No. 372." Australian Institute of Criminology. 2009. Accessed 18 October 2010. http://www.aic.gov.au/documents/6/F/F/%7B6FF03CB5-1EF7-43EE-84FC-F0997C5C84C9%7Dtandi372_001.pdf
74 Toni Makkai & Jason Payne. "Key Findings from the Drug Use Careers of Offenders (DUCO) Study. Trends & Issues in Crime and Criminal Justice no. 267." Australian Institute of Criminology. 2003. 18 October 2010. http://www.aic.gov.au/publications/tandi2/ tandi267.html
75 United States Department of Justice, Office of Justice Programs, Bureau of Justice Assistance. *Alcohol and Violent Crime: What is the Connection? What can be Done?* 2006. United States. Accessed 18 October 2010. http://www.nllea.org/documents/Alcohol_and_Crime.pdf

76 H. Wesley Perkins. "Surveying the damage: A Review of Research on Consequences of Alcohol Misuse in College Populations." Last Reviewed 2005. Accessed 18 October 2010. http://www.collegedrinkingprevention.gov/supportingresearch/Journal/perkins.aspx

77 Morbidity and Mortality Weekly Report . Vital Signs: Binge Drinking Prevalence, Frequency and Intensity among Adults—United States 2010. Last Modified 1 January 2012. Accessed December 19, 2012. http://www.cdc.gov/mmwr/pdf/wk/mm6101.pdf

78 Kenneth D. Kochanek, M.A.; Jiaquan Xu, M.D.; Sherry L. Murphy, B.S.; Arialdi M. Minino, M.P.H.; and Hsiang-Ching Kung, Ph.D., "Deaths: Final Data for 2009." Division of Vital Statistics. Centers for Disease Control, 60 (3) (201): 11. http://www.cdc.gov/nchs/data/nvsr/nvsr60/nvsr60_03.pdf

79 C.A. Youngers, & E. Rosin. "Drugs and Democracy in Latin America. The Impact of U.S. Policy. A Washington Office of Latin America Report. 2004." Accessed 23 August 2010. http://www.seguridadregional-fes.org/upload/2433-001_g.pdf

80 K. Klostermann, & M.L. Kelley. "Alcoholism and Intimate Partner Violence: Effects on Children's Psychological Adjustment. 2009." *International Journal of Environmental Research and Public Health*, 6. (2009): 3156-3168. doi:10.3390/ijerph6123156. Print.

81 Glenda Kaufman Kantor & Murray A. Strauss. (1987). "The 'Drunken Bum' Theory of Wife Beating." *Social Problems*, 34.3 (1987): 214-234.13 October 2010. Print. http://pubpages.unh.edu/~mas2/VB4.pdf

82 National Institute on Alcohol Abuse and Alcoholism (2011). *Alcohol Across the Lifespan*. Accessed 25 November, 2012. http://pubs.niaaa.nih.gov/publications/StrategicPlan/NIAAASTRATEGICPLAN.htm

83 Nutrition Information Center-University of Stellenbosch (n.d). *What is Fetal Alcohol Syndrome?* Accessed 25 November, 2012. http://sun025.sun.ac.za/portal/page/portal/Health_Sciences/

English/Centres%20and%20Institutions/Nicus/Nutrition_Facts_sheets/Fetal%20Alcohol%20Syndrome.pdf

84 Teratogen. Webster's New World Medical Dictionary 3rd ed. 2008.
85 C. Lupton, L. Burd, & R. Harwood. "Cost of Fetal Alcohol Spectrum Disorders." *American Journal of Medical Genetics*, 127C (2004):42-50
86 S.I. McMillen, S.I. & David Stern. *None of These Diseases (3rd ed)*. Grand Rapids, MI: Flemming H. Revell, 2000.pp. 47
87 Harvey A. Skinner & Stephen Holt. "Early Intervention for Alcohol Problems." *Journal of the Royal College of General Practitioners*, 33 (1983): 787-791. Print.

CHAPTER 8

88 William F. Dankenbring. "Bible Laws-The Foundation of Good Health." 1972. Accessed 25 November, 2012. http://home.sprynet.com/~pabco/tw0172_health.htm
89 Eugenia Tognotti. "The Dawn of Medical Microbiology: Germ Hunters and the Discovery of the Cause of Cholera. *Journal of Medical Microbiology, 60* (4), (2011): 555-558
90 Laura Del Col. "Chadwick's Report on Sanitary Conditions." 2002. Web. 7 September 2010, http://www.victorianweb.org/history/chadwick2.html
91 Annette Pruss-Ustum, Robert Bos, Fiona Gore & Jamie Bartram. "Safer Water, Better Health: Costs, Benefits and Sustainability of Interventions to Protect and Promote Health." Accessed 13 September, 2010. http://whqlibdoc.who.int/publications/2008/9789241596435_eng.pdf
92 Donald T. Atkinson. *Magic, Myth and Medicine*. New York. (The World Publishing Company. New York. 1950). Accessed 20 December, 2012. http://thehealingproject.net.au/wp-content/uploads/2009/10/ATKINSON-Donald-_1956_-Magic-Myth-and-Medicine.pdf

93   United Nations Water Statistics (n.d.).Drinking Water and Sanitation. United Nations, United States. Accessed 25 November, 2012. http://www.unwater.org/statistics_san.html

94   United Nations. *International Year of Sanitation Global Launch.* Press Release 21 November 2007. United Nations Headquarters, New York. Accessed 21 December 2012. http://esa.un.org/iys/iys_launch.shtml

95   Brendan Walsh & Marcus Grant. "Public Health Implications of Alcohol Production and & Trade." World Health Organization-1985. Accessed 14 December 2010. http://whqlibdoc.who.int/offset/WHO_OFFSET_88.pdf

96   Mukesh Yadav. "Hospital Waste-A Major Problem." *JK-Practitioner* 8 (4), (2001): 276-202

97   Mary-Jane Schneider. *Introduction to Public Health.* Sadbury, Massachusetts. Jones and Bartlett Publishers. Inc. 2004. pp. 339.

98   Interstate Technology & Regulatory Council (ITRC). *Characterization, Design, Construction, and Monitoring of Bioreactor Landfills*.2005. ALT-3. Washington, D.C.: Interstate Technology & Regulatory Council, Alternative Landfill Technologies Team. Accessed December 2012. www.itrcweb.org.

99   Mary-Jane Schneider. *Introduction to Public Health.* Sadbury, Massachusetts. Jones and Bartlett Publishers, Inc. 2004. pp.341.

100 Olar Zerbock. "Urban Solid Waste Management Waste Reduction in Developing Nations 2." (Apr., 2003), (unpublished paper written to meet the requirements of the Master's International Program, Michigan Technological University. Requirements of CE 5993, 2003). *Masters Thesis.* Michigan Technological University.

101 Hisashi Ogawa. "Sustainable Waste Management in Developing Countries." WHO Western Pacific Regional Environmental Health Centre (EHC), Kuala Lumpur, Malaysia. (Paper Presented at the 7the ISWA International Congress of Exhibition. Parallel Session 7. International Perspective. Yokohama, Japan. October/November 1996). Accessed 21 December 2012. http://www.gdrc.org/uem/waste/swm-fogawa1.htm

102 CalRecovery, Inc. and UNEP International Environmental Technology Center. *Solid Waste Management, Volume II: Regional Overviews and Information Sources*. 2005. Accessed 26 November, 2012. http://www.unep.org/ietc/Portals/136/SWM_Vol-II.pdf

103 Lars Mikkel Johannessen & Gabriela Boyer. "Observations of Solid Waste Landfills in Developing Countries: Africa, Asia and Latin America." Urban and Local Government Working Paper, Series no. 3. Washington DC: Urban Development Waste Management Team. 1999. The World Bank. Accessed 21 December 2012. http://www.worldbank.org/urban/solid_wm/erm/CWG%20folder/uwp3.pdf

104 United Nations Environment Programme. *Training Modules: Closing of an Open Dumpsite and Shifting from Open Dumping to Controlled Dumping and to Sanitary Land Filling*. 2005. Accessed 18 August 2011. http://www.unep.or.jp/ietc/Publications/spc/SPC_Training-Module.pdf

CHAPTER 9

105 Centers for Disease Control and Prevention (CDC). Etiologic Agent Import Permit Program (EAIPP). 2011. Accessed 26 November, 2012. http://www.cdc.gov/od/eaipp/

106 O. Morgan. "Infectious Disease Risks from Dead Bodies Following Natural Disasters." *Pan American Journal of Public Health*, 15 (5) (2004): 307-312

107 "Nosocomial Infection." Webster's New World Medical Dictionary. 3er ed. 2008.

108 M.J. Richards, J.R. Edwards, D.H. Culver, & R.R. Gaynes. "Nosocomial Infections in Medical Intensive Care Units in the United States. National Nosocomial Infections Surveillance System." *Critical Care Medicine* 27.5: (1999): 853-854.

109 John D. Keyser. "Ancient Bible Health Secrets Revealed Today." n.d. Accessed 18 August 2010. http://www.hope-of-israel.org/bihealth.htm.

110 Cwikel, J. "Lessons from Semmelweis: A social epidemiologic update on safe motherhood." *Social Medicine*, 3.1 (2008): 19-31. Print.
111 Centers for Disease Control and Prevention. *2007 Guideline for Isolation Precautions: Preventing Transmission of Infectious Agents in Healthcare Settings*. Atlanta. State of Georgia. 2010.
112 Collins, A. S. (n.d.) Preventing Health Care-Associated Infections. Retrieved November 26, 2012 from http://www.ahrq.gov/qual/nurseshdbk/docs/CollinsA_PHCAI.pdf
113 Lisa R. Delaney, & Richard B. Gunderman. "Hand hygiene." *Radiology*, 246.1(2008):15-19: doi: 10.1148/radiol.2461061676.
114 R. K. Albert, & M.S. Condie. "Hand-Washing Patterns in Medical Intensive-Care Units." *The New England Journal of Medicine*, 304 (1981): 1465-1466.
115 Kyle Butt, K. "Scientific Foreknowledge and Medical Acumen of the Bible." 2006. Accessed 25 August 2010. http://apologeticspress.org/apcontent.aspx?category=13&article=2024
116 Shelov, Stephen, P., & Altmann,Tanya.R. (Eds.). Caring for Your Baby and Young child. Birth to age 5. The Complete and Authoritative Guide. New York. American Academy of Pediatrics (5th ed.). Bantam Books. 2009. ISBN 978-0-553-38630-1
117 BBC News. "Boy Babies 'Boost Appetite." British Broadcasting Corporation. Thursday June 5, 2003. Accessed 21 December 2012. http://news.bbc.co.uk/2/hi/health/2962130.stm
118 Emelia Del Bono, & John Ermisch, (2009). "Birth Weight and the Dynamics of Early Cognitive and Behavioral Development." [Institute for Study of Labor (IZA) Discussion Paper No. 4270]. Accessed 21 December 2012. http://ftp.iza.org/dp4270.pdf
119 Academy for Educational Development. Facts for Feeding. 2012. Accessed 26 November, 2012. http://rehydrate.org/breastfeed/facts-birth-7days.htm
120 Torngren, P. "The Needs of the Newborn in the First Few Hours of Life."2004. International Primal Association. Accessed 14 June 2013. http://www.primals.org/articles/torngren04.html

121 Robinson, L., Saisan, J., Smith, M., & Segal, J. "Building a Secure Attachment Bond With Your Baby: Parenting Tips for Creating a Strong Attachment Relationship."2013. Accessed 14 June 203. http://www.helpguide.org/mental/parenting_attachment.htm

122 Ray, R. "A Detailed Look at Parental Leave Policies in 21 OECD Countries," 2008. Center for Economic and Policy Research. Accessed 14 June 2013. http://www.lisdatacenter.org/wp-content/uploads/parent-leave-details1.pdf

123 American Public Health e-Newsletter. Get Ready Now: Fall 2010 Issue. Get Ready Newsletter. Accessed16 December 2010. http://www.getreadyforflu.org/enewsletter/NewsFall10.htm

124 Myers-Smith, C. "After Birth: The First Six Weeks." American College of Nurse-Midwives. n.d. Accessed 8 September 2010, http://www.mymidwife.org/After-Birth-The-First-Six-Weeks

125 Craig Lambert, C. (2005).Deep into Sleep. Harvard Magazine. Accessed 26 November, 2012. http://harvardmagazine.com/2005/07/deep-into-sleep.html

126 National Institute of Neurological Disorders and Stroke. Brain basics: Understanding Sleep. United States. 2007. Accessed 12 September 2010 http://www.ninds.nih.gov/disorders/brain_basics/understanding_sleep.htm

CHAPTER 10

127 R. Bartlett, et al. "Emerging and Re-emerging Infectious Diseases: The Third Epidemiologic Transition." *Annual Review of Anthropology*, 27 (1998): 247-271. Print.

128 Gro Harlem Brundtland. "World Health Organization Report on Infectious Diseases: Removing Obstacles to Healthy Development."1999. Accessed 14 June 2013. http://www.who.int/infectious-disease-report/pages/textonly.html

129 National Center for Biotechnology Information, U.S. National Library of Medicine *Understanding Emerging and Re-emerging Infectious Disease*, 2007. Accessed 14 June 2013. http://www.ncbi.nlm.nih.gov/books/NBK20370/

130 George Santayana. "The Life of Reason," 1905 In National Churchill History *War Is Glorious,* Blog. November 16, 2012. Accessed 20 June 2013. http://www.nationalchurchillmuseum.org/blog/

131 Steve Mirsky. Re-emerging Diseases: Gone today, here tomorrow? 1997. Accessed 20 June 2013. http://www.columbia.edu/cu/21stC/issue-2.3/mirsky.html

132 Lloyd F, Novick & Cynthia B. Morrow. "Defining Public Health: Historical and Contemporary Developments" in Public Health Administration : Principles for Population-Based Management, ed. Novick, L.F., Morrow, C. B., & Mays, G.P.. 2nd ed. 2008. Electronic copy, pp. 2

133 G. Clark, "*Microbes and Markets: was the Black Death an Economic Revolution?* Accessed 21 September 2010. http://www.econ.ucdavis.edu/faculty/gclark/papers/black1.pdf

134 Stefan Riedel. "Edward Jenner and the History of Smallpox and Vaccination." *Baylor University Medical Center Proceedings,* 18:1(2005): 21-25. PMCID: PMC1200696. Print.

135 WHO, UNICEF, World Bank (2009). *State of the World's Vaccines and Immunization (3rd ed.) World Health Organization.* New York. United States. Accessed 27 November 2012 http://www.unicef.org/immunization/files/SOWVI_full_report_english_LR1.pdf

136 Molly Billings. (2005). "The influenza Pandemic of 1918." 2005. Accessed 11 January 2011. http://virus.stanford.edu/uda

137 M.I. Meltzer, N.J. Cox, & K. Fukuda, "The Economic Impact of Pandemic Influenza in the United States: Priorities for Intervention." *Emerging Infectious Diseases,* 5 :5 (1999): 659-671. Print.

138 The Harvard University Library Open Collections Program. "Tuberculosis in Europe and North America, 1800-1922." Cambridge, United States. 2012. Accessed 27 November, 2012. http://ocp.hul.harvard.edu/contagion/tuberculosis.html

139 J. Croft, & N. Croft. "The History of Tuberculosis." In Justin Tanimoto: "Tuberculosis." Microbiology Fall. 2010. Accessed 2 December 2012. http://www.micklebring.com/oakwood/ch18.htm

140 David S. Jones. "The Persistence of American Indian Health Disparities." *American Journal of Public Health*, 96, (2006): 2122-2134

141 Peter D.O. Davies. "*Multidrug Resistant Tuberculosis.*" 1999. Accessed 11 January 2011. http://priory.com/cmol/TBMultid.htm

142 World Health Organization (2012). *Tuberculosis*. United States. Accessed 27 November, 2012. http://www.who.int/immunization/topics/tuberculosis/en/index.html

143 R.C.Cooksey, Morlock, G.P., Glickman, S. & Crawford, J.T. "Evaluation of a Line Probe Assay Kit for Characterization of *rpoB* Mutations in Rifampin-Resistant *Mycobacterium Tuberculosis* Isolates from New York City." *Journal of Clinical Microbiology*, 35:5 (1997): 1281-1283.

144 Peter D.O. Davies. "Drug Resistant Tuberculosis." *Journal of the Royal Society of Medicine*, 94.6. (2001):261-263

145 J. Delahanty & M. Johnson. "TB Reborn: An Old Disease Breathes New Life." *Review, 2* :1 (1998). Accessed 21September 2010. http://www.nsi-ins.ca/english/publications/review/v2n1/01.asp

146 National Institute of Drug Abuse (n.d.). *The Economic Costs of Alcohol and Drug Abuse in the United States-1992*. United States. Accessed 27 November, 2012. http://archives.drugabuse.gov/EconomicCosts/Chapter4b.html

147 World Health Organization. *Malaria is Alive and Well and Killing More Than 3000 African Children Every Day.* Accessed 22 September 2010. http://www.who.int/mediacentre/news/releases/2003/pr33/en/

148 World Health Organization (2012). *Malaria is Alive and Well and Killing More than 3,000 African Children Every Day.* Accessed 27 November, 2012. http://www.who.int/mediacentre/news/releases/2003/pr33/en/

149 Theobald C.E. Mosha, Devote Ntarukimana, & Matilda John. "Prevalence of Congenital Malaria among Neonates at Morogoro

Regional Hospital, Morogoro, Tanzania."*Tanzania Journal of Health Research*, 12 :4. (2010): 237-242. ISSN: 0856-6496. Print.

150 Roll Back Malaria. *The Global Malaria Action Plan for a Malaria Free World.* 2008 Geneva, Switzerland. Accessed 27, November, http://www.rollbackmalaria.org/gmap/gmap.pdf

151 Catholic Relief Services. *World Malaria Day is April 25: Accessed* 22 September 2010. http://crs.org/health/malaria-day/index.cfm

152 Claudia Torres Codeço, (2001). "Endemic and Epidemic Dynamics of Cholera: the Role of the Aquatic Reservoir." *BMC Infectious Diseases,* 1:1 (2001): doi: 10.1186/1471-2334-1-1

153 World Health Organization 2010. *Cholera.* Accessed 22 September 2010. http://www.who.int/mediacentre/factsheets/fs107/en/index.html

154 World Health Organization. *Ebola Hemorrhagic Fever: Fact Sheet No.103.* Accessed 22 December 2012. http://www.who.int/mediacentre/factsheets/fs103/en

155 Eurposurveillance. "Ebola Reston Virus Detected Pigs in the Philippines. European Center for Disease Prevention and Control. EuroSurveillance,14(4):pii=19105. Accessed 22 December 2012. http://www.eurosurveillance.org/ViewArticle.aspx?ArticleId=19105

156 World Health Organization. *Ebola.* 2012 United States. Accessed 21 December 2012. http://www.who.int/csr/don/archive/disease/ebola_haemorrhagic_fever/en/

157 John D. Keyser. "Ancient Bible Health Secrets Revealed Today." Accessed 21 December 2010. http://www.hope-of-israel.org/bihealth.htm

Chapter 11

158 Roderick McGrew. *Encyclopedia of Medical History.* In Kyle Butt."Scientific Foreknowledge and Medical Acumen of the Bible. Reason & Revelation, 26. (12): 89-96

159 S.I. McMillen, S.I. & David E. Stern. *None of These Diseases (3rd ed)*. Grand Rapids, MI: Flemming H. Revell, 2000, pp. 15

160 Merck Manual Home Health Handbook. *Leprosy*. Merck Sharp & Dohme Corp. 2011. Accessed 9 September 2012. http://www.merckmanuals.com/home/infections/tuberculosis_and_leprosy/leprosy.html

161 Atkinson, D. T. *Magic, myth and medicine*. In John D. Keyser. "Ancient Bible health secrets revealed today." Accessed 21 December 2011. http://www.hope-of-israel.org/bihealth.htm

162 Wendy E. Parmet. "Health Care and the Constitution: Public Health and the Role of the State in the Framing Era." *Hastings Constitutional Law Quarterly* 267-335, 285-302 (Winter, 1992)

163 Vernellia R. *Randall. Public Health Practices in the Colonial and Federalist Periods. Bioterrorism, Public Health and the Law*. Law 801: Health Care Law Seminar. Accessed 21 December 2012. http://academic.udayton.edu/health/syllabi/bioterrorism/4phealthlaw/PHLaw00c.htm

164 World Health Organization. *Initiative for Vaccine Research (IVR): Acute Respiratory Infections*. Geneva, Switzerland. Accessed 21 December 2012. http://www.who.int/vaccine_research/diseases/ari/en/index.html

165 J.R. Gwilt. "Public Health in the Bible." *Journal of the Royal Society of Health*. (1987): 247-248

166 Angus Nicoll. *Consensus Document on the Epidemiology of Severe Acute Respiratory Syndrome (SARS). Department of Communicable Disease Surveillance and Response. Global Health Security*. World Health Organization. 2003. Accessed 10 November 2010. http://www.who.int/csr/sars/en/WHOconsensus.pdf

Chapter 12

167 Christine A. Courtois. "Healing the Incest wound: A Treatment Update with Attention to Recovered-Memory Issues." *American Journal of Psychotherapy*, 51:4 (1997): 464-496.

168 Edwards, W. & Hensley, C. Contextualizing Sex Offender Management Legislation and Policy: Evaluating the Problem of Latent Consequences in Community Notification Laws. 2001. *International Journal of Offender Therapy and Comparative Criminology, 45* (1), 83-101.

169 Ho, J. "Incest and Sex Offender Registration: Who is Registration Helping and Who is it Hurting?" 2008. *Cardozo Journal of Law & Gender, 14,* 429-457

170 D.M. Buckley. "Child Sexual Offenders: How They Select, Manipulate and Groom Their Victims." 2008. John E. Reid Associates. Accessed 16 June 2013. http://www.reid.com/training_programs/buckley-sexual_offenders.pdf

171 J.A. Bushnell, J.E. Wells & M.A. Oakley-Browne (1992). Long-Term Effects of Intrafamilial Sexual Abuse in Childhood. *Acta Psychiatrica Scandinavica, 85* (2), 136-142

172 New York City Alliance against Sexual Assault. *Fact Sheet Incest,* 1997. New York, United States. Accessed 30 August 2010. http://www.svfreenyc.org/survivors_factsheet_37.html#1

173 J. Read, & N. Argyle, N. "Hallucinations, Delusions, and Thought Disorder among Adult Psychiatric Inpatients with a History of Child Abuse." *Psychiatric Services,* 50:11 (1999): 1457-1472.

174 Hadar Lubin, David Read Johnson, & Steven M. Southwick. "Impact of Childhood Abuse on Adult Psychopathology: A Case Report." *Dissociation,* 9:2 (1996):134-139.

175 Oliver Onyama, Catherine Paltoo & Julian Greengold . "Somatoform Disorders." *America Family Physician, 1.* 76 (2007):1333-1338

176 D.J. Gelinas. "The Persisting Negative Effects of Incest." *American Journal of Psychiatry,* 46 (1983): 313-332. Print.

177 L.S. Coker. "A Therapeutic Recovery Model for the Female Adult Incest Survivor." *Issues in Mental Health Nursing,* 11:2 (1990):109-123: doi: 10.3109/01612849009014548.

178 Hal Herzog. "The Problem with Incest: Evolution, Morality and the Politics of Abortion," 2012. Accessed 16 June 2013.

http://www.psychologytoday.com/blog/animals-and-us/201210/the-problem-incest

179 Bert Thompson, & Trevor Major. *Where Did Cain Get His Wife?* Apologetics Press Article Reprint. 1987. Accessed 13 *January 2011. http://www.apologeticspress.org/rr/reprints/cain.pdf*

CHAPTER 13

180 Gillian C. Mezey. "Treatment of Rape Victims." *Advances in Psychiatric Treatment*, 3 (1997): 197-203. Print.

181 World Health Organization. *Rape: How women, the Community and Health Sector Respond. Sexual Violence Initiative.* Geneva, Switzerland. 2007. Accessed 18 November 2010 http://www.svri.org/rape.pdf

182 Tara Gingerich, & Jennifer Leaning. *The Use of Rape as a Weapon of War in the Conflict in Darfur, Sudan. Program on Humanitarian Crises and Human Rights.* 2004. Accessed 13 January 2011. http://physiciansforhumanrights.org/library/documents/reports/the-use-of-rape-as-a-weapon.pdf

183 J. Robert Lilly. "Counterblast. Soldiers and rape: The other Band of Brothers." *The Howard Journal of Criminal Justice*, 46.1(2007):72-75. doi:10.1111/j.1468-2311.2007.00455.x Key: citeulike:1056318

184 Anthony Beevor. *Berlin: The Downfall 1945.* 2002. New York. New York. Penguin Books.

185 Elisabeth Jean Wood. "Variation in Sexual Violence During War."*Politics and Society*, 34.3 (2006). 307-34: doi: 10.1177/0032329206290426

186 Hua-Ling W. Hu. "Don't Forget the Chinese Women Under the Rape of Nanking." *Chinese American Forum*, 7.4 (1992):20 -23.

187 Inger Skjelsbæk. *The Elephant in the Room: An Overview of How Sexual Violence Came to be Seen as a Weapon of War.* Report to the Norwegian Ministry of Foreign Affairs. Peace Research Institute of Oslo. 2010. Accessed 18 November 2012. http://

www.peacewomen.org/assets/file/Resources/NGO/vas_ sexualviolencewarweapon_prio_may2010.pdf

188 Genocide Intervention Fund (n.d.). *Darfur: Gendered Violence and Rape as a Weapon of Genocide.* Accessed 23 December 2012. http:// www.ncdsv.org/images/darfurgenderedviolencerapeweapon.pdf

189 John A. Hules. *The Traditional Values of Sex Offenders and Their Victims: What the Research Shows.* 2005. Accessed 18 November 2011. http://www.hules.us/CS_ch02.pdf

190 Holly Burkhalter. *Gender-Based Violence, Health and the Role of the Health Sector*, In The World Bank Group, 2011. Accessed 21 December 2012. http://go.worldbank.org/C1UQRGBCE0

191 Dean G. Kilpartrick. *Rape and Sexual Assault.* 2000. National Violence Against Women Prevention Center. Medical University of South Carolina. Accessed 15 November 2010. http://www. musc.edu/vawprevention/research/sa.shtml

192 Dean G. Kilpatrick. & Benjamin E. Saunders. (1996) *Prevalence and Consequences of Child Victimization: Results from the National Survey of Adolescents.* Final Report (Revised).1996. Accessed 18 November 2011. http://www.ncjrs.gov/pdffiles1/nij/ grants/181028.pdf

193 Dean G. Kilpatrick. *Rape and Sexual Assault.* National Violence Against Women Prevention Research Center Medical University of South Carolina. Accessed 23 December 2012.

194 United Nations Theme Group on HIV and AIDS. *Violence against Women and Girls in the Era of HIV and AIDS. A Situation and Response Analysis in Kenya.* UNAIDS and the Global Coalition on Women and AIDS. UNAIDS, Kenya. 2006. Accessed 19 November 2011 http://data.unaids.org/pub/Report/2006/20060630_gcwa_re_ violence_women_girls_kenya_en.pdf

195 Mike Earl-Taylor. *HIV/AIDS, the Stats, the Virgin Cure and Infant Rape.* Science in Africa-Africa's First On-Line Science Magazine. Janice Limson. Accessed 23 December 2012. http:// www.scienceinafrica.co.za/2002/april/virgin.htm

196 Doug McIntosh. *Deuteronomy: Holman Old Testament Commentary (HOTC)*, Vol. 3. 2002. B & H Publishing Group.
197 James B. Jordan. *The Law of the Covenant In Bahnsen: An Exposition of Exodus 21-23*. Institute for Christian Economics. Tyler, Texas. 1984. Accessed August 30, 2011. http://www.biblicalhorizons.com/pdf/jjlc.pdf
198 Philip Yancey. *Reaching for the Invisible God: What Can We Expect to Find?* Zondervan Publishing Company, Grand Rapids, Michigan, 2002, pp. 119.

CHAPTER 14

199 Richard V. Milani, & Carl J. Lavie. Stopping Stress at its Origins. Editorial Commentary. *Hypertension*, 49. (2007): 268-269
200 D. Hasson, U.M. Anderberg, T. Theorell, & B.B. Arnez. "Psychophysiological Effects of a Web-Based Stress Management System: A Prospective, Randomized Controlled Intervention Study of IT and Media Workers." *BMC Public Health* 5.78 (2005): doi:10.1186/1471-2458-5-78. Print.
201 American Institute of Stress. *Reminiscences of Hans Selye, and the Birth of "Stress."* The Newsletter of the American Institute of Stress.1997. Park Avenue, New York. Accessed 01 September 2011. http://www.stress.org/hans.htm
202 Hans Selye. *The Stress of Life*. New York: McGraw-Hill. 1976 (Rev. ed.).
203 A.C. Healey, D.M. Rutledge, & D. Bluestein. "Validation of the Insomnia Treatment Acceptability Scale (ITAS) in Primary Care." *Journal of Clinical Psychology in Medical Settings, 18* (3) (2011):234-242, PMID 21671011
204 K. Kim, M. Uchiyama, M. Okawa, X. Liu, & R. Oqihara. An Epidemiological Study of Insomnia among the Japanese General Population. *Sleep*, 23. 1. (2000): 41-47
205 Ruth Benca. *The Impact of Stress on Insomnia and Treatment Considerations.* n.d. Accessed 24 December 2012. http://www.

behaviormanagementsystems.org/docs/The%20Impact%20 of%20Stress%20on%20Insomnia.pdf

206 J. Vignau, D. Bailly, A. Duhamel, P Vervaecke, R. Beuscart, & C. Collinet. "Epidemiologic Study of Sleep Quality and Troubles in French Secondary School Adolescents." *Journal of Adolescent Healthcare*, 21.5 (1997): 343-350.Print.

207 Sonia Ancoli-Israe, & T. Roth. "Characteristics of insomnia in the United States: results of the 1991 National Sleep Foundation Survey. Sleep. *Suppl.* 1 (22) (1999): S347-353. PUBMED PMID: 10394606.

208 S.I. McMillen, & David E. Stern. *"None of These Diseases."* Grand Rapids. Flemming H. Revell. 2000. Print.

209 Caroll Bedell Thomas, & Edmond A. Murphy. "Further Studies on Cholesterol Levels in the Johns Hopkins Medical Students: The Effect of Stress at Examinations." *Journal of Chronic Diseases,* 8.6 (1958): 661-668. doi:10.1016/j.physletb.2003.10.071

210 Feroza Hamid Wattoo, Muhammad Saleh Memon, Allah Nawaz Memon, Muhammad Hamid Sarwar et al. "Quantitative Analysis of Stress and Cholesterol Levels in University Teachers and Housewives of Hyderabad-Pakistan." *Pakistan Journal of Medical Research*, 46:2 (2007): 42-45. Accessed 24 December 2012. http://www.pmrc.org.pk/QACHOLESTEROL.htm

211 Meyer Friedman, Ray H. Rosenman, Vernice Caroll & Russell J. Tat. "Changes in the Serum Cholesterol and Blood Clotting Time in Men Subjected to Cyclic Variation of Occupational Stress." *Circulation*, 17 (1958): 852-861. Print.

212 Mika Kivimäki, Päivi Leino-Arjas, Ritva Luukkonen, Hilkka Riihimäi, Jussi Vahtera, & Juhani Kirjonen . "Work Stress and Risk of Cardiovascular Mortality: Prospective Cohort Study of Industrial Employees." *British Medical Journal* (2002): *325*, 857. doi: 10.1136/bmj.325.7369.857.Print.

213 T. Alteman, R.B.Shekelle, & K.D. Burau. "Decision Latitude, Psychologic Demand, Job Strain, and Coronary Heart Disease

in the Western Electric Study." *American Journal of Epidemiology*, 139.6 (1994): 620-627.

214 Hans Bosma, Richard Peter, Johannes Siegrist, & Michael Marmot. "Two Alternative Job Stress Models and the Risk of Coronary Heart Disease." *American Journal of Public Health*, 88.1(1998): 68-74.

215 Weixian Xu, Yiming Zhao, Lijun Guo, Yanhong Guo, Wei Gao. "Job Stress and Coronary Heart Disease: A Case-Control Study Using a Chinese Population." *Journal of Occupational Health*, 51 (2009):107-113

216 Roger Dobson "Stress due to mounting debt costs NHS millions," The Telegraph, October 25, 2008, 8:50 PM. Accessed 17 June 2013. http://www.telegraph.co.uk/health/3257875/Stress-due-to-mounting-debt-costs-NHS-millions.html

217 Mark Meyer *Consumer Debt Stress and Credit Cards*. 2008. Research Brief. Filene Research Institute. Accessed 10 January 2011. http://www.mcul.org/files/cucorp/744/file/News_and_Publications/Information%20Services/Filene%20Reports/170_Meyer_Credit_Card_CFM.pdf

218 Tim Westrich, & Christian E. Weller. *House of Cards: Consumers Turn to Credit Cards Amid the Mortgage Crisis, Delaying Inevitable Defaults*. 2008. Center for American Progress. Accessed 18 January 2011 http://www.americanprogress.org/issues/2008/02/pdf/house_of_cards.pdf

219 Meyer, M. *Consumer Debt Stress and Credit Cards*. 2008. Research Brief. Filene Research Institute. Accessed 10 January 2011. http://www.mcul.org/files/cucorp/744/file/News_and_Publications/Information%20Services/Filene%20Reports/170_Meyer_Credit_Card_CFM.pdf

220 M. Kalia. "Assessing the Economic Impact of Stress--the Modern Day Hidden Epidemic." *Metabolism*, 51:6 Suppl. 1. (2002): 49-53.

221 Medibank Private. *The Cost of Workplace Stress in Australia*. 2008. Accessed 23 December 2012. http://www.medibank.com.au/Client/Documents/Pdfs/The-Cost-of-Workplace-Stress.pdf

222 American Institute of Stress. *Workplace Stress.* n.d. Fortworth, Texas. Accessed 23 September 1, 2011. http://www.stress.org/workplace-stress/
223 S.L. Sauter, L.R. Murphy, & J.J.Hurrell, Jr. "Prevention of Work-Related Psychological Disorders." *American Psychologist. 45.*10 (1990):1146-1153

CHAPTER 15

224 Christian Perring "Mental Illness", *The Stanford Encyclopedia of Philosophy (Spring 2010 Edition)*, Edward N. Zalta (ed.). Accessed 24 December 2012. http://plato.stanford.edu/archives/spr2010/entries/mental-illness/
225 Steven Hyman, Dan Chisholm, Ronald Kessler, Vikram Patel,& Harvey Whiteford. *Mental Disorders.* 2006. Accessed19 January 19, 2011.http://www.ncbi.nlm.nih.gov/books/NBK11766/pdf/ch31.pdf
226 National Alliance on Mental Illness.*Mental Illness.*2003.Arlington, Virginia. Accessed December 23, 2012 from http://www.nami.org/Template.cfm?Section=By_Illness&Template=/TaggedPage/TaggedPageDisplay.cfm&TPLID=54&ContentID=23049
227 The National Institute of Mental Health. *Mental Health Information.* 2009.Accessed 23 December, 2012. http://www.nimh.nih.gov/index.shtml
228 Christopher J. L. Murray, & Alan. D. Lopez, Majid Ezzati, & Dean T. Jamison (eds). The Global Burden of Disease and Risk Factors. Co-publication of Oxford University Press, Madison Avenue, New York and the World Bank.Washington, D.C. 2006. Accessed 23 December 2012. http://files.dcp2.org/pdf/GBD/GBD.pdf
229 National Institute of Mental Health. *Generalized anxiety disorder.* 2009. Accessed 23 December, 2011. http://www.nimh.nih.gov/health/topics/generalized-anxiety-disorder-gad/index.shtml

230 National Institute of Mental Health (NIMH). The Numbers Count: Mental Disorders in America. 2012. Accessed 23 December 2012. http://www.nimh.nih.gov/health/publications/the-numbers-count-mental-disorders-in-america/index.shtml

231 National Alliance on Mental Illness. *Mental Illness: Panic Disorder.* 2012. Arlington, Virginia. Accessed 23 December 2012. http://www.nami.org/Template.cfm?Section=By_Illness&Template=/TaggedPage/TaggedPageDisplay.cfm&TPLID=54&ContentID=23050

232 Steven Hyman, Dan Chisholm, Ronald Kessler, Vikram Patel, & Harvey Whiteford. *Mental Disorders.* 2006. Web. 19 January 19, 2011. http://www.ncbi.nlm.nih.gov/books/NBK11766/pdf/ch31.pdf

233 Gro Harlem Brundtland, "WHO/China Mental Health Awareness Raising Event."(Speech at Beinjing on Mental Illness. 11 November 1999.) Accessed 23 December 2012. http://www.who.int/director-general/speeches/1999/english/19991111_beijing.html

234 Gro Harlem Brundtland, "Mental Health in the 21st Century." Editorials. Special Theme-Mental Health. Bulletin of the World Health Organization, 78 (4), (2000): 411. Accessed 23 December 2012. http://www.who.int/bulletin/archives/78%284%29411.pdf

235 Charles W. Schmidt, "Environmental Connections: A Deeper Look into Mental Illness." *Environmental Health Perspectives* 115.8 (2007): doi:10.1289/ehp.115-a404

236 J.S. Bell, S.E. Aaltonen, M.S. Airaksinen, D. Volmer et al. "Determinants of Mental Health Stigma among Pharmacy Students in Australia, India, Finland, Belgium, Estonia and Latvia." *International Journal of Social Psychiatry*, 56.1 (2010): 3-14. doi: 10.1177/0020764008097621

237 Oye Gureje, Benjamin Oladapo Olley, Ephraim-Oluwanuga Olusola, & Lola Kola. "Do beliefs about Causation Influence Attitudes to Mental Health?" *World Psychiatry*, 5 (2) (2006): 104-107

238 A. Kapungwe, S. Cooper, J. Mwanza, L. Mwape et al. "Mental illness-Stigma and Discrimination in Zambia." *African Journal of Psychiatry*, 13 (2010): 192-203

239 David Satcher, "Mental Health: A Report of the Surgeon General–Executive Summary. Surgeon General, United States. 2000. Accessed 23 December 2012. http://www.psychosocial.com/policy/satcher.html

240 Thomas R. Insel. "Assessing the Economic Costs of Serious Mental Illness". *American Journal of Psychiatry*, 165.6 (2008): 663-665. doi:10.1176/appi.ajp.2008.08030366

241 National Alliance on Mental Illness (2012). Mental Illness. 2012. Arlington, Virginia. Accessed 23 December 2012. http://www.nami.org/template.cfm?section=about_mental_illness

242 J. Cecil3 (2003). On Mental Illness (blog), October 8, 2003 (3:14 pm). Accessed 23 December 2012. http://outofmind1.blogspot.com/

243 The Pastoral Counseling Center. *Pastoral Counseling: A National Mental Health Resource.* 2010. Accessed 5 September 5, 2011 http://www.pccmidvalley.org/mental-health-resource.html

244 Professional Pastoral-Counseling Institute. *What is Pastoral Counseling?* 2012. Accessed 23 December, 2012. http://www.pastoral-counseling.org/asp/page.asp?ID=1003

245 Archibald D. Hart. *The Anxiety Cure.* Thomas Nelson, Inc. Publishers. 1999, pp. 217.

246 Mayo Clinic (2012). *"Positive Thinking: Reduce Stress by Eliminating Negative Self-Talk."* Stress Management. 2012. Accessed 23 December, 2012. http://www.mayoclinic.com/health/positive-thinking/SR00009

247 S.I. McMillen, S.I. & Davide Stern. *None of These Diseases. (3rd ed).* Grand Rapids, MI: Flemming H. Revell, 2000.pp. 169, 171

248 Carl Gustav Jung. *Modern Man in Search of a Soul.* Kegan Paul, Trench, Trubner & Co., pp. 234. 1933.

249 David R. Williams, David B. Larson, Robert E. Buckler, Richard C. Heckman & Caroline M. Pyle. "Religion and Psychosocial

Distress in a Community Sample." *Social Science Medicine*, 32 (1991, pp. 1261): 1257-1262

250 Ronna Casar Harris, Mary Amand Dew, Ann Lee, Michael Amaya et al. "The Role of Religion in Heart-Transplant Recipients' Long-Term Health and Well Being." *Journal of Religion and Health*, 34.1 (1995, Abstract): 17-32. DOI: 10.1007/BF02248635

251 H. G. Koenig, *The Healing Power of Faith: Science Explores Medicine's Last Great Frontier*. New York: Simon & Schuster, 1999, pp. 24. Print.

252 World Health Organization Summary Report. *Prevention of Mental Illness: Effective Intervention and Policy Options*. 2004. Geneva, Switzerland. Accessed 22 October 2011. http://www.who.int/mental_health/evidence/en/prevention_of_mental_disorders_sr.pdf

CHAPTER 16

253 World Health Organization. *WHO Guidelines for Indoor Air Quality. Dampness and Mould*. 2009. Geneva, Switzerland. Accessed 14 September 2010 http://www.euro.who.int/__data/assets/pdf_file/0017/43325/E92645.pdf

254 Lewis G. Harriman III, Michael J. Witte, Marek Czachorski & Douglas R. Kosar. "Evaluating Active Desiccant Systems for Ventilating Commercial Buildings." *American Society of Heating, Refrigerating and Air Conditioning Engineers, Inc.(SHRAE) Journal, (1999):* 28-34

255 Armin F. Rudd, Joseph W. Lstiburek, P. Eng, Kohta Ueno. "Residential Dehumidification Systems Research for Hot-Humid Climates, September 1, 2001-December 30, 2003." Research Report-0505, February 2005. U.S. Department of Energy. Westford, MA. Accessed 25 December 2-12. http://www.buildingscience.com/documents/reports/rr-0505-residential-dehumidification-systems-research-for-hot-humid-climates

256 National Capital Poison Center. *Indoor Mold and Effects on Health.* 2011. Accessed 25 December 2012. http://www.poison.org/current/indoor%20mold.htm

257 Institute of Medicine. *Damp Indoor Spaces and Health. Consensus Report.* The National Academy of Sciences, 2004. Accessed 25 December 2012. http://www.iom.edu/Reports/2004/Damp-Indoor-Spaces-and-Health.aspx

258 Edmond D. Shenessa, Constantine Daskalakis, Allison Liebhaber, Matthias Braubach, & MaryJean Brown. "Dampness and Mold in the Home and Depression: An Examination of Mold-Related Illness and Perceived Control of One's Home as Possible Depression Pathways." *American Journal of Public Health*, 97.10 (2007): 1893-1899. doi: 10.2105/AJPH.2006.093773.

259 Robert E. Dales, Harry Zwanenburg, Richard Burnett & Claire A. Franklin. "Respiratory Health Effects of Home Dampness and Molds among Canadian Children." *American Journal of Epidemiology*, 134.2 (1991): 196-203.

260 W.J. Fisk, Q. Lei-Gomez, & M.J.Mendell. "Meta-Analyses of the Associations of Respiratory Health Effects with Dampness and Mold in Homes." *Indoor Air*, 17.4 (2007): 284-296. PMID: 17661925 [PubMed - indexed for MEDLINE].

261 Nelson, B.D. 2001. *Stachybotrys chartarum*: The Toxic Indoor Mold. APS*net* Features. Online. doi: 10.1094/APSnetFeature-2001-1101

262 Berlin D. Nelson. "Stachybotrys chartarum: The Toxic Indoor Mold." American Phytopathological Society. 2012. Accessed 25 December 2012. http://www.apsnet.org/publications/apsnetfeatures/Pages/Stachybotrys.aspx

263 William A. Croft, Bruce C. Jarvis, & C.S. Yatawara. "Airborne Outbreak of Trichothecene Toxicosis." *Atmospheric Environment* 20 (1986): 549-552. Print.

264 Elisabeth Heseltine and Jerome Rosen. Eds. *Guidelines for Indoor Air Quality. Dampness and Mould.* World Health Organization, 2009. Europe. Accessed 23 September 2012. http://www.euro.who.int/__data/assets/pdf_file/0017/43325/E92645.pdf

265 Jay Romano. "Your Home: Managing Mold, and Law Suits." The New York Times Archives. January 26, 2003. Accessed 25 December 2012. http://www.nytimes.com/2003/01/26/realestate/your-home-managing-mold-and-lawsuits.html?pagewanted=all&src=pm

266 David Mudarri, & William J. Fisk. "Public Health and Economic Impact of Dampness and Mold." *Indoor Air Journal*, 17.3 (2007): 226-235. DOI: 10.1111/j.1600-0668.2007.00474.x. Print.

267 Ronald E. Wright. "The Mold Challenge in Construction." n.d. Accessed 6 September 2011. http://www.buric.com/Mold_Challenge.pdf

268 BLR-Business and Legal Resources. "Court Finds Toxic Mold Caused Worker's Health Problems." Workplace Safety News. November 30, 2007. Accessed 23 December 2012. http://safety.blr.com/workplace-safety-news/hazardous-substances-and-materials/air-contaminants/Court-Finds-Toxic-Mold-Caused-Workers-Health-Probl/

269 Nathan Albright, March 11, 2011, Comment on Leviticus 14: 33-53, "On Mold Addendums and Leprous Houses." Edge Induced Cohesion. Blog at WordPress.com. March 11, 2011. Accessed 23 December 2012. http://edgeinducedcohesion.wordpress.com/2011/03/11/leviticus-14-33-53-on-mold-addendums-and-leprous-hous/

270 Steven Martens, S. "Bettendorf Home with Mold Problems Torn Down." Quad-City Times. January 8, 2012 (9:00 am). Accessed 23 December 2012. http://qctimes.com/news/local/bettendorf-home-with-mold-problems-torn-down/article_45db24e0-b0ff-11e1-b5b2-0019bb2963f4.html

271 David Silverman "The Curse of the Curse of the Pharaohs," 1923. Expedition, 29 (2), 56-63. Accessed 17 June 2013. http://www.penn.museum/documents/publications/expedition/PDFs/29-2/The%20Curse.pdf

Chapter 17

272 Jeremy Greenwood, & Nezih Guner. "Social Change: The Sexual Revolution. Population Studies Center Working Paper Series." 2009. Population Studies Center. Accessed 29 September 2010 http://repository.upenn.edu/cgi/viewcontent.cgi?article=1011&context=psc_working_papers

273 Greenwood, J., & Guner, N. "Social Change: The Sexual Revolution," 2010. International Economic Review, 51 (4), 893-923. Accessed 19 June 2013. http://pareto.uab.es/nguner/gg-ier.pdf

274 Jesus Fernandez-Villaverde, Jeremy Greenwood & Nezih Guner "From Shame to Game in One Hundred Years: A Macroeconomic Model of the Rise in Premarital Sex and its De-Stigmatization." 2011. Accessed 19 June 2013. http://repository.upenn.edu/cgi/viewcontent.cgi?article=1016&context=psc_working_papers

275 Margaret Sanger (1917). *Family Limitation (6th ed.).* London: Rose Witcop, (Pref. 1924). Electronic Copy. Accessed 4 December, 2012 from http://archive.lib.msu.edu/DMC/AmRad/familylimitations.pdf

276 Sheetal Malhotra. "Impact of the Sexual Revolution: Consequences of Risky Sexual Behaviors." *Journal of American Physicians and Surgeons,* 13. 3 (2008): 88-90. Print.

277 Centers for Disease Control and Prevention (2012). *Sexually Transmitted Diseases (STDs): Syphilis-CDC Fact Sheet.* Accessed 23 December http://www.cdc.gov/std/syphilis/stdfact-syphilis.htm

278 Aletha C. Huston, Ellen Wartella, & Edward Donnerstein. "Measuring the Effects of Sexual Content in the Media.: A Report to the Kaiser Family Foundation." 1998. Accessed 30 September 2010. http://www.kff.org/insurance/loader.cfm?url=/commonspot/security/getfile.cfm&PageID=14624

279 Anita Chandra, Steven C. Martino, Rebecca L. Collins, & Marc N. Elliott. "Does Watching Sex on Television Predict Teen Pregnancy? Findings from a National Longitudinal Survey

of Youth." *Pediatrics*, 122 (2008): 1047-1054.doi: 10.1542/peds.2007-3066. Print.

280 Centers for Disease Control and Prevention. *Sexually Transmitted Diseases (STDs). Genital Herpes—CDC Fact Sheet*. Accessed 23 December September 2012. http://www.cdc.gov/std/herpes/stdfact-herpes.htm

281 Centers for Disease Control and Prevention. *Sexually Transmitted Diseases in the United States, 2008. National Surveillance Data for Chlamydia, Gonorrhea, and Syphilis*. November 2009. Accessed 26 January2011.http://www.cdc.gov/std/stats08/2008survFactSheet.PDF

282 Eileen F. Dunne, & Lauri E. Markowitz."Genital Human Papillomavirus Infection." *Clinical Infectious Diseases*, 43 (2006): 624-629. Print.

283 Ray Bohlin. "The Epidemic of Sexually Transmitted Diseases."1993. Probe Ministries International. Accessed 29 September. 2011. http://www.leaderu.com/orgs/probe/docs/epid-std.html

284 D.S. Meyers, H. Halvorson, & S. Luckhaupt. "Screening for Chlamydia Infection: An Evidence Update for the U.S. Preventive Services Task Force." *Annals of Internal Medicine*, 147.2 (2007): 135-142. Print.

285 Centers for Diseases Control and Prevention. *STD is Adolescents and Young Adults*. Atlanta, Georgia. Updated 2011. Accessed 26 December 2012. http://www.cdc.gov/std/stats10/adol.htm

286 Centers for Disease Control and Prevention. *Sexually Transmitted Diseases. Gonorrhea- CDC Fact Sheet*. 2012. Atlanta, Georgia. Accessed 26 December 2012. http://www.cdc.gov/std/gonorrhea/stdfact-gonorrhea.htm

287 Williams College Health Center. *Male Latex Condoms and Sexually Transmitted Diseases. 2012*. Accessed 23 December 2012. http://health.williams.edu/ephnotes-newsletter/sexual-and-reproductive-health/male-latex-condoms-and-sexually-transmitted-diseases/

288 Gypsyamber D'Souza, Aimee R. Kreimer, Raphael Viscidi, Michael Pawlita," et al. "Case–Control Study of Human Papillomavirus and Oropharyngeal Cancer," *The New England Journal of Medicine*, 356.19 (2007): 1944-1956. Print.

289 Liviu Feller, Niel H. Wood, Razia A.G. Khammissa, Johan Lemmer, et al. "Human Papillomavirus-Mediated Carcinogenesis and HPV-Associated Oral and Oropharyngeal Squamous Cell Carcinoma. Part 2: Human Papillomavirus Associated Oral and Oropharyngeal Squamous Cell Carcinoma." *Head & Face Medicine*, 6.15 (2010). doi: 10.1186/1746-160X-6-14

290 Peter A. Hall, Maxine Holmqvist, & Simon B. Sherry. "Risky Adolescent Sexual Behavior: A Psychological Perspective for Primary Care Clinicians." *Advanced Practice Nursing eJournal*, 4.1. (2004).

291 Sheetal Malhotra. "Impact of the Sexual Revolution: Consequences of Risky Sexual Behaviors." *Journal of American Physicians and Surgeons*, 13. 3 (2008): 88-90. Print.

292 Hillard Weinstock, Stuart Berman, & Willard Cates, Jr. "Sexually Transmitted Diseases among American Youth: Incidence and Prevalence Estimates, 2000." *Perspectives on Sexual and Reproductive Health*, 36.1(2004): 6-10. Print.

293 Centers for Disease Control and Prevention. HIV/AIDS Surveillance Report, 2000. Year-end Edition, 12, 2. Accessed 26 December 2012. http://www.cdc.gov/hiv/topics/surveillance/resources/reports/pdf/hasr1202.pdf

294 Office of the Surgeon General (US); Office of Population Affairs (US). *The Surgeon General's Call to Action to Promote Sexual Health and Responsible Sexual Behavior*.2001. A Letter from the Surgeon General U.S. Department of Health and Human Services. Rockville (MD): Office of the Surgeon General (US); 2001 Jul. Accessed 26 December 2012. http://www.cdc.gov/hiv/topics/surveillance/resources/reports/pdf/hasr1202.pdf

295 Rex Russell. *What the Bible Says about Healthy Living*. Regal Book Publishers. Ventura, CA. 1996, pp.80.

296 Dewitt S. Williams, & Donna D. Cameron. *Black Seventh-day Adventists and Health Issues.* 1996. Accessed 17 January 2011. http://www.oakwood.edu/goldmine/ldoc/perspectives/perspective18.pdf

Chapter 18

297 Africa Health and Development International. *Making Sex Work Safer.* 2012. Accessed 23 December 2012. http://www.ahadi.org/index.php?option=com_content&view=article&id=131:making-sex-work-safer
298 J. Cribb. "The Origin of Acquired Immune Deficiency Syndrome: Can Science Afford to Ignore It?" *Philosophical Transactions of the Royal Society,* 356. 1410. (2001); 935-938
299 N.D. Wolfe, W.M. Switzer, J.K. Carr, V.B. Bhullar, et al. "Naturally Acquired Simian Retrovirus Infections in Central African Hunters." *Lancet,* 363. 9413. (2004): 932-937
300 Baffour Ankomah. "Monkey Business Over AIDS." 1998. Accessed 23 December 2012. http://www.virusmyth.com/aids/news/namonkey.htm
301 Mary-Jane Schneider. *Introduction to Public Health.* Jones and Bartlett Publishers, Inc. Sudbury, MA, 2004. pp.146. Print.
302 Alan Cantwell, Jr. "AIDS: Who is to Blame?" *New Dawn Magazine.* 2002. Accessed 23 December 2012. http://www.newdawnmagazine.com/Articles/AIDS_Who_is_to_Blame.html
303 Alan Cantwell, Jr. "The Secret Origin of AIDS and HIV: How Scientists Produced the Most Horrifying Plague of All Time- and then Covered it Up." 2000. Accessed 23 December 2012. http://www.whale.to/v/cantwell3.html
304 Boyd E. Graves. (2003). AIDS/Graves. Accessed 23 December 2012. http://members.iimetro.com.au/~hubbca/aids.htm
305 Philippe Denis & Charles Becker (Eds). October 2006. *The HIV/AIDS Disease in sub-Saharan Africa in a Historical Perspective. Twenty Years of Intervention and Controversy.* 2006. Web. 1 June 1, 2010 http://rds.refer.sn/IMG/pdf/AIDSHISTORYALL.pdf

306 Kaiser Family Foundation. *The Global HIV/AIDS Timeline*. 2007. Menlo Park, CA. Accessed 23 September 2012. http://www.kff.org/hivaids/timeline/hivtimeline.cfm

307 Holly Hannam, Rachel Mackie, Sarah Smith, Rich Williams, et al. "*HIV/AIDS: A Global Epidemic*." 11 September 2011. http://web.clark.edu/tkibota/240/Disease/AIDS.pdf

308 Dallas Swendeman, Mary Jane Rotheram-Borus, Scott Comulada, Robert Weiss, et al. "Predictors of HIV-Related Stigma among Young People Living with HIV. Nation Institutes of Health Public Access." *Health Psychology*, 25.4 (2006): 501-509. doi: 10.1037/0278-6133.25.4.501. Print.

309 Gregory M. Herek, Keith F. Widaman, John P. Capitanio."When sex equals AIDS: Symbolic Stigma and Heterosexual Adults' Inaccurate Beliefs about Sexual Transmission of AIDS". *Social Problems*, 52.1(2005):15–37. doi 10.1525/sp.2005.52.1.15. Print.

310 Melinda F. Gates, "Prepared Remarks by Melinda Gates, Co-Chair," (presentation, 16th International AIDS Conference in Toronto, Canada, March 13, 2006). Accessed 23 December 2012. file:///C:/Users/Reigh/AppData/Local/Temp/speech.html and http://dawn.thot.net/aids2006_day1.html

311 Li Li, Zunyou Wu, Yu Zhao, Chunqing Lin, et al. "Using Case Vignettes to Measure HIV-Related Stigma among Health Professionals in China." *International Journal of Epidemiology*, 36 (2007): 178-184. doi: 10.1093/ije/dyl256. Print.

312 B. Forsyth, A. Vandormae, T. Kershaw, J. Grobbelaaret. "The political Context of AIDS-Related Stigma and Knowledge in a South African Township Community." *Journal of Social Aspects of HIV/AIDS*, 5.2 (2008): 74-82. Print.

313 Joanne Csete. "Missed Opportunities: Human Rights and the Politics of HIV/AIDS." *Development, 47* .2. (2004): 83-90

314 Ngianga-Bakwin Kandala, Eugene K Campbell,[2] Serai Dan Rakgoasi,[2] Banyana C Madi-Segwagwe, et al. "The Geography of HIV/AIDS Prevalence Rates in Botswana." *Research and Palliative Care*, 4, (2012): 95-102

315 USAID. *HIV/AIDS Multisector: Development Challenges.* 2011. Accessed 23 December 2012. http://transition.usaid.gov/zm/hiv/hiv.htm

316 UNICEF and UNAIDS. "Africa's Orphaned and Vulnerable Generations." August, 2006. New York, United States and Geneva Switzerland. Accessed 23 December 2012. http://www.unicef.org/publications/files/Africas_Orphaned_and_Vulnerable_Generations_Children_Affected_by_AIDS.pdf

317 S.I. McMillen & David E. Stern *None of These Diseases. (Millennium 3 edition).* Grand Rapids, MI: Flemming H. Revell, 2000. Print. pp.115

318 World Vision. *Violence against children affected by HIV/AIDS.* June, 2005. Accessed 11 September 2011. http://www.wvi.org/wvi/wviweb.nsf/8ACB216444EC63D3882579680069B44D/$file/children_violence-uganda_study.pdf

319 Tiaji Salaam. "AIDS Orphans and Vulnerable Children (OVC): Problems, Responses, and Issues for Congress. Congressional Research Service Report. 2005. Accessed 23 December 2012. http://www.law.umaryland.edu/marshall/crsreports/crsdocuments/RL3225202112005.pdf

320 Hoosen M. Coovadia, & Jacqui Hadingham. "HIV/AIDS: Global Trends, Global Funds and Delivery Bottlenecks." *Globalization and Health*, 1.13 (2005): doi:10.1186/1744-8603-1-13. Print.

321 Nicole Marie Mason. "A Test of the New Variant Famine Hypothesis: Panel Survey Evidence from Zambia." (Masters Thesis, Michigan State University, 2008).

Chapter 19

322 *Universal Declaration of Human Rights*, General Assembly Resolution. 217A (III), United Nations Document A/810 at 71 (1948). The Circumcision Reference Library. File Revised 25 September 2006. Accessed 26 December 2012. http://www.cirp.org/library/ethics/UN-human/

323 United Nations Children's Fund (UNICEF). *Children have Rights.* Updated June 2003, Accessed 5 November, 2012. http://www.unicef.org/why/why_rights.html

324 Brian M. Willis, & Barry S. Levy. "Child Prostitution: Global Health Burden, Research Needs, and Interventions." *The Lancet*, 359 (2002): 1417-1422. Print.

325 International Labor Organization, UNICEF and UN.GIFT. *Training Manual to Fight Trafficking in Children for Labour, Sexual and Other Forms of Exploitation.*2009. Accessed 1 February 2011. http://www.unicef.org/protection/files/CP_Trg_Manual_Textbook_1.pdf

326 Jennifer L. Kennedy. ""Shrouded Sins: An Exploration of Child Sex Trafficking in South Africa" (2010). *Pell Scholars and Senior Theses.* Paper 43." Accessed 23 December 2012. http://escholar.salve.edu/cgi/viewcontent.cgi?article=1043&context=pell_theses

327 Sibnath Deb. "Child trafficking in South Asia: Dimensions, Roots, Facets & Interventions." *Social Change*, 35.2 (2005): 143-155. doi:10.1177/004908570503500211. Print.

328 BBC News. "UN Warns on South Asia Child Sex."BBC News, 29 September 2004. Accessed 23 December 2012. http://news.bbc.co.uk/2/hi/south_asia/3700110.stm

329 Sigma Huda "Sex trafficking in South Asia." *International Journal of Gynecology and Obstetrics*, 94 (2006): 374-381. Print.

330 United Nations Interregional Crime and Justice Research Institute (UNICRI) *Child Protection from Violence, Exploitation and Abuse.* Accessed 24 December 2012. http://www.unicef.org/protection/index.html

331 Laura J. Lederer Comment on September 9, 2010, "Sex trafficking and illegal pornography: Is there a link? Part 2. The Enough is Enough. Educating, Equipping and Empowering Adults to Protect Kids Online Blog. Accessed 23 December 2012. October 2010 http://pornharms.com/Sex_Trafficking_and_Illegal_Pornography_Statement.pdf

332 Sandro Calvani, UNICRI Director, "Children's Exploitation and Women's Condition: The Issue of Human Trafficking." Speech presented at Scuola d'Applicazione, Institute of Military Studies, Turin. 12 June 2009. Accessed 23 December 2012. http://www.sandrocalvani.it/docs/Speeches_090612.pdf

333 Jay G. Silverman, Michele R. Decker, Heather L. McCauley, & Katelyn P. Mack. "A regional Assessment of Sex Trafficking and STI/HIV in Southeast Asia: Connections Between Sexual Exploitation, Violence and Sexual Risk." July 2009. UNDP Regional Centre in Colombo. Accessed 23 December 2012. http://www.snap-undp.org/elibrary/Publications/SexTrafficking.pdf

334 University of Colorado Boulder "Child Sex Trafficking Study by CU-Boulder Sociologist Reveals Misperceptions." February 28, 2005. News Release. Accessed 23 December 2012. http://www.colorado.edu/news/releases/2005/02/28/child-sex-trafficking-study-cu-boulder-sociologist-reveals-misperceptions

335 Nicole Lindstrom "Regional Sex Trafficking in the Balkans: Transnational Networks in an Enlarged Europe." May/June 2004. *Problems of Post-Communism*, 51.3 (2004): 45-52. Accessed 23 December 2012. http://lastradainternational.org/lsidocs/lindstrom_04reg_sex_tra_0408.pdf

336 Integrated Regional Information Networks (IRIN) (2012). *Kenya: Drought, Poverty Forcing Young Women into Risky Commercial Sex*. Humanitarian News and Analysis. Accessed 23 December, 2012. http://www.irinnews.org/Report/39462/KENYA-Drought-poverty-forcing-young-women-into-risky-commercial-sex

337 United States Department of State Publication 11407 Office of the Under Secretary for Democracy and Global Affairs Bureau of Public Affairs. Trafficking in Persons Report. June 2007. Accessed 23 December 2012. http://www.state.gov/documents/organization/82902.pdf

338 Donna M. Hughes,"The Demand: Where Sex Trafficking Begins." June 2004. Accessed 23 December 2012. http://www.uri.edu/artsci/wms/hughes/demand_rome_june04.pdf

339 United Nations Population Fund. *Gender Inequality: Ending Widespread Violence against Women.* n.d. Accessed 12 September 2011. http://www.unfpa.org/gender/violence.htm

340 DEMAND Shared Hope International. *Demand. A Comparative Examination of Sex Tourism and Trafficking in Jamaica, Japan, the Netherlands, and the United States.* European Network against Trafficking in Human Beings. (n.d). Accessed 23 December 2012. http://sharedhope.org/wp-content/uploads/2012/09/DEMAND.pdf

341 Department of Justice and Constitutional Development, Republic of South Africa. Amendment Act, 2007. *The New Sexual Offenses Act Protecting Our Children from Sexual Predators.* Accessed December 24 2012. http://www.justice.gov.za/docs/InfoSheets/2008%20 02%20SXOactInsert_web.pdf

342 Kevin Bales, & Steven Lize "Trafficking in Persons in the United States." A Report of the National Institute of Justice- Final Report. 2005. Accessed December 5, October 2012. https://www.ncjrs.gov/pdffiles1/nij/grants/211980.pdf

343 Sally Terry Green. "Protection for Victims of Child Sex Trafficking in the United States: Forging the Gap Between U. S. Immigration Laws and Human Trafficking Laws." *UC Davis Journal of Juvenile Law & Policy, 12.2.2006.* Accessed 23 December February 2012. http://jjlp.law.ucdavis.edu/archives/vol-12-no-2/06_Article-Green.pdf

344 U.S. Department of State (2009). *U.S. Government Domestic Anti-Trafficking Efforts.* Accessed 23 December 2012. http://www.state.gov/j/tip/rls/tiprpt/2009/123133.htm

345 Chris Beyrer, & Julie Stachowiak, "Health consequences of trafficking of women and girls in Southeast Asia." *Brown Journal of World Affairs,* 10.1(2003): 105-117. Print.

346 Jonathan Martens, Maciej 'Mac'Pieczkowski, & Bernadette van Vuuren-Symth, "Seduction, Sale and Slavery: Trafficking in Women and Children for Sexual Exploitation in Southern Africa." International Organization for Migration. 2003.

Accessed 12 September 2011. http://www.queensu.ca/samp/migrationresources/gender/documents/martens.pdf
347 Cable News Network, *"Woman Fighting Sex Slavery Named CNN Hero of the Year."*CNN News, November 22, 2010. Hosted by Anderson Cooper. Accessed 23 December 2012. http://www.cnn.com/2010/LIVING/11/21/cnnheroes.hero.of.year/index.html
348 Melissa Faley, "Prostitution: Factsheet on Human Rights Violation." Prostitution Research & Education. 2004. Accessed 5 October, 2011. http://www.prostitutionresearch.com/factsheet.html
349 United Nations Children's Fund (or UNICEF) *Reference Guide on Protecting the Rights of Child Victims of Trafficking in Europe.* 2003. Accessed 18 June 2013. http://www.unicef.org/ceecis/UNICEF_Child_Trafficking_low.pdf

CHAPTER 20

350 David I. Macht, "An Experimental Pharmacological Appreciation of Leviticus XI & Deuteronomy XIV." *Bulletin of the History of Medicine,* 27.5 (1953): 444-450. Print.
351 Joe C. Guthrie, Jr. "Experimental Relationship Between Leviticus XI, Deuteronomy XIV, and Poor Health of Louisiana Population." April 2007. Accessed 11 November 2012. http://www.wonmp.us/resources/Documents/Louisiana%20Health%20Problem%20thesis.pdf
352 World Health Organization/Food and Agricultural Organization Technical Report Series, 916. *Diet, Nutrition and the Prevention of Chronic Diseases Report of the Joint WHO/FAO Expert Consultation.* Geneva, Switzerland 2003. Accessed 9 November 2011. http://whqlibdoc.who.int/trs/WHO_TRS_916.pdf
353 The International Federation of Red Cross and Red Crescent Societies (2011). World Disaster Report 2011: Focus on Hunger and Malnutrition. Accessed 23 December 2012. http://www.

ifrc.org/PageFiles/89755/Photos/307000-WDR-2011-FINAL-email-1.pdf

354 Heather Pringle, "The Curse of the Mummies' Arteries. American Association for the Advancement of Science." 2011. Accessed 23 December 2012. http://news.sciencemag.org/sciencenow/2011/04/the-curse-of-the-mummies-arteries.html?ref=hp

355 Sir Marc Armand Ruffer. Edited by Roy L. Moodie. "Studies in the Palaeopathology of Egypt." University of Chicago Press. Chicago, Illinois. 1921. Accessed 23 December 2012. http://archive.org/stream/studiesinpalaeop00ruff/studiesinpalaeop00ruff_djvu.txt

356 Jeffery Hays, (2008). "Health and Health Care in Ancient Egypt." Facts and Details. Accessed 23 December 2012. http://factsanddetails.com/world.php?itemid=1927&catid=56&subcatid=365

357 World Health Organization (2012). *Zoonoses and Veterinary Public Health: Bovine Spongiform Encephalopathy (BSE)*. Accessed 23 December 2012. http://www.who.int/zoonoses/diseases/bse/en/

358 Trichinosis Annual Report. *"Trichinosis (Trichinellosis). Louisiana Office of Public Health-Infection Disease Epidemiology Section-Annual Report."* 2010. Accessed15 November 2011. http://www.dhh.louisiana.gov/assets/oph/Center-PHCH/Center-CH/infectious-epi/Annuals/LaIDAnnual_Trichinosis.pdf

359 Centers for Disease Control and Prevention. *Parasites-Trichinellosis (also known as Trichinosis): Epidemiology and Risk Factors*. 2012. Georgia, Atlanta. Accessed 2 February 2012. http://www.cdc.gov/parasites/trichinellosis/epi.html

360 Rex Russell. *What the Bible Says About Healthy Living: Three Biblical Principles That Will Change Your Diet and Improve Your Health. Regal Books.* Ventura, CA.1996. Print.

361 Rex Russell. *What the Bible Says about Healthy Living. Three Biblical Principles That Will Change Your Diet and Improve Your Health* Regal Book. Ventura, CA, 1996.pp. 31-21

362 World Health Organization. *Global Alert: and Response (GAR): Severe Acute Respiratory Syndrome.* October, 2004. Accessed12 September 2011. http://www.who.int/csr/sars/en/
363 Murrell, K.D., ed., Dorny, P., Flisser, A., Geerts, A., et al. eds. "WHO/FAO/OIE Guidelines for the surveillance, prevention and control of taeniosis/cysticercosis." 2005. Accessed 18 June 2013. http://www.oie.int/doc/ged/d11245.pdf
364 Ma, W., Kahn, R.E., & Richt, J.A. "The pig as a mixing vessel for influenza viruses: Human and veterinary implications," 2009. *Journal of Molecular and Genetic Medicine,* 3 (1): 158–166.
365 Ibid
366 European Food Safety Authority *New influenza A (H1N1).* 2011. Accessed 18 June 2013. http://www.efsa.europa.eu/en/topics/topic/h1n1.htm
367 Centers of Disease Control and Prevention *Marine Toxins.* 2005. Accessed 18 June 2013. http://www.cdc.gov/ncidod/dbmd/diseaseinfo/marinetoxins_g.htm

CHAPTER 21

368 Patrick Mathieu, Paul Poirier, Philippe Pibarot, Isabelle Lemieux,. et. al. "Brief Review, Visceral Obesity: The Link among Inflammation, Hypertension, and Cardiovascular Disease." *Hypertension,* 53 (2009): 577-584. doi: 10.1161/HYPERTENSIONAHA.108.110320
369 Frank W. Booth, Scott E. Gordon, Christian J. Carlson & Marc T. Hamilton. "Waging War on Modern Chronic Diseases: Primary Prevention through Exercise Biology." *Journal of Applied Physiology,* 88. (2000): 774-787
370 American Heart Association. *1999 Heart and Stroke Statistical Update.* In President's Council on Physical Fitness and Sports. Cost and Consequences of Sedentary Living: New Battleground for an Old Enemy. Research Digest Series 3, 16. 2002. Accessed 23

December 2012. https://www.presidentschallenge.org/informed/digest/docs/200203digest.pdf
371 J.P.Kassirer, & M. Angell, "Losing Weight: An Ill-Fated New Year's Resolution." *New England Journal of Medicine*, 338.1. (1998): 52-54. Medline
372 L. Qi, L. Parast, T. Cai, C. Powers, et al. "Genetic Susceptibility to Coronary Heart Disease in Type 2 Diabetes." *Journal of the American College of Cardiology*, 58. 25. (2011): 2675-2682
373 S.I. McMillen, & David Stern. *None of These Diseases (3rd ed.)*. Flemming H. Revell. Grand Rapids, MI. 2000. Print.
374 Rex Russell. *What the Bible Says About Healthy Living: Three Biblical Principles That Will Change Your Diet and Improve Your Health*. Regal Books. Ventura, CA. 1996. Print.
375 Stephen Allender, Peter Scarborough, Viv Peto & Mike Rayer. (2008). European Cardiovascular Disease Statistics (2008 Edition. British Heart Foundation Health Promotion Research Group. Department of Public Health. University of Oxford. Accessed 9 December, 2012. Ht)tp://www.herzstiftung.ch/uploads/media/European_cardiovascular_disease_statistics_2008.pdf
376 World Health Organization/Food and Agricultural Organization Joint Report. *Global Strategy on Diet, Physical Activity and Health: Diet, Nutrition and the Prevention of Chronic Diseases*. 2003. Geneva, Switzerland. Accessed 14 September 2012. http://whqlibdoc.who.int/trs/WHO_TRS_916.pdf
377 Maarten L. Simoons."Cardio-Vascular Disease in Europe: Challenges for the Medical Profession. Opening Address of the 2002 Congress European Society of Cardiology." *European Heart Journal*, 24 (2002): 8-12. doi:10.1016/S0195-668X(02)00751-0
378 Jacqueline Partarrieu, "The human and economic cost of heart disease in Europe." February 2008. European Society of Cardiology. Accessed 14 September 2011. http://www.eurekalert.org/pub_releases/2008-02/esoc-tha022008.php
379 Jose´ Leal, Ramo´n Luengo-Ferna´ndez, Alastair Gray, Sophie Petersen et al. "Economic Burden of Cardiovascular Diseases

in the Enlarged European Union." *European Heart Journal*, 27 (2006): 1610-1619. doi:10.1093/eurheartj/ehi733

380 Rachel Nugent "Chronic diseases in developing countries: Health and economic burdens." *Annals of the New York Academy of Sciences*, 1136 (2008): 70-79. doi: 10.1196/annals.1425.027

381 L. Fezeu, E. Minkoulouet, B. Balkau, A.P.Kengne, et. al. "Association Between Socioeconomic Status and Adiposity in Urban Cameroon." *International Journal of Epidemiology*, 35 (2005): 105-111. Print.

382 Rachel Nugent "Chronic diseases in developing countries: Health and economic burdens." *Annals of the New York Academy of Sciences*, 1136 (2008): 70-79. doi: 10.1196/annals.1425.027

383 K. Srinath Reddy, & Salim Yusuf, "Emerging Epidemic of Cardiovascular Disease in Developing Countries." American Heart Association. *Journal of the American Heart Association. Circulation*, 97 (1998): 596-601. Print.

384 Claude Lenfant, "Can We Prevent Cardiovascular Diseases in Low-and Middle-Income Countries?" *Bulletin of World Health Organization*, 79, 10 (2001): 980-987 Accessed 23 December 2012. http://www.who.int/bulletin/archives/79%2810%29980.pdf

385 Margaret E. Bentley, Amy L. Corneli, Ellen Piwoz, Agnes Moses, et. al. "Perceptions of the Role of Maternal Nutrition in HIV-Positive Breast-Feeding Women in Malawi. The American Society of Nutritional Sciences." *The Journal of Nutrition*, 135 (2005): 945-949.

386 John C. LaRosa, "Understanding Risk in Hypercholesterolemia." *Clinical Cardiology*, 26 (2003): (Supplementary I), 1-3–1-6

387 J. H. O'Keefe Jr., L. Cordain, W.H. Harris, R.M. Moe, et al. "Optimal Low-Density Lipoprotein in 50 to 70 mg/dl: Lower is Better and Physiologically Normal." *Journal of American College of Cardiology*, 43.11 (2004): 2142-2146. doi:10.1016/j.jacc.2004.03.046.

Chapter 22

388 Centers for Disease Control and Prevention. *Healthy Weight, Overweight, and Obesity among U.S. adults.* 2003. Georgia, Atlanta. National Health and Nutrition Examination Survey. Accessed 23 November 2012. http://www.cdc.gov/nchs/data/nhanes/databriefs/adultweight.pdf

389 World Health Organization. Obesity and Overweight. 2003. Geneva, Switzerland. Accessed 23 December, 2012. http://www.who.int/dietphysicalactivity/media/en/gsfs_obesity.pdf

390 Centers for Disease Control and Prevention. *National diabetes fact sheet: general information and national estimates on diabetes in the United States, 2007.* Atlanta, GA: U.S. Department of Health and Human Services, Centers for Disease Control and Prevention, 2008. Accessed 27 December 2012. http://www.cdc.gov/diabetes/pubs/pdf/ndfs_2007.pdf

391 Simon R. Heller, "A Summary of the ADVANCE Trial." Diabetes and Cardiovascular Disease. American Diabetes Association. *Diabetes Care*, 32, Supplement 2 (2009): S357-S361

392 Action in Diabetes and Vascular Disease (*ADVANCE*) *Clinical Trial.* Backgrounder. Type 2 Diabetes. n.d. Accessed 24 November 2012. http://www.advance-trial.com/static/upload/BGLA/ServierADVANCEType_II_Diabetes_Backgrounder_FINAL.pdf

393 American Heart Association. *Cardiovascular Disease & Diabetes.* Accessed 27 December 2012. http://www.heart.org/HEARTORG/Conditions/Diabetes/WhyDiabetesMatters/Cardiovascular-Disease-Diabetes_UCM_313865_Article.jsp

394 National Institute of Health. *New Survey Results Show Huge Burden of Diabetes.* 2009. U.S. Department of Health and Human Sciences. Accessed 23 November 2012. http://www.nih.gov/news/health/jan2009/niddk-26.htm

395 Catherine C. Cowie, Keith F. Rust, Earl S. Ford, Mark S. Eberhardt, et al. Full Accounting of Diabetes and Pre Diabetes in the United

States. Population in 1988-1994 and 2005-2006. *Diabetes Care, 32* (2). (2008): 287-294

396 Pan American Health Organization. The U.S.-Mexico Border Diabetes Prevention and Control Project (n.d.). First Report of Results. Accessed 27 December 2012. http://www.borderhealth.org/files/res_719.pdf

397 Anna Glayzer, & Jessica Mitchell. "*Ignorance is Not Bliss When Eating Out: The Need for Nutrition Labeling at Fast Food and Other Chain Restaurants.*" December 2008. Accessed 1 December 2011. http://www.cspinet.org/new/pdf/food_commission_menu_labelling_report.final.pdf

398 Hiroyasu Iso, Chigusa Date, Kenji Wakai, Mitsuru Fukui, et. al. "The Relationship Between Green Tea and Total Caffeine Intake and Risk for Self-Reported type 2 Diabetes among Japanese adults." American College of Physicians. *Annals of Internal Medicine,* 144.8 (2006): 554-562. Print.

399 Wenying Yang, Juming Lu, Jianping Weng, Weiping Jia, et al. Prevalence of Diabetes among Men and Women in China. Massachusetts Medical Society. *The New England Journal of Medicine,* 362 (2010): 1090-1101. Doi: 10.1056/NEJMoa0908292.

400 City of Los Angeles Public Health. *Trends in Diabetes: A Reversible Public Health Crisis.* L.A. Health . November 2010. Accessed 16 December 2011 http://www.publichealth.lacounty.gov/ha/reports/habriefs/2007/diabetes/Diabetes_Secure/Diabetes_2010_6pg_Sfinal.pdf

401 Diabetes.co.uk. *Cost of Diabetes.* 2012. The Global Diabetes Community. Accessed 23 December 2012. http://www.diabetes.co.uk/cost-of-diabetes.html

402 International Insulin Foundation. *Diabetes in sub-Saharan Africa.* (n.d.) London, United Kingdom. Accessed 23 December 2011. http://www.access2insulin.org/uploads/4/9/1/0/4910107/factsheet.pdf

403 Paul Rheeder, "Type 2 Diabetes: The Emerging Epidemic." *South African Family Practice, 48.* 10, (2006): 20.

404 Thandi Puoane, Krisela Steyn, Debbie Bradshaw, Ria Laubscher, et al. "Obesity in South Africa: the South African Demographic and Health Survey." *Obesity Research*, 10 (2002):1038-1048. doi: 10.1038/oby.2002.141

405 V. Radha, & V. Mohan, "Genetic Predisposition to Type 2 Diabetes among Asian Indians." *Indian Journal of Medical Research*, 125 (2006): 259-274. Print.

406 Ambady Ramachandran, A. "Urban India: A Breeding Ground for Diabetes." Health Delivery. *Diabetes Voice*, 47.1(2002): 18-20. Print.

407 V. Mohan, S. Sandeepet, R. Deepa, B. Shah et al. "Epidemiology of Type 2 Diabetes: Indian Scenario." *Indian Journal of Medical Research*, 125 (2007): 217-230. Print.

408 Sarah Wild, Gojka Roglic, Anders Green, Richard Sicree, et al. "Global Prevalence of Diabetes: Estimates for the Year 2000 and Projections for 2030." *Diabetes Care*, 27.5 (2004): 1047-1453. Print.

409 Arnab Ghosh, Minakshi Bhagat, Mithun Das, Sanjib Kumar Bala et al. "Prevalence of cardiovascular disease risk factors in people of Asian Indian origin: Age and sex variation." Journal of Cardiovascular Disease Research, 1, 2, (2010):81-85.

410 Economist Intelligence Unit. *The Silent Epidemic: An Economic Study of Diabetes in Developed and Developing Nations*. June 2007. The Economist. Accessed 8 December 2011. http://viewswire.eiu.com/report_dl.asp?mode=fi&fi=1882281973.PDF&rf=0

411 Alberto Barcelo, Cristian Aedo, Swapnil Rajpathak, & Sylvia Robles. "The cost of Diabetes in Latin America and the Caribbean." *Bulletin of the World Health Organisation* 81.1(2003): 19-28. Accessed 23 December 2012.

412 Laura Fraser. "Ten Pounds in Ten Days: A sampler of Diet Fads and Abuse." 2012. LimeHealth. News for Healthier Living. Accessed 5 December 2011. http://consumer.healthday.com/encyclopedia/article.asp?AID=644429

413 Aabha Jain, & Ashley Schneider. "*Diet, Media Representation, and Public Health Policy (rewrite).*" Updated April 2007. Accessed 6 December 2012. http://www.cwru.edu/med/epidbio/mphp439/Diet.pdf
414 National Alliance on Mental Illness. *What is Anorexia Nervosa?* 2012. Arlington, Virginia. Accessed 28 December 2012. http://www.nami.org/Template.cfm?Section=Other_Mental_Illnesses&template=/ContentManagement/ContentDisplay.cfm&ContentID=102975
415 Aabha Jain, & Ashley Schneider. "*Diet, Media Representation, and Public Health Policy (rewrite).*" Updated April 2007. Accessed 6 December 2012. http://www.cwru.edu/med/epidbio/mphp439/Diet.pdf
416 Stein, J. *Amish paradox: Simpler, Active Lifestyles Help Keep the Weight Off.* January 2004. HighBeam Research. Accessed 6 December 2011. http://www.highbeam.com/doc/1P1-89868519.html
417 Walter Willet. "Lessons from Dietary Studies in Adventists and Questions for the Future." *American Journal of Clinical Nutrition*, 78.3 (2003): 5395-5435. Print.
418 U.S. Department of Health and Human Services Office of the Assistant Secretary for Planning and Evaluation. *Physical Activity Fundamental to Preventing Disease.* June 2002. Accessed 14 December 2011. http://aspe.hhs.gov/health/reports/physicalactivity/physicalactivity.pdf
419 Mary Ruth Swope. "Science and the Bible agree on nutrition." n.d. Accessed 6 December 2011. http://www.kingdomkalories.org/docs/science_and_the_bible.pdf
420 Karl Marx. "A Contribution to the Critique of Hegel's Philosophy of Right. Introduction. December 1843-January 1844. Proofed and Corrected by Andy Blunden, 2005. Corrected by Matthew Carmody, 2009. Accessed 28 December 2012. http://www.marxists.org/archive/marx/works/1843/critique-hpr/intro.htm

421 R.R. Reno. "An Error Worse than an Error." July 2010. First Things. Accessed 28 December 2012. http://www.firstthings.com/onthesquare/2010/07/an-error-worse-than-error/rr-reno
422 Ann Lamont. "Great Creation Scientist: Blaise Pascal (1623-1662). Outstanding Scientist and Committed Christian. December 1997. Accessed 28 December 2012. http://www.answersingenesis.org/articles/cm/v20/n1/pascal
423 Philip Yancey. *Reaching for the Invisible God: What Can We Expect to Find?* Zondervan Publishing Company, Grand Rapids, Michigan. 2002. pp. 154

CHAPTER 23

424 Eugene Rogot, & James L. Murray."Smoking and Causes of Death Among U.S. Veterans: 16 Years of Observation." *Public Health Reports*, 95.3 (1980): 213-222
425 Harold F. Dorn "Tobacco Consumption and Mortality from Cancer and Other Diseases." *Public Health Reports*, 74, (1959): 581-593.
426 Jonathan M. Samet, & Frank E. Speizer, "Sir Richard Doll 1912-2005." *American Journal of Epidemiology, 164*. 1, (2006): 95-100
427 Richard Doll, & A. Bradford Hill. "The mortality of Doctors in Relation to Their Smoking Habits." *British Medical Journal*, 328, (1954):1529-1533.
428 Centers for Disease Control and Prevention. *Smoking and Tobacco Use: Fast Facts.* Atlanta, Georgia. Accessed 29 December, 2012. http://www.wpro.who.int/media_centre/fact_sheets/fs_20020528.htm
429 American Cancer Society. *Cigarette Smoking.* 2012 United States. Accessed 29 December 2012. http://www.cancer.org/acs/groups/cid/documents/webcontent/002967-pdf.pdf
430 U.S. Department of Health and Human Services. *The Health Consequences of Smoking: A Report of the Surgeon General. Atlanta.* U.S. Department of Health and Human Services, Centers for

Disease Control and Prevention, National Center for Chronic Disease Prevention and Health Promotion, Office on Smoking and Health, 2004. Accessed 29 December 2012. http://www.ncbi.nlm.nih.gov/books/NBK44695/pdf/TOC.pdf

431 S. I. McMillen, & David E. Stern. *None of These Diseases*. Flemming H. Revell. Grand Rapids, MI. 2000. pp. 56Pr. int.

432 Florentina R. Salvail, "Exposure to Second Hand Smoke at Home." The Hawaii Behavioral Risk Factor Surveillance System Special Report. 2003. Accessed 19 October 2011. http://hawaii.gov/health/statistics/brfss/reports/2ndhandsmoke02.pdf

433 Donald F. Behan, Michael P. Eriksen, & Yijia Lin. "Economic Effects of Environmental Tobacco Smoke." March 2005. Accessed 5 November 2011. http://www.soa.org/research/research-projects/life-insurance/research-economic-effect.aspx

434 U.S. Department of Health and Human Services. *The Health Consequences of Involuntary Exposure to Tobacco Smoke: A Report of the Surgeon General.* Atlanta, GA: U.S. Department of Health and Human Services, Centers for Disease Control and Prevention, Coordinating Center for Health Promotion, National Center for Chronic Disease Prevention and Health Promotion, Office on Smoking and Health, 2006.

435 U.S. Department of Health and Human Services. The Health Consequences of Involuntary Exposure to Tobacco Smoke: A Report of the Surgeon General. Atlanta, Georgia: U.S. Department of Health and Human Services, Centers for Disease Control and Prevention, Coordinating Center for Health Promotion, National Center for Chronic Disease Prevention and Health Promotion, Office on Smoking and Health, 2006. Accessed 29 December 2012. http://www.ncbi.nlm.nih.gov/books/NBK44324/pdf/TOC.pdf

436 Centers for Disease Control and Prevention. *Smoking Attributable Mortality, Years of Potential Life Lost, and Productivity Losses-United States, 2000-2004.* Morbidity and Mortality Weekly Report. 2008. Accessed 5 November 2011. http://www.cdc.gov/mmwr/preview/mmwrhtml/mm5745a3.htm

437 U.S. Department of Health and Human Services (HHS), *Preventing Tobacco Use Among Youth and Young Adults.* A Report of the Surgeon General. Atlanta, Georgia. U.S. Department of Health and Human Services. Centers for Disease Control and Prevention. National Center for Chronic Disease Prevention and Health Promotion Office on Smoking and Health. 2012. Accessed 29 December 2012. http://www.surgeongeneral.gov/library/reports/preventing-youth-tobacco-use/full-report.pdf

438 World Health Organization Fact Sheet. *Smoking Statistics. Fact Sheet.* Geneva, Switzerland. May 2002. Accessed 29 December 2012. http://www.wpro.who.int/mediacentre/factsheets/fs_20020528/en/index.html

439 World Health Organization Fact Sheet. *Smoking Statistics. Fact Sheet.* Geneva, Switzerland. May 2002. Accessed 29 December 2012. http://www.wpro.who.int/mediacentre/factsheets/fs_20020528/en/index.html

440 Ross Hammond. "Tobacco Advertising & Promotion: The Need for a Coordinated Global Response. World Health Organization Conference on Global Tobacco Control Law" (paper presented at the WHO Conference on Global Tobacco Control Law: Towards a WHO Framework Convention on Tobacco Control, New Delhi, India, 7 to 9 January 2000). Accessed 29 December 2012. http://www.who.int/tobacco/media/ROSS2000X.pdf

441 D.H.O. Kwamanga, J.A. Odhiambo, & E.I. Amukoye. "Prevalence and Risk Factors of Smoking Among Secondary School Students in Nairobi." *East African Medical Journal,* 80.4 (2003): 207-212.

442 Niels Schoenmaker, Jeroen Hermanides, &GailDavey, "Prevalence and Predictors of Smoking in Butajira Town, Ethiopia." *Ethiopian Journal of Health Development,* 19, 3, (2005): 182-187

443 A. Hawamdeh, F.A. Kasasbeh, & M.A. Ahmad, "Effects of Passive Smoking on Children's Health: a Review." *Eastern Mediterranean Health Journal,* 9.3 (2003): 441-447.

444 Susan Harlap & A. Michael Davies, "Infant Admissions to Hospital and Maternal Smoking." *Lancet, 303,* 7857, (1974): 529–32. doi.org/10.1016/S0140-6736(74)92714-7

445 Jouni J.K. Jaakkola, & Mika Gissler. "Maternal Smoking in Pregnancy, Fetal Development, and Childhood Asthma." *American Journal of Public Health*, 94.1 (2004): 136-140. Print

446 L. Hogberg, & S. Cnattingius. "The influence of Maternal Smoking Habits on the Risk of Subsequent Stillbirth: Is There a Causal Relation?" *International Journal of Obstetrics and Gyaecology*, 114 (2007): 699-704. DOI: 10.1111/j.1471-0528.2007.01340.x.

447 European Commission. Health Effects of Smokeless Tobacco Products.2008.Scientific Committee on Emerging and Newly Identified Health Risks (SCENIHR). 2008. Accessed 29 December 2012. http://ec.europa.eu/health/ph_risk/committees/04_scenihr/docs/scenihr_o_013.pdf

Chapter 24

448 S.I. McMillen, & David E. Stern, David. *None of These Diseases*. Flemming H. Revell. Grand Rapids, MI. 2000. Print.

449 Abraham L. Wolbarst. "Circumcision and Penile Carcinoma." *The Lancet, 1* (5655). (1932): 150-153

450 R. Dagher, M. L. Selzer, & J. Lapides. "Carcinoma of the Penis and the Anti-Circumcision Crusade." *Journal of Urology*, 110 (1). (1973): 79-80.

451 Hiram N. Wineberg. *The Rare Occurrence of Cancer of the Womb Among Jewish Women*, In S.I. McMillen. "*None of These Diseases*: Science—4000Years Behind Times! Sacred Writings Predate Modern Science. n.d. Accessed 29 December 2012. http://www.trosch.org/the/circumcision-cancer.pdf

452 I.I. Kaplan, & R. Rosh. "Cancer of the Cervix: Belleveu Hospital Method of Treatment Over a Period of Twenty-One Years." *American Journal of Roentgenology*, 57(6) (1947): 659-664

453 William B. Ober, & Leopold Reiner. "Cancer of the Cervix in Jewish Women." *New England Journal of Medicine*, 251(1954): 555-559. Print.

454 W.K.C. Morgan. "Penile Plunder." The Circumcision Reference Library. *The Medical Journal of Australia,* 1(1967): 1102-1103. Print.

455 John P. Warren, &Jim Bigelow. "The Case Against Circumcision." The Circumcision Reference Library. *British Journal of Sexual Medicine,*(1994): 6-8. Print.

456 Circumcision and Human Rights. *The United Nations Convention on the Rights of the Child, Article 13, Part 1.* Accessed 29 December 2012. http://www.circumstitions.com/Rights.html#UDHR

457 Thompson, H.C. American Academy of Pediatrics, Committee on Fetus and Newborn. Evanston, IL: *American Academy Standards and Recommendation for Hospital Care of Newborn infants.* 5th ed. *of Pediatrics,* 1971:110. Accessed 29 December 2011. http://www.cirp.org/library/statements/aap/

458 H. C. Thompson, L.R. King, E. Knox, & S.B. Korones. "Report of the Ad Hoc Task Force on Circumcision." American Academy of Pediatrics, Committee on Fetus and Newborn. *Pediatrics*;56(4) (1975):610-111

459 American Academy of Pediatrics. "Report of the Taskforce on Circumcision". *Pediatrics 84 (1989):388–391*

460 American Academy of Pediatrics. Circumcision Policy Statement. Pediatrics, 103,3, (1999): 686-693

461 American Academy of Pediatrics. Circumcision Policy Statement. Pediatrics, 103 (3) (1999): 686-693

462 Aaron A. R. Tobian, Ronald H. Gray & Thomas C. Quinn. "Male Circumcision for the Prevention of Acquisition and Transmission of Sexually Transmitted Infections: The Case for Neonatal Circumcision." *Archives of Pediatrics and Adolescent Medicine, 164* (1) (2010): 78-84. doi: 10.1001/archpediatrics.2009.232

463 S.I. McMillen. None of These Diseases: Science-4000 Years Behind Times! n.d. Accessed 29 December 2012. ttp://www.trosch.org/the/circumcision-cancer.pdf

464 Johannes van Dam, & Marie-Christine Anastasi, "Male Circumcision and HIV Prevention." 2000. Accessed 29 December 2011. http://pdf.usaid.gov/pdf_docs/PNACK848.pdf

465 World Health Organization (WHO). *Male Circumcision for HV Prevention.* 2012. Accessed 26 December 2011. http://www.who.int/hiv/topics/malecircumcision/en/index.html

466 Andy Coghlan. A. "Bill Gates helps fund mass circumcision programme." NewScientist. 2009. Accessed 29 December 2012. http://www.newscientist.com/article/dn17312-bill-gates-helps-fund-mass-circumcision-programme.html

467 Zambia National Broadcasting Company News Report, (Thursday, June 18, 2009), "Universal Circumcision: Mandatory Circumcision for Zambia Police Recruits." Accessed 29 December 2012. http://mandatorycircumcision.blogspot.com/2009/06/mandatory-circumcision-for-zambia.html

468 Integrated Regional Information Networks (IRIN). Humanitarian News and Analysis. *Africa: Tracking the Male Circumcision Roll-Out.* 2010. Accessed 12 December 2012. Accessed 29 December 2011. http://www.irinnews.org/printreport.aspx?reportid=88286

469 Tom Zeigler, & John Oakes. *"Medical Evidence from the Bible."* 2011. Accessed 17 August 2011. http://www.docstoc.com/docs/885166/MEDICAL-EVIDENCE-FOR-THE-BIBLE

470 Rex Russell. *What the Bible Says About Healthy Living: Three Biblical Principles That Will Change Your Diet and Improve Your Health.* Regal Books. Ventura, CA. pp. 21, 22. 1996. Print.

CHAPTER 25

471 Conference of European Churches. *Ageing and Care for the Elderly.* June 2007. Accessed October 2011. http://csc.ceceurope.org/fileadmin/filer/csc/Ethics_Biotechnology/AgeingandCareElderly.pdf

472 World Health Organization. *Elder Abuse and Alcohol Fact Sheet.* Geneva, Switzerland. n.d. Accessed 23 October 2011 http://

www.who.int/violence_injury_prevention/violence/world_report/factsheets/ft_elder.pdf

473 Encyclopedia of Aging. *Elder abuse and Neglect*. 2002. HighBeam Research. Accessed 23 December 2011. http://www.encyclopedia.com/topic/Elder_abuse.aspx

474 Hilary Brown, *Safeguarding Adults and Children with Disabilities against Abuse*. Council of Europe Publishing, 2003. ISBN 92-871. Accessed 29 December 2012. http://www.coe.int/t/e/social_cohesion/soc-sp/Abuse%20_E%20in%20color.pdf

475 Lawrence Robinson, Tina de Benedictis, & Jeanne Segal. (2012). "Elder Abuse and Neglect: Warning Signs, Risk Factors, Prevention and Help."2012. Accessed 14 December 2012. http://www.helpguide.org/mental/elder_abuse_physical_emotional_sexual_neglect.htm

476 Lawrence Robinson, Tina de Benedictis, & Jeanne Segal. "Elder Abuse and Neglect: Warning Signs, Risk Factors, Prevention and Help." 2011. Accessed 24 October 2012. http://www.helpguide.org/mental/elder_abuse_physical_emotional_sexual_neglect.htm

477 Jane A. Raymond. "Facts about Domestic Violence in Later Life and Elder Sexual Assault Occurring in Residential Care Facilities. Wisconsin Department of Health Services. Accessed 30 December 2012. http://www.dhs.wisconsin.gov/dsl_info/infomemos/ddes/cy_2004/InfoMemo2004-03_appendixA.htm

478 Anna Mae Kobbe. "Preventing Abuse and Neglect of the Elderly." n.d. Accessed 25 October 2011. http://utextension.tennessee.edu/publications/Documents/pb1414.pdf

479 Kelly Johnson. "Financial Crimes against the Elderly." Guide No. 20 (2003): 2012. Center for Problem-Oriented Policing. Accessed 30 December 2012. http://www.popcenter.org/problems/crimes_against_elderly/

480 Economic and Social Commission for Western Asia (ESCWA). *Literature Review on Social Exclusion in the ESCWA Region*. July 2007. Accessed 23 October 2010. http://www.escwa.un.org/information/publications/edit/upload/sdd-07-wp4-e.pdf

481 HelpAge International and HelpAge Kenya. *Elder Abuse in the Healthcare Services in Kenya.* 2001. Accessed17 February 2011. http://www.who.int/ageing/projects/elder_abuse/alc_ea_ken.pdf

482 Help-Age International and HelpAgeKenya. *Elder Abuse in the Health Care Services in Kenya.* 2001. December 13, 2012. Accessed 30 December 2012. http://www.who.int/ageing/projects/elder_abuse/alc_ea_ken.pdf

483 National Center on Elder Abuse. *Elder Abuse Prevalence and Incidence.* Fact Sheet. 2005. Accessed 23 October 2010. http://www.ncea.aoa.gov/NCEAroot/main_site/pdf/publication/FinalStatistics050331.pdf

484 The Anti-Ageism Taskforce at the International Longevity Center. *Ageism in America.* 2006. Accessed 26 September 26, 2011. http://www.graypanthersmetrodetroit.org/Ageism_In_America_-_ILC_Book_2006.pdf

485 Office of the District Attorney-Lancaster County, Pennsylvania. Elder Abuse Response Protocol. Accessed 31 December 2012. http://www.umaine.edu/mainecenteronaging/documents/issuebriefelderabuse.pdf

486 Ron Acierno, Melba A. Hernandez, Ananda B. Amstadter, Heidi S. Resnick, et al. "Prevalence and Correlates of Emotional, Physical, Sexual, and Financial Abuse and Potential Neglect in the United States: The National Elder Mistreatment Study." *American Journal of Public Health*, 100 (2010): 292-297. doi:10.2105/ AJPH.2009.163089

487 A.R. Hamilton. *Elder Abuse, Neglect, and Financial Exploitation. A Power Point Presentation at Community Solutions Conference, 15 April 2003, Rockport, Maine*, In Jason C. Charland, "Elder Abuse, Neglect, and Exploitation," (paper prepared for Blaine House Conference on Aging, The University of Main Center on Aging, Orono, Maine, September 2006). Accessed 31 December 2012. http://umcoa.siteturbine.com/uploaded_files/mainecenteronaging.umaine.edu/files/issuebriefelderabuse.pdf

488 Associated Press Maine High in Suicides of Elderly: State Officials to Study Cause of Phenomenon, Bangor Daily News, pp. B1. July 8, 2002, In Jason C. Charland, "Elder Abuse, Neglect, and Exploitation," (paper prepared for Blaine House Conference on Aging, The University of Main Center on Aging, Orono, Maine, September 2006). Accessed 31 December 2012. http://umcoa.siteturbine.com/uploaded_files/mainecenteronaging.umaine.edu/files/issuebriefelderabuse.pdf

489 Lawrence Robinson, Tina de Benedictis, & Jeanne Segal. "Elder abuse and neglect: Warning Signs, Risk Factors, Prevention and Help." 2012. Accessed 31 December 2012. http://helpguide.org/mental/elder_abuse_physical_emotional_sexual_neglect.htm

490 Nursing Home Abuse News. *Institutional Elder Abuse*. n.d. Accessed 31 December 2012. http://www.nursinghomeabuse-news.com/html/institutional.html

491 Elaine Lies "Ageing Japan Wakes Up to the Problem of Elder Abuse." 2004. Reuters Foundation. Accessed 25 October 2010. http://www.globalaging.org/elderrights/world/2004/japanabuse.htm

492 Conference of European Churches. *Ageing and Care for the Elderly*. 2007. Accessed 26 October 2011. http://www.cec-kek.org/pdf/AgeingandCareElderly.pdf

CHAPTER 26

493 Global Initiative for Asthma. *Global Strategy for Asthma Management and Prevention*. 2012. Accessed 31 December 2012. http://www.ginasthma.org/uploads/users/files/GINA_Report_2012.pdf

494 Ibid.

495 Emily Rosenbaum."Racial/ethnic Differences in Asthma Prevalence: The Role of Housing and Neighborhood Environments."*Journal of Health and Social Behavior*, 49. 2 (2008): 131-135. doi: 10.1177/002214650804900202

496 T.D. Hill, L.M. Graham, & V. Divqi. "Racial Disparities in Pediatric Asthma: A Review of the Literature." *Current Allergy and Asthma Reports*, 11 (1) (2011): 85-90. doi: 10.1007/s11882-010-0159-2

497 Vinod Mishra. "Effect of Obesity on Asthma among Adult Indian Women." *International Journal of Obesity*, 28 (2004): 1048-1058. Print.

498 S. H. Arshad. "Primary Prevention of Asthma and Allergy." *The Journal of Allergy and Clinical Immunology*, 116.1(2005): 3-14. Print.

499 Thomas F. Bateson, & Joel Schwartz. "Children's Response to Air Pollutants." *Journal of Toxicology and Environmental Health, Part A*, 71 (2008): 238-243. doi: 10.1080/15287390701598234. Print.

500 G.L. Ginsberg, B. P. Foos, & M.P. Firestone. "Review and Analysis of Inhalation Dosimetry Methods for Application to Children's Risk Assessment." *Journal of Toxicology and Environmental Health A* 6 8 (2005):573–615. Print

501 M. Studnicka, E. Hackl, J. Pischinger, C. Fangmeyer, et. al. "Traffic Related NO2 and the Prevalence of Asthma and Respiratory Symptoms in Seven Year Olds." *European Respiratory Journal*, 10 (1997): 2275-2278. doi: 10.1183/09031936.97.10102275. Print.

502 Ursula Kramer, Thilo Koch, Ulrich Ranft, Johannes Ring, et al. "Traffic Related Air Pollution is Associated with Atopy in Children Living in Urban Areas." *Epidemiology*, 11.1 (2000): 64-70. Print.

503 Patricia van Vliet, Mirjam Knape, Jeroen de Hartog, Nicole Janssen, et al. "Motor Vehicle Exhaust and Chronic Respiratory in Children Living Near Freeways." *Environmental Research* 74.2 (1997): 122-132. doi.org/10.1006/enrs.1997.3757

504 U.S. Environmental Protection Agency. What are the Trends in Indoor Air Quality and Their Effects on Human Health? 1989. Report on the Environment. 2011. Accessed 31 December 2012. http://cfpub.epa.gov/eroe/index.cfm?fuseaction=list.listBySubTopic&ch=46&s=343

505 Lawrence E. Gelber, Leonard H. Seltzer, James K. Bouzoukis, Susan M. Pollart, et al. "Sensitization and Exposure to Indoor

Allergens as Risk Factors for Asthma among Patients Presenting to Hospital. *American Review of Respiratory Disease,*147, (1993): 573–578.

506 D.P. Garcia, M. L. Corbett, J. L. Sublett, S.J. Pollard, et al. Cockroach Allergy in Kentucky: A Comparison of Inner City, Suburban, and Rural Small Town Populations. *Annals of Allergy,* 72,3. (1994):203–208

507 James E. Gern, & William W. Busse. "Relationship of Viral Infections to Wheezing Illnesses and Asthma." *Nature Reviews Immunology* 2 (2002): 132-138. doi: 10.1038/nri725. Print.

508 Matthew M. Huckabee, & R. Stokes Peebles, Jr. "Novel Concepts in Virally Induced Asthma." *Clinical and Molecular Allergy* 2009, 7:2 doi:10.1186/1476-7961-7-2

509 P. Wu, W. D. Dupont, M. R. Griffin, K.N. Carroll, et. al. "Evidence of Causal Role of Winter Virus Infection during Infancy in Early Childhood Asthma." *American Journal of Respiratory and Critical Care Medicine,* 178 (2008): 1123-1129. doi: 10.1164/rccm.200804-579OC

510 Riny Janssen, Louis Bont, Christine L. Siezen, Hennie M. Hodemaekers, et al "Genetic Susceptibility to Respiratory Syncytial Virus Bronchiolitis Is Predominantly Associated with Innate Immune Genes." *The Journal of Infectious Diseases,* 196 (2007): 826-834. Doi: 10.1086/520886. Print.

511 World Health Organization. *Occupational Health: The Workplace. Protection of the Human Environment.* 1997. Geneva, Switzerland. Accessed 22 December 2010. http://www.who.int/peh/Occupational_health/occupational_health2.htm

512 Jean Bousquet, Philippe J. Bousquet, Philippe Godard, & Jean-Pierre Daures. "The Public Health Implications of Asthma." Bulletin of the World Health Organization, 83 (7) (2005): 548-554. Accessed 22 December, 2011. http://www.who.int/bulletin/volumes/83/7/548.pdf

513 Mayo Clinic (2012). *Occupational Asthma: Causes.* Accessed 31 December 2012. http://www.mayoclinic.com/health/occupational-asthma/DS00591/DSECTION=causes

514 Thomas Rémen, Vincent Coevoet, Dovi-Stéphanie Acouetey, Jean-Louis Guéant, et. al. "Early Incidence of Occupational Asthma among Young Bakers, Pastry Makers and Hairdressers: Design of a Retrospective Cohort Study." *BMC Public Health*, 10 (2010): 206. doi:10.1186/1471-2458-10-206

515 Gianna Moscato, Patrizia Pignatti, Mona-Rita Yacoub, Canzio Romano, et. al. "Occupational Asthma and Occupational Rhinitis in Hairdressers." *Chest*, 128 (2005): 3590-3598. doi: 10.1378/chest.128.5.3590. Print.

516 Jane A. Hoppin, "Chronic Disease Epidemiology Group." 2012. National Institute of Environmental Health Science. Accessed 31 December 2012. http://www.niehs.nih.gov/research/atniehs/labs/epi/chronic/staff/hoppin/index.cfm

517 J. A. Hoppin, D.M. Umbach, S.J. London, M.C. Alavania, et al. (2002). Chemical predictors of wheeze among farmer pesticide applicators in the Agricultural Health Study. *American Journal of Respiratory and Critical Care Medicine*, 165, 5. (2002):683-689

518 Carlos E. Baena-Cagnani, R. Maximiliano Gomez, Rodrigo Baena-Cagnani, &Walter Canonica. "Impact of Environmental Tobacco Smoke and Active Tobacco Smoking on the Development and Outcomes of Asthma and Rhinitis." *Current Opinion in Allergy and Clinical Immunology*, 9, 2. (2009): 136-140. doi: 10.1097/ACI.0b013e3283294038

519 S.I. McMillen & David Stern,. *None of These Diseases*. 3rd ed. Flemming H. Revell. Grand Rapids, MI. 2000. pp. 58. Print

520 Neil C.Thomson, R. Chaudhuri, & E. Livingston. "Asthma and Cigarette Smoking." *European Respiratory Journal*, 24 (2004): 822-833. doi: 10.1183/09031936.04.00039004. Print.

521 Saskia M. Willers, Alet H. Wijga, Bert Brunekreef, Marjan Kerkhof, et. al. "Maternal Food Consumption during Pregnancy and the Longitudinal Development of Childhood Asthma." *American Journal of Respiratory and Critical Care Medicine*, 178 (2008): 124-131. doi: 10.1164/rccm.200710-1544OC . Print.

522 European Food Information Council. *Diet May Help Prevent Allergies and Asthma.* 2012. Accessed 20 December 2011. http://www.eufic.org/page/en/show/latest-science-news/fftid/diet-allergies-asthma/

523 Friedman, N. J., & Zeiger, R. S. *The Role of Breast-Feeding in the Development of Allergies and Asthma In Global Initiative for Asthma.* In Global Initiative for Asthma. *Global Strategy for Asthma Management and Prevention.* 2012. Accessed 31 December 2012. http://www.ginasthma.org/uploads/users/files/GINA_Report_2012.pdf

524 Devereux G, Seaton A. *Diet as a Risk Factor for Atopy and Asthma. In* Global Initiative for Asthma. *Global Strategy for Asthma Management and Prevention.* 2012. Accessed 31 December 2012. http://www.ginasthma.org/uploads/users/files/GINA_Report_2012.pdf

525 World Health Organization. *Indoor Pollution and Health.* Media Centre. Fact Sheet, No. 292. 2011. Accessed 21 December 2011. http://www.who.int/mediacentre/factsheets/fs292/en/index.html

526 S. Padmavati, & B. Joshi (1964). "Incidence and Etiology of Chronic Cor Pulmonale in Delhi: A Necropsy Study." *Chest Journal, 46* (4), 457-463. doi:10.1378/chest.46.4.457

527 Manish Desai, Sumi Mehta & Kirk R. Smith. "Indoor Smoke from Solid Fuels: Assessing the Environmental Burden of Disease at National and Local Levels." 2004. Geneva, Switzerland. World Health Organization. Accessed 31 December 2012. http://www.who.int/quantifying_ehimpacts/publications/en/Indoorsmoke.pdf

528 Carlos Torres-Duque, Dario Maldonado, Rogelio Pérez-Padilla, Majid Ezzati, et. al. "Biomass Fuels and Respiratory Diseases. A Review of the Evidence." *The Proceedings of the American Thoracic Society,* 5,5. (2008): 577-590. doi: 10.1513/pats.200707-100RP. Print.

529 Johns Hopkins University-Women and Children's Health Policy Center. *Asthma Interventions and Cost Consequences-Synthesis of*

Research Findings. 2007. Accessed 26 December 2011. http://www.jhsph.edu/sebin/y/v/Asthma.pdf

530 David M. Mannino, David M. Homa, Lara J. Akinbami, Jeanne E. Moorman, et al. *Surveillance for Asthma—United States, 1980-1999.* Centers for Disease Control and Prevention. *MMWR* 51(SS01) (2002): 1-13. Accessed 31 December 2012. http://www.cdc.gov/mmwr/preview/mmwrhtml/ss5101a1.htm

531 Phaedra Corso, & Angela Pertig. "The Long-Term Economic Costs of Asthma." Partnership for America's Economic Success. Issue Paper # 13. (2004): 2-12. Accessed 26 December 2011. http://www.partnershipforsuccess.org/uploads/20090708_asthmafinalformatted.pdf

532 JHU–WCHPC. Asthma Interventions and Cost Consequences—Synthesis of Research Findings. 2007. http://www.jhsph.edu/research/centers-and-institutes/womens-and-childrens-health-policy-center/publications/Res_Syntheses/Asthma.pdf

533 Jean Bousquet, Philippe J. Bousquet, Philippe Gordad, & Jean-Pierre Daurtes. "The Public Health Implications of Asthma." *Bulletin of the World Health Organization,* 83 (2005): 548-554. Accessed 22 December 2011. http://www.who.int/bulletin/volumes/83/7/548.pdf

534 C.K.W. Lai, Y-Y. Kim, S-H. Kuo, M. Spencer, et.al. "Cost of Asthma in the Asia-Pacific Region." *European Respiratory Review,* 15.98 (2006): 10-16. doi: 10.1183/09059180.06.00009802.

535 Matthew Masoli, Denise Fabian, Shaun Holt & Richard Beasley (n.d.). Global Burden of Asthma-Summary. Accessed 31 December 2012. http://www.ginasthma.org/pdf/GINABurdenReport.pdf

536 Christopher Granger, C. "Hair and Skin Care: No Wrinkles-Can You Make it Happen?" 2012. Accessed 31 December 2012. http://www.livingfithealthyandhappy.com/hair-and-skin-care/

537 Intercommunity Peace & Justice Center. *Six Session Process for Faith Communities are All for Creation.* 2008. Accessed 31 December 2012. http://www.showyourimpact.org/files/project_files/ab2009/CareForAllOfCreation.pdf

Chapter 27

538 Alan G. Kraut. "APS Calls for Change in Behavioral Science at NIH." 2009. Observer. Association for Psychological Science. Accessed 1 January 2013. https://aps.psychologicalscience.org/observer/getArticle.cfm?id=2465

539 Ibid.

540 Centers for Disease Control and Prevention. *Chronic Diseases and Health Promotion*. 2012. Atlanta, Georgia. Accessed 23 December 2012. http://www.cdc.gov/chronicdisease/overview/index.htm

541 Ross DeVol, & Armen Bedroussian. "An Unhealthy America: The Economic Burden of Chronic Disease." 2007. Milken Institute. Accessed 23 December 2012. http://www.milkeninstitute.org/healthreform/pdf/AnUnhealthyAmericaExecSumm.pdf

542 Thomson Medstat (2006). *Health and Productivity Management Benchmarking Project*. Centers of Disease Control and Prevention Association of Chronic Disease Program Directors. Accessed 23 December 2012. http://www.ihwsolutions.com/pdf/cdcsummary.pdf

543 Ross DeVol, & Armen Bedroussian. "An Unhealthy America: The Economic Burden of Chronic Disease." 2007. Milken Institute. Accessed 23 December 2012. http://www.milkeninstitute.org/healthreform/pdf/AnUnhealthyAmericaExecSumm.pdf

544 Alan G. Kraut. "APS Calls for Change in Behavioral Science at NIH." 2009. Observer. Association for Psychological Science. Accessed 1 January 2013. https://aps.psychologicalscience.org/observer/getArticle.cfm?id=2465

545 John T. Cohen, Peter J. Neumann, & Milton C. Weinstein. "Does Preventive Care Save Money? Health Economics and the Presidential Candidates." *New England Journal of Medicine*, 358.7 (2008): 661-663. doi: 10.1056/NEJMp0708558

546 Sarah Goodell, Joshua Cohen, & Peter Neumann. "Cost Savings and Cost-Effectiveness of Clinical Preventive Care." The Synthesis Project. Policy Brief No. 18. The Robert Wood Johnson

Foundation. 2009. Accessed 9 December 2011. http://www.rwjf.org/content/dam/farm/reports/issue_briefs/2009/rwjf46045

547 Ulrich Laaser, & Leon Epstein."Threats to Global Health and Opportunities for Change: A New Global Health. " Public Health Reviews. ISSN 2107-6952. 2011. Accessed 29 December 2012. http://www.publichealthreviews.eu/show/f/32

548 Population Reference Bureau. *Improving the Health of the World's Poorest People*. 2004. Accessed 12 December 2011. http://www.prb.org/pdf04/improvingtheHealthbrief_Eng.pdf

549 Robert Sharpe. "Better Than Cure." n.d. International Association Against Painful Experiments on Animals. Accessed 23 December 2012. http://www.iaapea.com/pdf/better_than_cure.pdf

550 Brian Inglis, *Diseases of Civilization: We Need a New Approach to Medical Treatment*, In Robert Sharpe. "Better Than Cure." n.d. International Association against Painful Experiments on Animals. Accessed 23 December 2012. http://www.iaapea.com/pdf/better_than_cure.pdf

551 Centers for Disease Control and Prevention. *Chronic Disease Prevention and Health Promotion*. 2012. Atlanta, Georgia. Accessed 23 December 2012. http://www.cdc.gov/chronicdisease/overview/index.htm

552 Preetha Anand, Ajaikumar B. Kunnumakara, Chitra Sundaram, Kuzhuvelil B. Harikumar, et al. "Cancer is Preventable Disease that Requires Major Lifestyle Changes." *Pharmaceutical Research Journal*, 25 (9) (2008): 2097-2116. doi: 10.1007/s11095-008-9661-9

553 Susan Brink. "The Diabetes Prevention Program: How the Participants Did It." *Health Affairs*, 28.1 (2009): 57-61. doi: 10.1377/hlthaff.28.1.57

554 Janet R. Hankin "Protecting the Next Pregnancy: Maternal Drinking and Infant Developmental Outcomes" (presentation, The Annual Meeting of the American Sociological Association, Atlanta Hilton Hotel, Atlanta, Georgia. May 26, 2009). Accessed 29 December 2012. http://citation.allacademic.com/meta/p_mla_apa_research_citation/1/0/7/4/9/p107492_index.html

www.ingramcontent.com/pod-product-compliance
Lightning Source LLC
Chambersburg PA
CBHW030315100526
44592CB00010B/435